Neonatal EEG

Mary Payne • David Gloss II
Editors

Neonatal EEG

A Clinical Guidebook

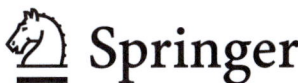

Editors
Mary Payne
Department of Pediatrics, Division of
Pediatric Neurology, Joan C. Edwards
School of Medicine, Hoops Family
Children's Hospitaly
Marshall University
Huntington, WV, USA

David Gloss II
The Neuromedical Center
Baton Rouge, LA, USA

ISBN 978-3-031-92555-9   ISBN 978-3-031-92556-6   (eBook)
https://doi.org/10.1007/978-3-031-92556-6

© The Editor(s) (if applicable) and The Author(s), under exclusive license to Springer Nature Switzerland AG 2025

This work is subject to copyright. All rights are solely and exclusively licensed by the Publisher, whether the whole or part of the material is concerned, specifically the rights of translation, reprinting, reuse of illustrations, recitation, broadcasting, reproduction on microfilms or in any other physical way, and transmission or information storage and retrieval, electronic adaptation, computer software, or by similar or dissimilar methodology now known or hereafter developed.
The use of general descriptive names, registered names, trademarks, service marks, etc. in this publication does not imply, even in the absence of a specific statement, that such names are exempt from the relevant protective laws and regulations and therefore free for general use.
The publisher, the authors and the editors are safe to assume that the advice and information in this book are believed to be true and accurate at the date of publication. Neither the publisher nor the authors or the editors give a warranty, expressed or implied, with respect to the material contained herein or for any errors or omissions that may have been made. The publisher remains neutral with regard to jurisdictional claims in published maps and institutional affiliations.

This Springer imprint is published by the registered company Springer Nature Switzerland AG
The registered company address is: Gewerbestrasse 11, 6330 Cham, Switzerland

If disposing of this product, please recycle the paper.

Dedicated to our smallest patients with the biggest hearts and the most fascinating brains.

Preface

I have been privileged to take care of the youngest patients in my state and to be a part of the medical teams who devote their all to these babies. We, as medical staff, are fortunate to have the ability and toolset to provide support for their developing brains. I, myself, am continuously learning from these patients as each neonate is so unique and their medical path is unpaved. I hope this guidebook can be helpful for those who care for neonates. Using basic science and fundamentals of neurophysiology, I have tried to clarify some complicated but important topics through figures, charts and practical examples.

Huntington, WV, USA Mary Payne
Baton Rouge, LA, USA David Gloss II

Acknowledgments

Ana Maria Gonzalez Cadavid, MD, FAAP
Marshall University Joan C. Edwards School of Medicine
Department of Pediatrics
Section of Neonatal-Perinatal Medicine
Huntington, WV

Bobby Miller, MD, FAAP
Senior Assistant Dean for Education Projects
Executive Director for Medical Education and Continuous Quality Improvement
Professor, Department of Pediatrics
University of South Carolina School of Medicine
Columbia, South Carolina

Rankin Payne, BS
Morgantown, West Virginia

Joseph Werthammer, MD, FAAP
Professor, Neonatology
Senior Associate Dean for Clinical Affairs
Marshall University Joan C. Edwards School of Medicine
Huntington, WV

Natus Medical Incorporated

Competing interests—none

Neurodiagnostic departments at Cabell Huntington Hospital in Huntington, West Virginia, J.W. Ruby Memorial Hospital in Morgantown, West Virginia, and Women's and Children's Hospital in Charleston, West Virginia.

Contents

1. **Introduction and Technical Aspects of Neonatal EEGs**.............. 1
   Mary Payne and Dipali Nemade

2. **Developmental Maturation of the EEG in Neonates, from Preterm to Term Gestational Ages**........................ 25
   Mary Payne

3. **Abnormal Background Activity in Neonatal EEGs: Encephalopathy and Abnormal Frequency and Amplitude Findings**... 77
   Mary Payne

4. **Abnormal Background Patterns in Neonatal EEG Recordings: Sharp Waves**.. 105
   Mary Payne

5. **Electrographic Findings of Neonatal Seizures**.................... 129
   Mary Payne

6. **Seizures in Neonates: Clinical Manifestations and Etiology Timeline**... 155
   Jonathan Hanson and Mary Payne

7. **Common Artifacts of Neonatal EEG Recordings**................. 173
   Mary Payne and Kristen Newcomer

8. **Amplitude-Integrated EEG and Its Application for Neonates**...... 193
   Mary Payne, Rebecca Barnett, and Stefan R. Maxwell

9. **Case Examples in Neonates with Clinical Scenarios Using Electroencephalogram Recordings**............................. 205
   Christopher Luke Damron, Rebekah Fabela, Alicia Heyward, Cynthia Massey, Dustin Miller, Mary Payne, and Lauren Thompson

Glossary: Terminology Used in Describing Neonatal EEG's........... 237

Index... 245

Contributors

Rebecca Barnett Department of Pediatrics, Division of Neonatal-Perinatal Medicine, Joan C. Edwards School of Medicine, Hoops Family Children's Hospital, Marshall University, Huntington, WV, USA

Christopher Luke Damron Department of Pediatrics, Division of Neonatal-Perinatal Medicine, Joan C. Edwards School of Medicine, Hoops Family Children's Hospital, Marshall University, Huntington, WV, USA

Rebekah Fabela Department of Pediatrics, Division of Neonatal-Perinatal Medicine, Joan C. Edwards School of Medicine, Hoops Family Children's Hospital, Marshall University, Huntington, WV, USA

Jonathan Hanson University Hospital Center, Bridgeport, WV, USA

Alicia Heyward Department of Pediatrics, Division of Neonatal-Perinatal Medicine, Joan C. Edwards School of Medicine, Hoops Family Children's Hospital, Marshall University, Huntington, WV, USA

Cynthia Massey Department of Pediatrics, Division of Neonatal-Perinatal Medicine, Joan C. Edwards School of Medicine, Hoops Family Children's Hospital, Marshall University, Huntington, WV, USA

Stefan R. Maxwell Pediatrix Medical Group, WVU School of Medicine, WV Osteopathic School of Medicine, CAMC Women's and Children's Hospital, Charleston, WV, USA

Dustin Miller Department of Pediatrics, Division of Neonatal-Perinatal Medicine, Joan C. Edwards School of Medicine, Hoops Family Children's Hospital, Marshall University, Huntington, WV, USA

Dipali Nemade Orlando Health Neuroscience Institute, Orlando, FL, USA

Kristen Newcomer WVU Medicine Children's Hospital, Neurodiagnostic Clinical Preceptor, Morgantown, WV, USA

Mary Payne Department of Pediatrics, Division of Pediatric Neurology, Joan C. Edwards School of Medicine, Hoops Family Children's Hospital, Marshall University, Huntington, WV, USA

Lauren Thompson Department of Pediatrics, Division of Neonatal-Perinatal Medicine, Joan C. Edwards School of Medicine, Hoops Family Children's Hospital, Marshall University, Huntington, WV, USA

Introduction and Technical Aspects of Neonatal EEGs

Mary Payne and Dipali Nemade

1.1 What Is an Electroencephalogram (EEG)?

1.1.1 Introduction: History and Neurophysiology

The credit for the first neurophysiological detection of electrical activity of humans goes to Hans Berger, a German psychiatrist. He pioneered the first EEG for human use in 1924. EEG machines became commercially available in 1936.

Interpretation of the EEG requires knowledge of neurophysiology, clinical neurology, and EEG expertise. In particular, interpreting the neonatal EEG requires specialized understanding of the developing brain EEG and awareness of normal and abnormal state changes and behaviors in neonates. This book is meant to be a guide for those caring for these special patients to help clarify and bring understanding to the complexities of neonatal EEG findings in order to improve evaluation and treatment.

This chapter will discuss the basic principles of EEG technology and how the waveforms are displayed and can be visualized on the digital screen.

EEGs in general can tell you about the presence of

- Encephalopathy
- Seizures
- Abnormalities that might indicate areas of focal dysfunction and/or epileptic potential

M. Payne (✉)
Department of Pediatrics, Division of Pediatric Neurology, Joan C. Edwards School of Medicine, Hoops Family Children's Hospital, Marshall University, Huntington, WV, USA
e-mail: paynem@marshall.edu

D. Nemade
Orlando Health Neuroscience Institute, Orlando, FL, USA

EEG activity is the electrical signal from neuronal cell bodies, which is the gray matter, the outer cortex of the brain. These EEG signals from the gray matter traverse the meninges, skull, muscle, fat, and skin to represent the signal on the EEG recording. Beneath the cortex is the subcortical white matter, which is responsible for white matter tracts connecting pathways for the brain and spinal cord. Deeper gray matter exists in cases of cortical dysplasia (such as gray matter lining the ventricles) and is not often detected by scalp EEG recordings.

Signals responsible for EEG recordings are primarily generated by cortical pyramidal neurons that are oriented perpendicularly to the brain's surface. The neuronal activity detectable by the EEG is the summation of the excitatory and inhibitory postsynaptic potentials of large groups of neurons firing simultaneously (Fig. 1.1). Signals from cells oriented parallel to the brain's surface are not detected at the corresponding cortical electrode and, if detected at all, may be detected at other electrode regions (Fig. 1.2).

Figure Description:
The EEG waveforms seen represent the direction of the dipole. Current flows from positive to negative areas.

- When the electrode closer to the surface is more negative than the deeper electrode, a negative signal is produced, which is plotted as an upward deflection. (Convention of EEG)
- When the electrode closer to the surface is more positive than the deeper electrode, a positive signal is produced, which is plotted as a downward deflection. (Convention of EEG)

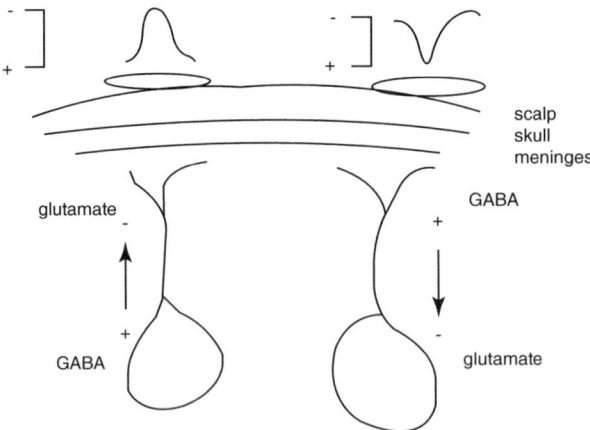

Fig. 1.1 Schematic showing electrical potentials and relation of the neurons to the scalp EEG electrodes and signal they produce

Fig. 1.2 Pictures of two different vectors showing electrical potential signals directed toward different directions

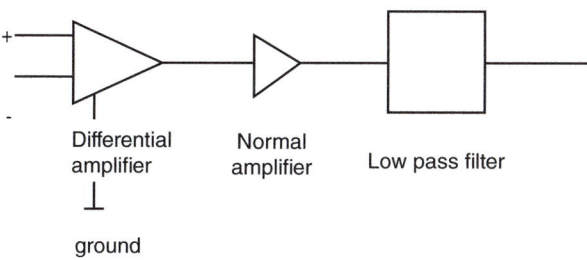

Fig. 1.3 Diagram of signals being processed through the EEG system

The potentials generated parallel to the scalp are not detected by the corresponding scalp EEG electrodes. In this case, such as in a cortical fissure, the signal is spread in a tangential manner and may be detected by EEG electrodes in other areas [3].

The actual signal detected by the scalp electrodes is very small, in the scale of a few microvolts. The EEG machine receives cortical potentials from the surface electrodes. When the signal is first processed, a differential amplifier calculates the difference in voltages between two electrodes, then amplifies this difference into a larger voltage. A standard amplifier further processes and increases that signal. A high-frequency (low pass) filter is then used to filter out high-frequency activity, which is usually electrical artifact (Fig. 1.3). The final signal seen on the EEG recording is a result of these manipulations [2].

1.2 Scalp Electrodes

Scalp electrodes are placed at standard positions on the head and a commonly used technique for placement is called the international 10–20 system, which is recommended by the International Federation of EEG Society (Fig. 1.4). EEG electrodes are placed in relation to anatomical landmarks, such as the nasion (bony depression in the middle of the face between the eyes), inion (occipital protuberance), and the preauricular area. The distances between these skull landmarks are measured and electrodes are spaced at a standardized 10% or 20% length of the total distances between them.

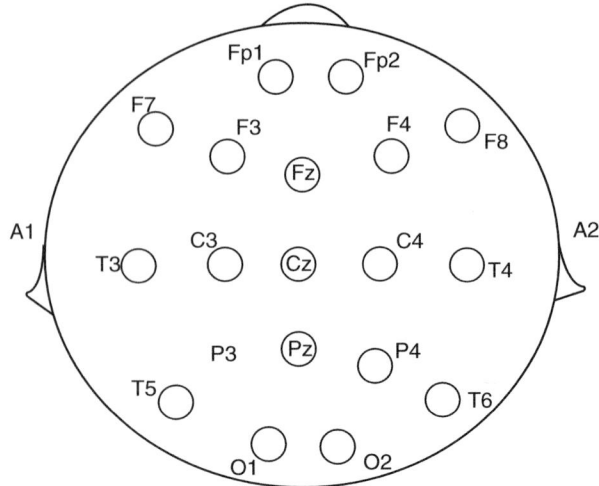

Fig. 1.4 Traditional EEG 10–20 electrode headset placement

The right side of the head has an even number electrodes, and the left side of the head has an odd number of electrodes.

Electrodes correspond to the first letter of the corresponding cortical region.

F—frontal
Fp—fronto-polar
C—central
P—parietal
T—temporal
O—occipital
A is for a reference electrode, commonly at the mastoid or ear lobe.

There are unique technical considerations for neonatal EEG placement because of the smaller head size. An abbreviated 10–20 system is used, in which the electrodes are measured based on the 10% and 20% format. However, not as many electrodes are placed (Fig. 1.5). If all electrodes were to be placed on a small head, interelectrode distance is likely to be too short, which could create an artifact. A salt bridge occurs when electrodes are close to each other and the signals from each electrode summate identically to both electrodes, creating a false flat line on the recording.

Most seizures in neonates occur in central and temporal head regions, so the central and temporal electrodes are included in the abbreviated headset [5]. Facilities have unique protocols for electrode use and placement. Specific electrodes used can vary, but the central and temporal regions are most consistently represented. Use of the abbreviated headset or full headset depends on each facility's head circumference criteria. The average newborn full-term head size is 35 cm, and this size can accommodate either the neonatal or standard headset. However, some facilities prefer to use a neonatal headset until 40 cm head size. Presence of a cephalic IV or post-surgical site may warrant an abbreviated headset as well.

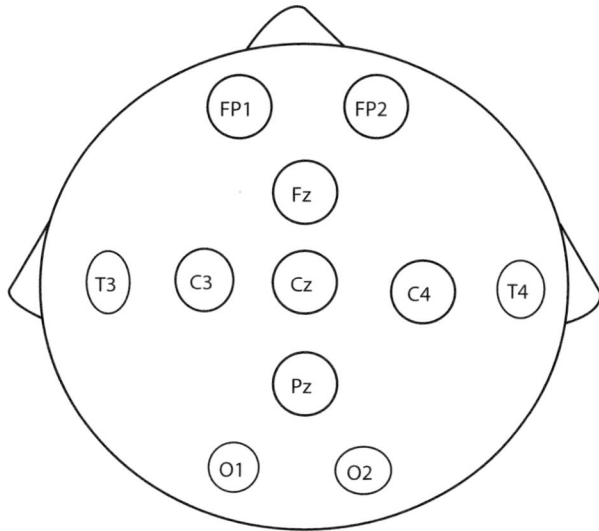

Fig. 1.5 Neonatal EEG example

1.3 Other Electrodes

Other measured parameters or extracerebral channels that are included in the neonatal EEG are

- Electrooculogram (EOC)—Two EOC electrodes are placed near the outer canthus of the eyes, one above the eye and the other below the eye. (Exact location of these electrodes may vary by facility.) Detecting eye movement allows for the identification of different behavioral stages, in particular the sleep stages. Eye movements can also be seen in seizures or nystagmus, so correlation with EEG activity can be helpful (Fig. 1.6).
- Electromyogram (EMG)—Electrodes that detect muscle activity placed on the chin. This aids in the identification of different behavioral stages: awake, active sleep, and quiet sleep.
- Electrocardiogram (ECG)—ECG leads on the chest to record variations of the heart rate and allow distinction of ECG artifact on the EEG.
- Respiratory belt—Monitors chest wall movement, which also helps identify sleep stages.

1.4 Impedance

When EEG electrodes are applied, the skin is often scrubbed and cleaned prior to the placement of the electrode. This is to minimize friction and other debris that could cause interference of the signal. The skin impedance is an indirect measure of the quality of the signal between the EEG electrode and the skin.

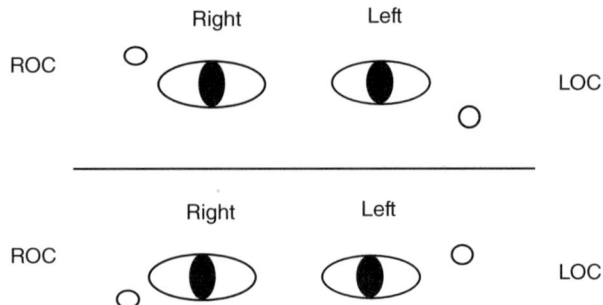

Fig. 1.6 Eye leads placement for electrooculogram that accompanies the neonatal EEG study. Eye lead placement varies based on the facility. For example, the right eye lead may be above or below the right eye but the left eye lead is always placed diagonal to the right eye lead. *ROC* right outer canthus, *LOC* left outer canthus

The unit detected by the EEG machine is an Ohm, which is a measure of electrical resistance. A type of glue or paste is applied to help conduct the signal as well. Babies have very thin and sensitive skin, which can be easily injured with cleaning or can be sensitive to certain glues and gels. However, the thin skin also has an advantage of allowing cortical signals to be more easily traversable. The recommendation is to keep the skin impedance around 5 kilo ohm (kΩ); however, an impedance up to 10 kΩ may produce a technically adequate recording, while avoiding severe skin abrasions.

1.5 Montage

A montage is a pattern in which the electrodes are linked, and this also determines how the signals are interpreted on the screen. This concept is similar to how a radiologist uses different anatomical views for interpreting a brain magnetic resonance image (MRI) via the sagittal, coronal, and axial viewpoints. The American Clinical Neurophysiological Society (ACNS) expects a standard EEG study to be run using three different montages. These may vary slightly from facility to facility but are overall similar. Using different montages can help localize an epileptiform discharge and evaluate artifacts. However, if a neonatal EEG is performed using the abbreviated headset, then typically the only montage used is the neonatal montage associated with that particular abbreviated headset. Fewer electrodes have fewer options for linkage and interelectrode comparisons.

A common montage is the longitudinal bipolar montage, also called double banana. The lines look like two bananas outlined (Fig. 1.7). The neonatal montage is partly longitudinal bipolar but may also have some electrodes linked as transverse (across the head) (Fig. 1.8). If an EEG reviewer prefers a certain montage with unique electrode linkages, the technicians can personalize this in the software.

1 Introduction and Technical Aspects of Neonatal EEGs

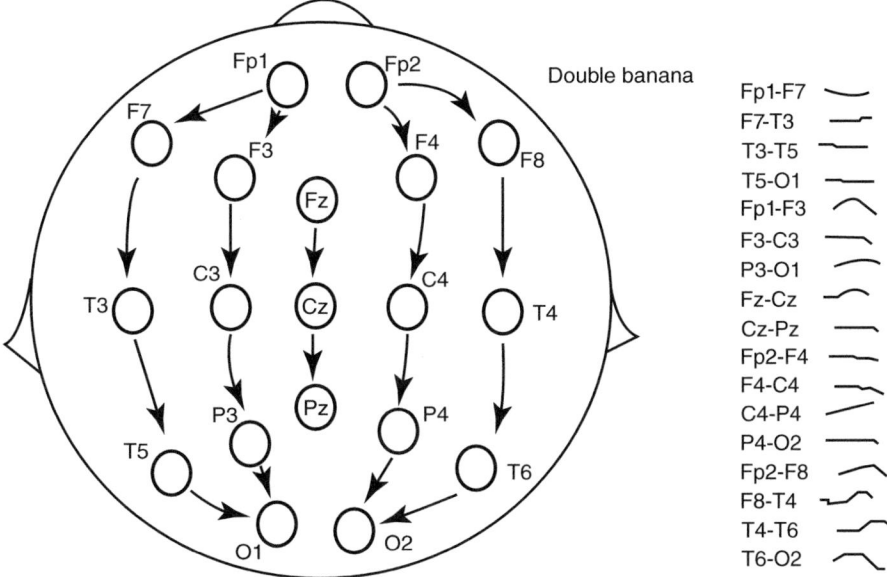

Fig. 1.7 Longitudinal bipolar montage example in a standard EEG headset

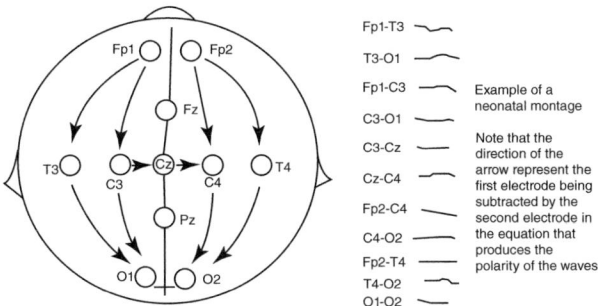

Fig. 1.8 Neonatal montage example

In each chain, an electrode's voltage is compared to that of the electrode above it, so each tracing line represents a pair of electrodes in which the voltage of the second electrode is subtracted from the voltage of the first. Because of this, in bipolar montage, if the first electrode in the tracing line is more positive or higher than the second, then there is a positive, downward deflection. If the second electrode is more positive or higher, then there is a negative, upward deflection. A phase reversal is created, where the downward and upward deflections meet, as if they touch. The electrode represents the region of maximal negativity in that particular chain of electrodes (Fig. 1.9). Using the example measurements in Fig. 1.9, we can see that within the chain F8 to T4 to T6, maximum negativity at T4 displays as a phase reversal at T4, the electrode in common.

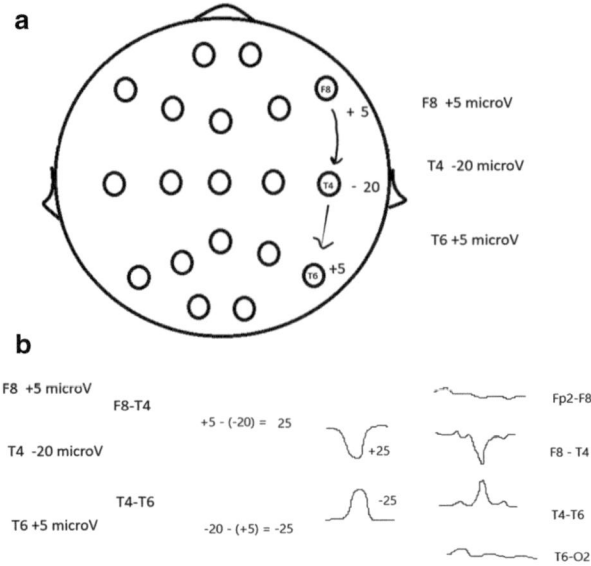

Fig. 1.9 Example of how the montage and electrode differences show the phase reversals as maximal negativity on the display. (**a**) electrode schematic; (**b**) calculations of electrical potential

1.6 EEG Tidbit

Negative and positive *phase reversals* are not the same as negative and positive *discharges*.

Negative discharge: Wave is upward deflection (EEG convention).
Positive discharge: Wave is downward deflection (EEG convention).
Negative phase reversal: Common electrode is most negative and waves point to each other.
Positive phase reversal: Common electrode is positive and waves point out from each other. Most of the time, this is caused by artifact and referred to as an "electrode pop" since it is usually due to a loose electrode. However, there are certain normal waveforms in neonates that have a positive polarity and thus a positive phase reversal.

What happens to the electrodes at the end of a chain?
Using the example above (Fig. 1.9), imagine the chain Fp1-F7-T3-T5-O1. We were able to identify the phase reversal for T4 when T4 had maximal negativity compared to F8 and T6. What happens if Fp1 or O1 have maximum negativity? This is called end of chain phenomenon, and only half of the phase reversal is displayed [3]. Montages can then be changed to one that incorporates the electrode of concern

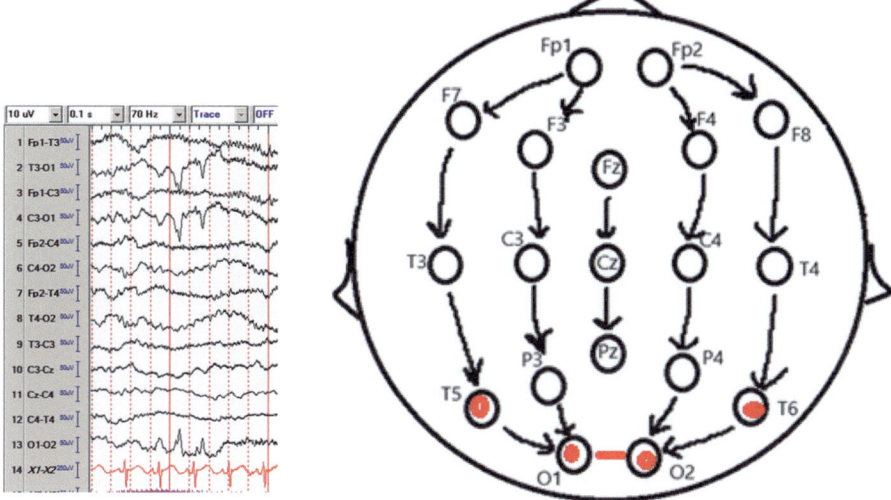

Fig. 1.10 (**a, b**) Example of the end of chain for O1: you can see there is only a downward deflection in the upper lines because O1 is at the end of the chain. However, the lowest line links O1 to O2, which helps identify the negative signal is maximal at O1 (upward deflection). Crossing from the left to the right hemisphere is a linkage used in transverse montages

to be within a chain, not at the end of the chain. For example, if a sharp wave is seen only in the O1 electrode in a bipolar montage, the reader can change the montage to one that shows the electrode (O1) to not be at the end of a chain (Fig. 1.10). A transverse montage links the order of electrodes T6-O2-O1-T5, so that the O1 electrode is not at the end and can be compared to its adjacent electrodes T5 and O2. O1 then shows a phase reversal, in the same way as T4 did in Fig. 1.9. Transverse montages link the left to the right hemispheres for these types of midline comparisons. Some neonatal montages also have an additional line linking the left and right occiput.

1.7 Parameters of EEG Waveforms

– Amplitude of Waves

Amplitude is the height of a wave and is measured in microvolts (Fig. 1.11).

– Frequency of Waves

The frequency of a waveform is its speed, or how many cycles of that wave occur per second. The unit is hertz (Hz) and terms have been assigned to certain frequency ranges (Table 1.1). The EEG display shows the screen divided by second intervals, so the frequency can be counted by how many cycles of that particular waveform occur within a 1 s duration (Figs. 1.12 and 1.13).

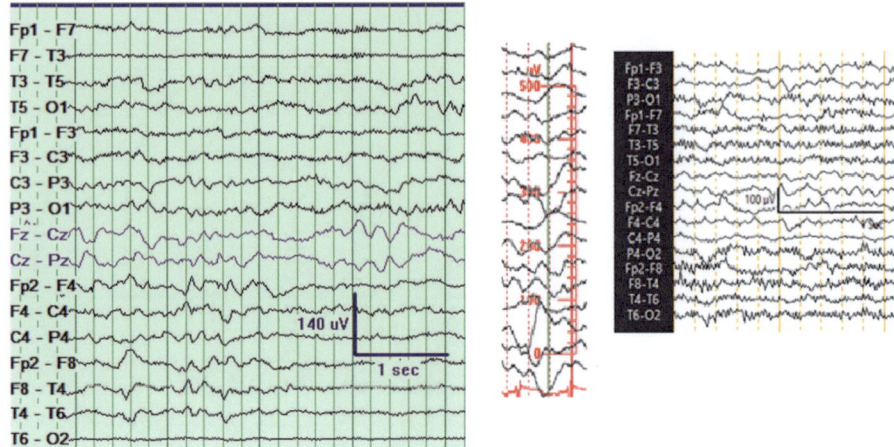

Fig. 1.11 The height of a wave is the amplitude. EEG software includes a ruler for measurement. Scale is in microvolts (μV)

Table 1.1 List of conventional terms for various frequencies in EEG

Defined frequency ranges:	
Delta	Less than 4 Hz
Theta	4–8 Hz
Alpha	8–12 Hz
Spindle[a]	11–16 Hz
Ripple[b]	16–20 Hz
Beta	12–30 Hz
Gamma	30–100 Hz

[a]Spindle is a particular type of waveform that is not a defined frequency but is mentioned in this chart for concept introduction. At 2 months of age (48 WGA) in sleep, sleep spindles begin to occur. These waveforms are low amplitude and are centrally located at a frequency of 11–16 Hz. Some premature neonatal background waveforms are described as having a "spindle-like" appearance, in which superimposed alpha frequencies are present on slower waveforms. This appearance may remind the reader of a sleep spindle, although not having any other similarities to a sleep spindle besides the frequency of 11–16 Hz. Using this term in neonatal EEGs can be very confusing and misleading

[b]Ripple, similar to spindle, is not a defined frequency but rather the occurrence of a fast frequency (16–20 Hz) that often occurs superimposed on a slow delta wave. Ripples are in the beta frequency range but the term ripple may be described in older textbooks as a "ripple of prematurity" when describing the more modern term *delta brush*

1 Introduction and Technical Aspects of Neonatal EEGs

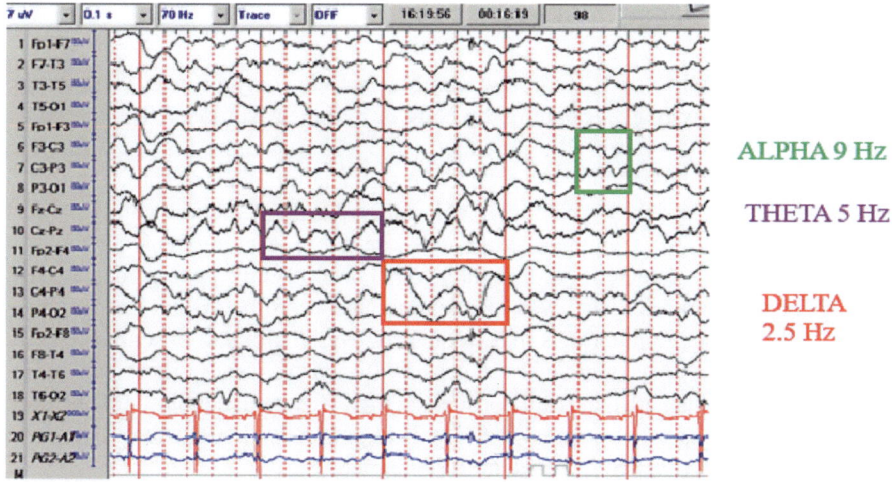

Fig. 1.12 Frequencies pictured: delta, theta, and alpha in a neonatal EEG recording. As in the example of alpha frequencies, the frequency may occur less than 1 s. In this case, the waves can be counted as if they continue for 1 s, which gives the appropriate number of Hertz

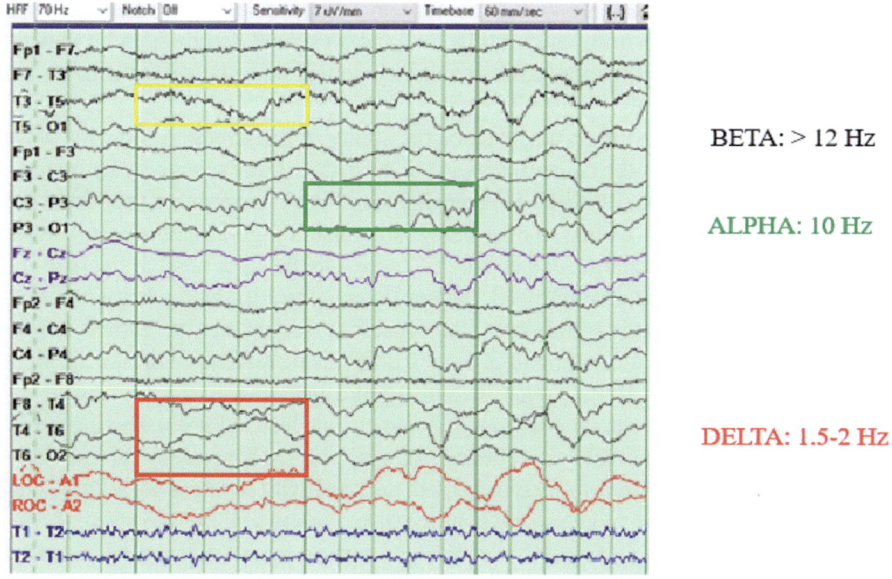

Fig. 1.13 Frequencies pictured in a neonatal EEG study: delta, alpha, and beta

1.8 Technical EEG Aspects

An unfortunate reality of EEG is that cerebral activity may be overwhelmed by other electrical activity generated by the body or in the environment. To be seen on the scalp surface, the cerebrally generated EEG voltages must first pass through multiple biological layers that both reduce the signal amplitude and spread the EEG activity out more widely than its original source vector. Cerebral voltages must traverse the brain, CSF, meninges, skull, and skin before reaching the recording site where they can be detected. Additionally, other biologically generated electrical activity by scalp muscles, the eyes, the tongue, and even the distant heart signals create massive voltage potentials that frequently overwhelm and obscure the cerebral activity. Being able to change the sensitivity and frequency filters can sometimes help distinguish artifact from cortical activity. However, caution must be used to not filter out important cortical activity. It is generally thought that it requires 5 cm^2 of cortical activity to generate an EEG signal.

– Sensitivity

The sensitivity setting changes the height of the waveform on the digital screen. A higher sensitivity (less sensitive) makes the waveform smaller and a lower sensitivity (more sensitive) makes the waveform higher. Standard setting for sensitivity is 7 μV per millimeter (μV/mm) and at this level most cortical activity can be viewed comfortably. For this guidebook, the sensitivity setting may be referred to as the microvolt (μV) value only.

A high-amplitude waveform may exceed the ability of the screen to show the wave in its totality. In this case, the reader may want to "turn down" the sensitivity by increasing the sensitivity setting: 10, then 15, then 30, then 50 μV to evaluate the waveform within a readable range. Doing so may help distinguish a high-amplitude wave from artifact, epileptiform discharge, or sleep architecture. On the other hand, if the baseline background activity is very suppressed, the reader may want to see the low-amplitude waveforms more distinctly. In this case, the sensitivity setting can be "turned up" by lowering the number of the setting to 5, 3, or 2 μV. This makes the environment more sensitive to show all waveforms, regardless of significance.

With any alteration of viewing settings, adjustment can lead to falsely viewing waveforms. For example, a low-voltage recording showing cortical suppression at a sensitivity setting of 7 μV. When sensitivity is increased, the sensitivity setting is set at 2 μV. This makes the recording view more sensitive, so the display shows all the waveforms better to the reader. However, waveforms that may not be cortical signals will also be increased in view and may give a false indication of cortical activity (Fig. 1.14).

On the other hand, very high-voltage activity can be difficult to interpret at the standard setting of 7 μV sensitivity. In this case, the sensitivity setting is turned down, which makes the recording less sensitive. High-amplitude waveforms will be minimized to appear smaller. The morphology can be discerned better when the entire waveform is viewable. In the below cases of extreme high-amplitude input, the signal is saturated and generates a flat max line. Lowering the sensitivity allows for the entire waveform to be seen. However, this change may cause the reader to overlook other high-amplitude activity as all the activity is overall lower in character (Fig. 1.15).

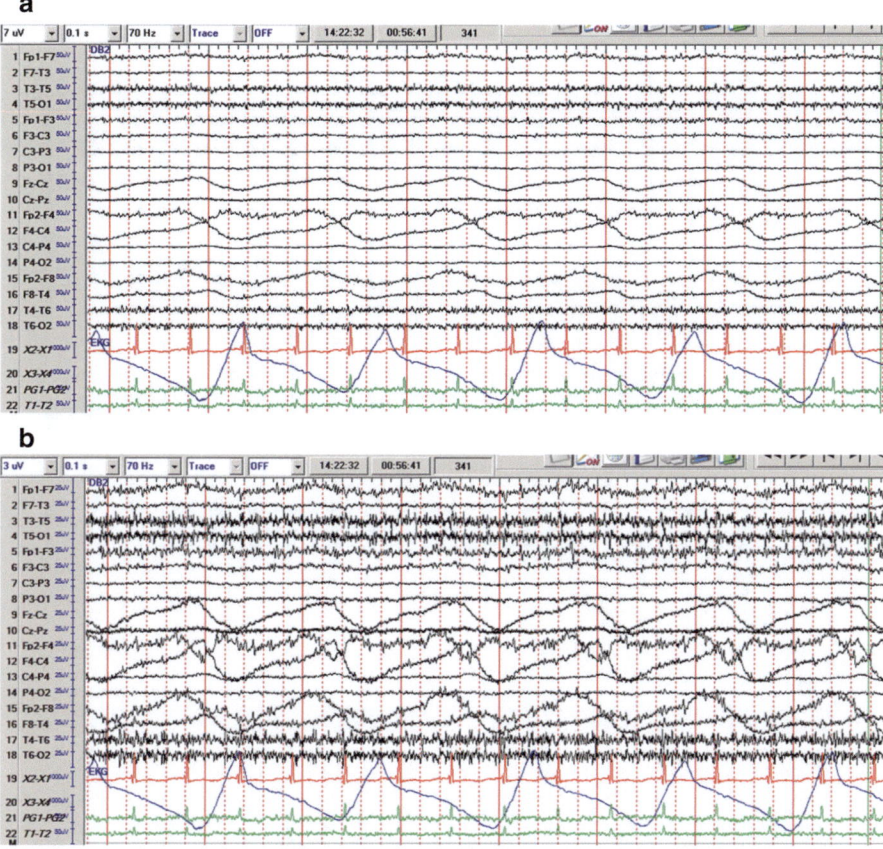

Fig. 1.14 Nearly isoelectric neonatal EEG. At a sensitivity setting of 7 μV (default), minimal change in waveforms is seen. With changes to 3 μV sensitivity, more waveforms are detected. However, this also shows many signals that are likely artifactual. (**a**) Sensitivity at 7 μV, (**b**) sensitivity 3 μV

High-voltage waveforms can be difficult to interpret using standard parameters. Below are the examples of high-amplitude activity, which can be better discerned at a lower sensitivity setting (Figs. 1.16 and 1.17). The ability to view the entire waveform allows the reader to distinguish between a high-amplitude epileptiform waveform and a high-amplitude movement-induced artifact waveform. In the case of myoclonic seizures in Fig. 1.16, the baby's movements occur synchronously with the high-amplitude epileptiform spikes, which causes artifact waves and epileptiform discharge waves concurrently. In Fig. 1.17, the baby's movements create a high-amplitude wave due to the movement artifact. This baby did not have an epileptic discharge associated with this movement. Lowering the sensitivity allows the reader to better discern the waveforms and look for an epileptic morphology.

– Filters

A low-frequency filter is also called a high-pass filter since higher frequencies are allowed to be viewed. A low-frequency filter is set lower in neonatal recordings than for

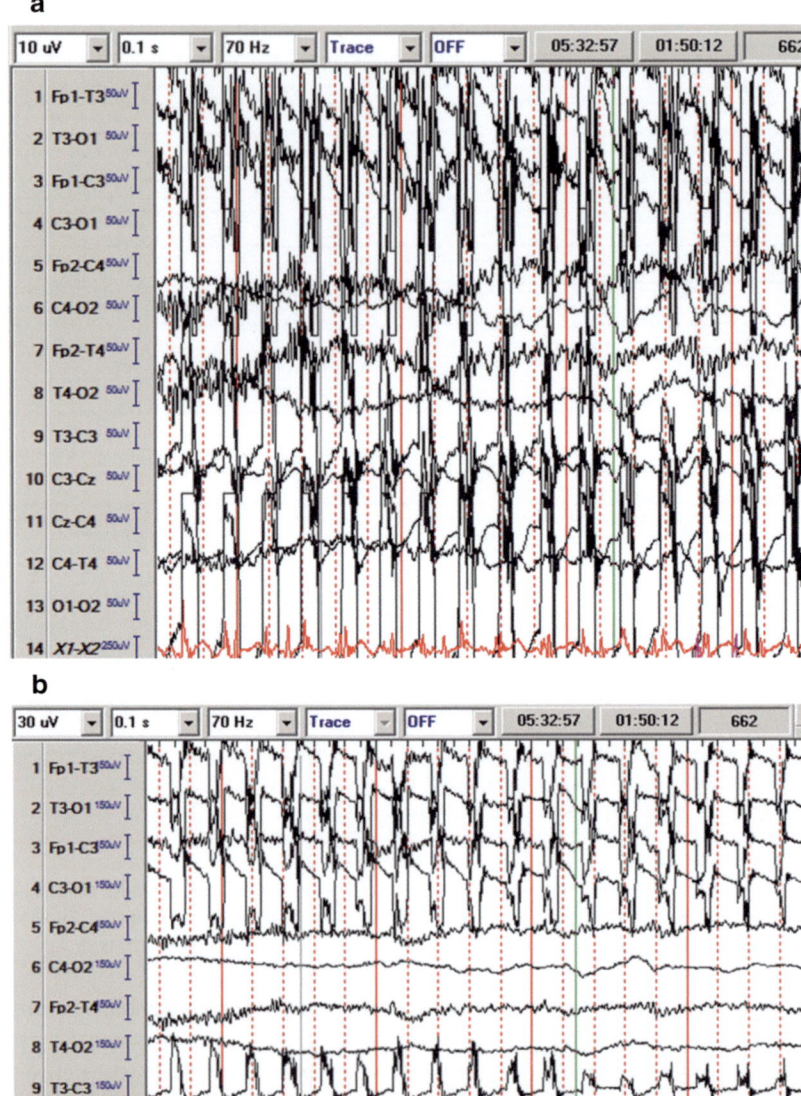

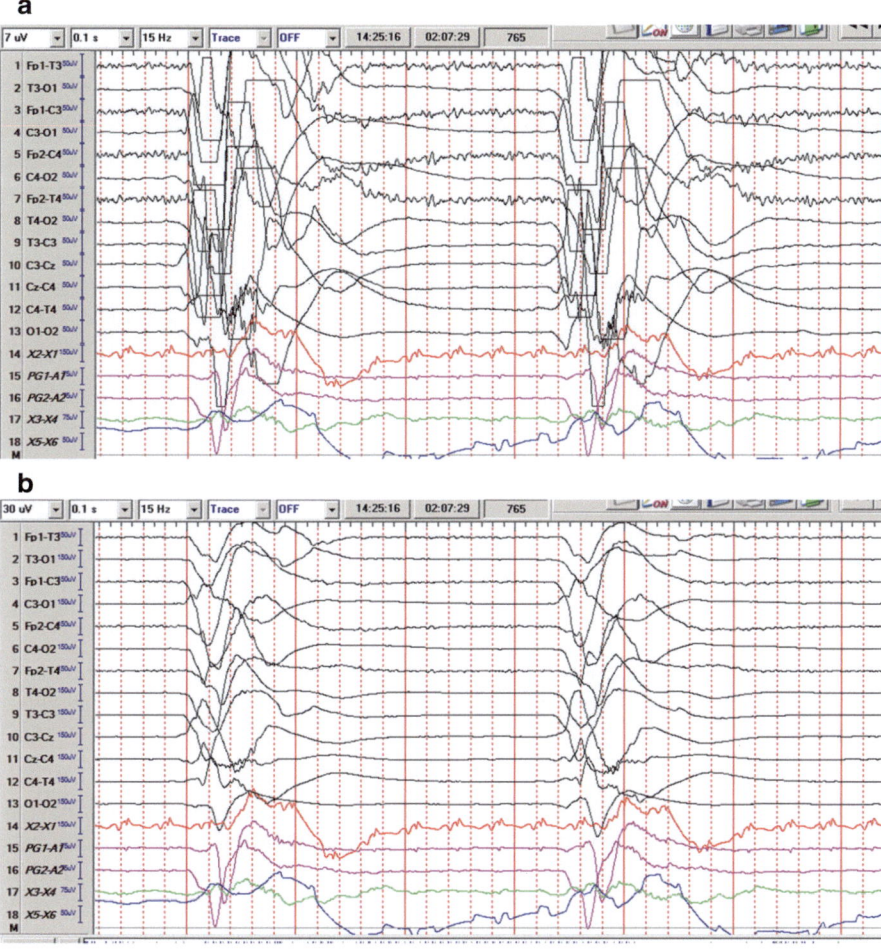

Fig. 1.16 (**a, b**) Examples of myoclonic seizures displayed at different sensitivities. (**a**) Sensitivity setting is at 7 μV and (**b**) 30 μV. The lower sensitivity of 30 μV setting allows for waveforms to appear smaller on the screen and the entire waveform morphology can be viewed. In this case, high-amplitude waveforms were generated from movement artifact only. (**a**) 7 μV/mm, (**b**) 30 μV/mm

Fig. 1.15 High-voltage waveforms can be difficult to interpret using standard parameters. The lower sensitivity setting allows for waveforms to appear smaller on the screen and the entire waveform morphology can be viewed. The ability to view the entire waveform allows the reader to distinguish between a high-amplitude epileptiform waveform and a high-amplitude movement-induced artifact waveform. (**a**) Sensitivity is set at 10 μV; (**b**) Sensitivity is set at 30 μV and the waveform shape is consistent with movement artifact

Above is an example in which high-amplitude waves saturate the output and cannot be interpreted wholly. Sensitivity is at a 10 μV setting (a) and a 30 μV setting (b), which allows for the interpretation of the waveform etiology

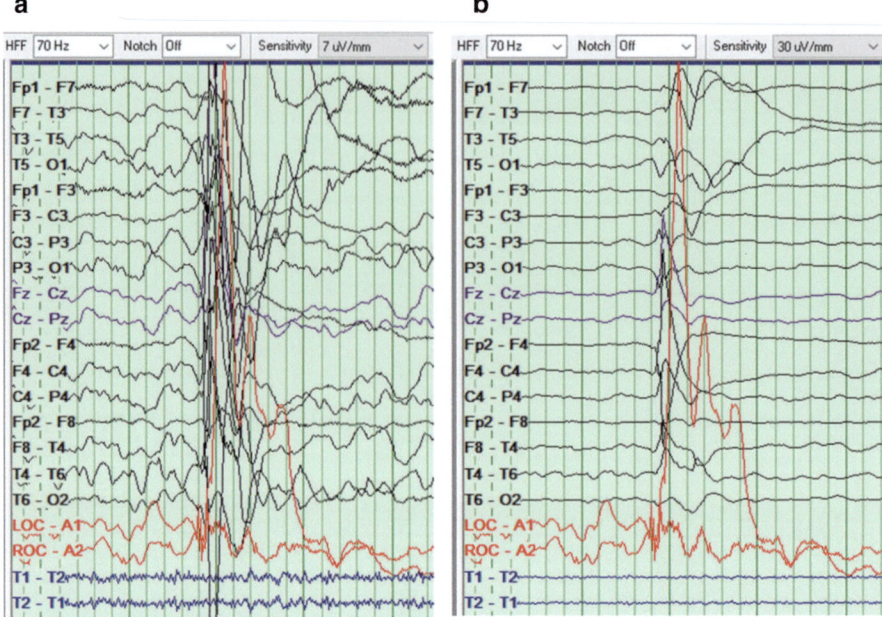

Fig. 1.17 High-voltage waveforms can be difficult to interpret using standard parameters. (**a**) Sensitivity setting is at 7 µV and (**b**) 30 µV. The lower sensitivity setting allows for waveforms to appear smaller on the screen and the entire waveform morphology can be viewed

EEG recordings in older children and adults to allow for the recording of slower frequencies at 0.005–0.01 Hz or 0.5 Hz, which are inherent in neonates. Neonates may have significant meaningful frequencies in this low range, whereas older children and adults do not. Having a filter set to show these lower frequencies in older patients may show signals that are more likely to be artifacts and then misinterpreted as cortical activity.

The high-frequency filter (low-pass filter) setting is similar to adult recordings at 35–70 Hz. High-frequency filter allows for signals to pass that are under the setting, so a high-frequency filter allows signals below 70 Hz. Electrical signal (artifact of electrical wires, computers) often occurs at frequencies of 60 Hz or greater (Fig. 1.18).

- Development of EEG technology into the digital and Internet age

Original machines that used paper
- Had a paper "speed" setting.
- Unable to change montage, sensitivity, filters after the recording.
- No video, relied on tech for comments, especially with mental status info and artifact info.
- Study was saved on paper recording, which was thick, bulky, not simple to transport.

Newer machines with digital technology
- Montages, sensitivity, filter settings easily changed during and after the recording.
- Video and audio recording.

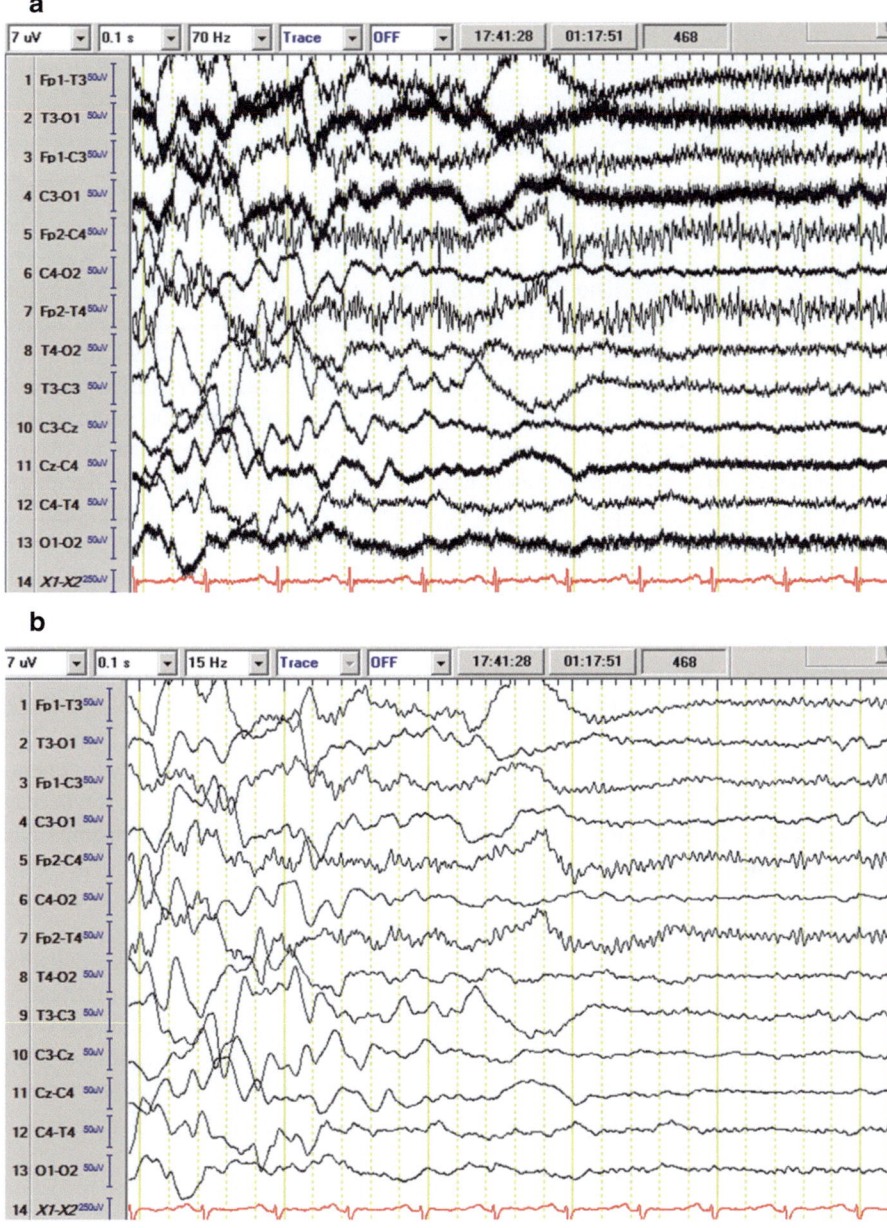

Fig. 1.18 (**a**, **b**) Figures showing how changing the high-frequency filter setting can lessen artifacts caused by high-frequency activity, such as muscle movements

Changing from 70 Hz (**a**) to 15 Hz (**b**), most of the muscle artifact activity is excluded. However, changing this setting also filters out potential high-frequency cortical sharp waves

- Ease of viewing (remotely, multiple medical personnel can view at same time from different places).
- Data stored, depending on lab, may be saved for a certain amount of time.
- Easier to do longer studies, digital data can later be clipped or deleted.
- Paper speed

Early EEG machines displayed the electrical signal display on rolls of paper. The paper fed through a rotating arm while needles with ink printed the EEG data. The paper page was standardized to a 10 s increment and typical EEG studies were run for 30 min. However, neonatal EEG recordings have always been at least a duration of 60 min because a normal term neonate should cycle between wakefulness, active sleep, and quiet sleep in this 60-min time frame. In the days of paper EEG, this study length of 60 min meant twice as much paper as the typical older child EEG study of 30 min. To accommodate for this difference and lessen the burden on supplies, the speed at which the paper moved around the rotating arm during a neonate recording was slowed by 50%, so twice as much data could be recorded on the same size page. A page showing 10 s of older child EEG data showed 20 s of neonatal EEG data.

As a result, neonatal electroencephalographers became accustomed to reviewing the EEG images containing 20 s of data per page. This speed produced a different appearance of the EEG; waveforms were shorter but with the same amplitude. The overall appearance gives the study a sharper character. With the onset of the digital age and EEG recordings then developed with computer technology, the advantage of saving paper was no longer needed. With a simple click of the mouse, it became very simple to switch from 10 s per viewing page to 20 s per viewing page. (The screen on a digital recording is still called a "page.") Over time, as a newer generation of electroencephalographers developed their skills in the digital age, the neonatal recordings defaulted to the same parameters of the other EEG recordings and were recorded and viewed at 10 s per page. However, in some of the older textbooks, the 20 s per page parameter has been used for figures and so the ability for EEG readers to interpret both parameters remains an important skill.

Some readers continue to favor the 20 s per page parameter since it is somewhat quicker to identify the state of the patient (Figs. 1.19 and 1.20). The amount of discontinuity can be easily assessed if the setting is changed to show a longer duration per computer screen view. Likewise, rhythmicity in seizure activity can sometimes be more apparent having a longer time frame within which to view (Fig. 1.21). The paper speed is generally chosen based on the reader's preference and experience.

- Justification for Long-Term EEG Monitoring

The invention of digital EEG recordings has not only changed how we can view and manipulate the recording data but has also improved our recording capacities. With digital data being easily stored and shared, longer recordings have become more common. However, any new technological advance may also yield some concerns and possible disadvantages for patient care.

The ACNS has established guidelines that outline the indications for long-term electroencephalography monitoring in neonates [4]. Reasons include

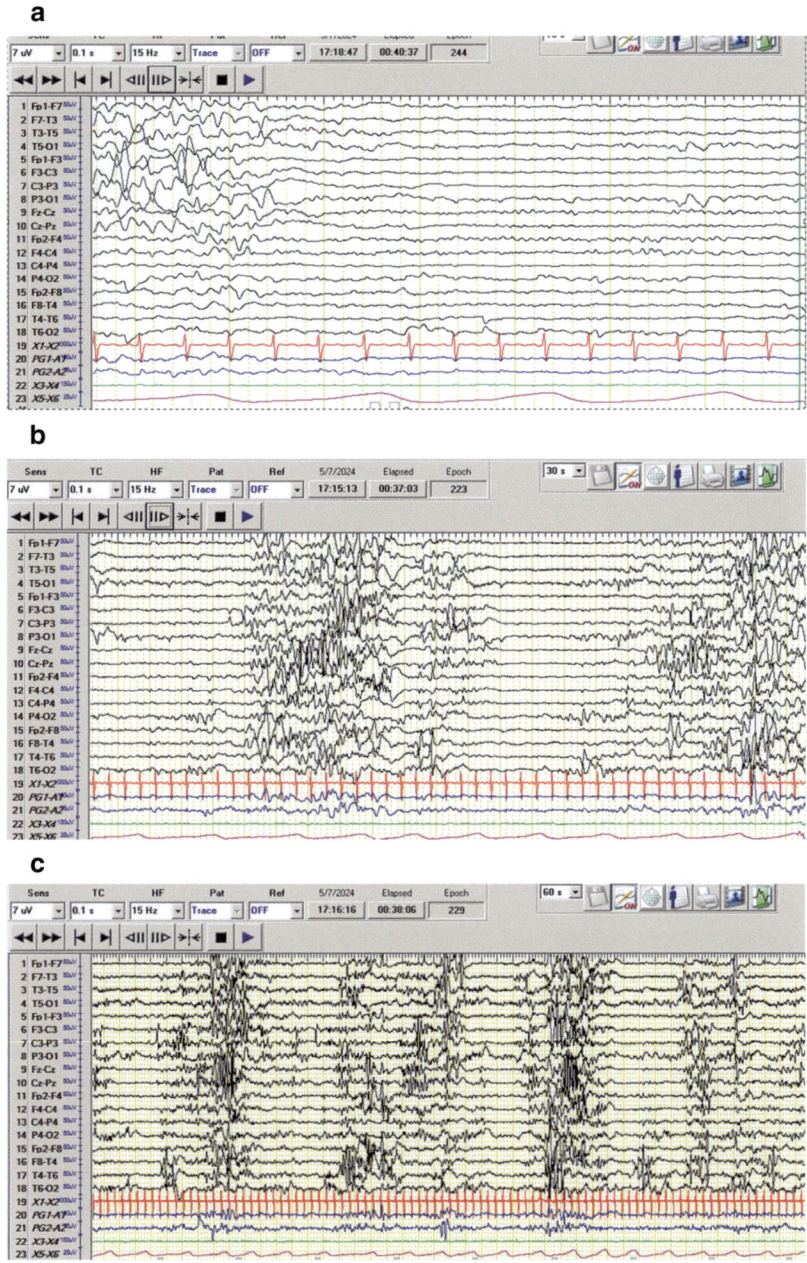

Fig. 1.19 (a–c) Advantages of viewing background activity as a longer duration of time within the same viewing page size when assessing neonatal background activity. (**a**) The screen is set at viewing 7 s per page, (**b**) 22 s, and (**c**) 45 s. This allows the reader to view the background activity well when there are long periods of attenuation. This patient's interburst interval was about 5 s in length

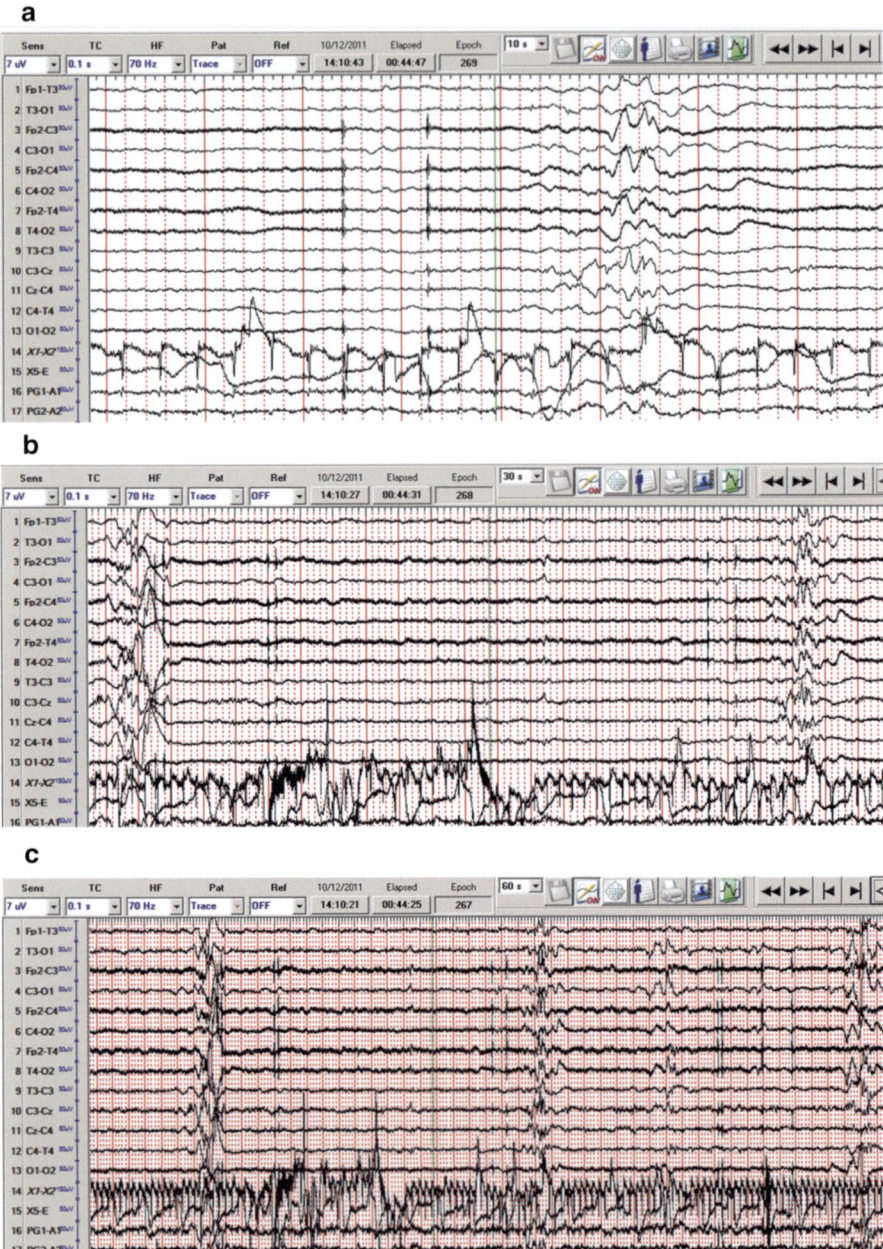

Fig. 1.20 (a–c) Advantages of viewing background activity as a longer duration of time within the same viewing page size when assessing neonatal background activity. (**a**) The screen is set at viewing 8 s per page, (**b**) 24 s, and (**c**) 48 s. This allows the reader to view the background activity well when there are long periods of attenuation. This patient's interburst interval was about 18 s in duration

1 Introduction and Technical Aspects of Neonatal EEGs

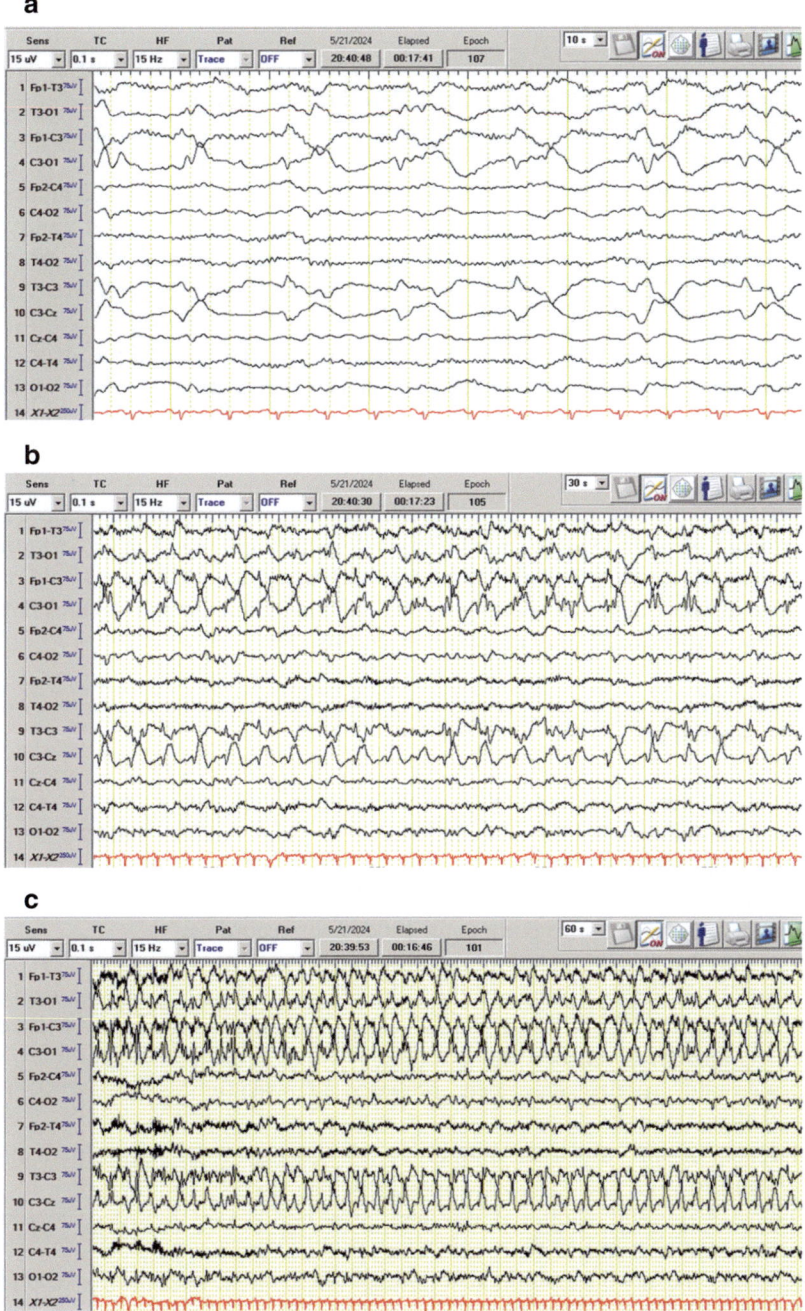

Fig. 1.21 (a–c) Advantages of viewing epileptic activity as a longer duration of time within the same screen size. A seizure located in the left central region is viewed using different page length parameters. (**a**) 8 s per page, (**b**) 16 s per page, and (**c**) 32 s per page

- Capture the events that are of concern and determine if the events are epileptic in nature.
    Goal is to treat epileptic events quickly and then to have the ability to monitor electrographic activity following initiation of treatment.
- Identify seizures in high-risk populations.
    This includes neonates with acute brain injury and neonates with encephalopathy. Neonates with cardiac or pulmonary compromise are at a higher risk of anoxic injury as well, thus leading to seizures. Infection and trauma can also cause focal areas of dysfunction and epileptogenicity. Known focal abnormalities such as infarction, vascular malformation, congenital cortical dysgenesis, or tumors can also lead to higher rates of seizures.
- Infants undergoing hypothermia protocols are also monitored with EEG recordings to evaluate for epileptic activity and monitor the degree of encephalopathy.
- Identification and treatment of subclinical seizures.

Concerns with overuse of recording are very controversial. Improved access to EEG recording can lead to more frequent recordings and longer recordings. Subclinical seizures are thus able to be detected, those that otherwise would not be identified. It is not clear how identifying and treating the subclinical seizures impacts the patient's overall care and long-term prognosis [1].

1.9   Reports

To provide an accurate interpretation of the neonatal EEG, reports need to provide

- Gestational age of the baby.
- Adjusted age of the baby.
- Medications the baby is taking at the time of the recording.
- Baby's response to stimulation, if performed.
- Optimally, behavioral states of the baby are either noted by the technician or observed on the video recording in order to correlate with EEG background activity and described as such.
- Background patterns described, presence of wakefulness, active sleep, or quiet sleep.
- Presence of any abnormal amplitudes, frequencies, symmetry patterns, or asynchrony.
- Clinical events and mention of any significant findings on the video recording.
- Electrographic events.
- Heart rate and any other significant findings based on the eye, chin, or respiratory monitoring leads.

References

1. Hunt RW, Liley HG, Wagh D, et al. Effect of treatment of clinical seizures vs electrographic seizures in full-term and near-term neonates: a randomized clinical trial. JAMA Netw Open. 2021;4(12):e2139604. https://doi.org/10.1001/jamanetworkopen.2021.39604.
2. Mizrahi E, Hrachovy R. Atlas of neonatal electroencephalography. 4th ed. New York: Demos Medical; 2016.
3. Niedermeyer E, De Silva FL. Electroencephalopagraphy, basic principles, clinical applications and related fields. Philadelphia: Williams and Wilkins; 1993.
4. Shellhaas R, Change T, Tsuchida T, et al. The American Clinical Neurophysiology Society's guideline on continuous electroencephalography monitoring in neonates. J Clin Neurophyiol. 2011;28:611–7.
5. Tekgul H, Bourgeois B, Gauvreau K, et al. Electroencephalopagraphy in neonatal seizures: comparison of a reduced and a full 10/20 montage. Pediatr Neurol. 2004;32:155–61. https://doi.org/10.1016/j.pediatrneurol.2004.09.014.

Developmental Maturation of the EEG in Neonates, from Preterm to Term Gestational Ages

Mary Payne

2.1 Introduction

As the use of EEG has become more commonplace and younger preterm neonates have been studied more frequently, it has become apparent that electrical brain activity develops according to conceptional age, not actual age. EEG baseline background activity changes as the neonate matures and advances accordingly with gestational age. The most extreme premature babies do not show a distinction between wakefulness and sleep. Their background pattern is discontinuous pattern with no state change or reactivity until about 30 WGA. As the baby matures, clear patterns of waking, active sleep, and quiet sleep can be seen. Maturation is thus a continuum, and obtaining an estimate of a neonate's gestational age can be made within a 2-week range based on EEG alone. This chapter outlines the typical patterns and findings in neonates based on their gestational age.

2.2 Age Definitions (Fig. 2.1)

Gestational age: Measured in weeks, based on 0 weeks gestational age (WGA) is the first day of last menstrual period. Term infant is 40 WGA. This is the most commonly used terminology.

Conceptual age: Measured in weeks, based on 0 weeks conceptional age (WCA) is time of conception. This is typically 2 weeks AFTER the first day of last menstrual period. Term infant is 38 WCA. This term is least often used.

Postmenstrual age (PMA): Gestational age plus chronological age.

Chronological age: Time since birth.

M. Payne (✉)
Department of Pediatrics, Division of Pediatric Neurology, Joan C Edwards School of Medicine, Hoops Family Children's Hospital, Marshall University, Huntington, WV, USA
e-mail: paynem@marshall.edu

© The Author(s), under exclusive license to Springer Nature Switzerland AG 2025
M. Payne, D. Gloss II (eds.), *Neonatal EEG*,
https://doi.org/10.1007/978-3-031-92556-6_2

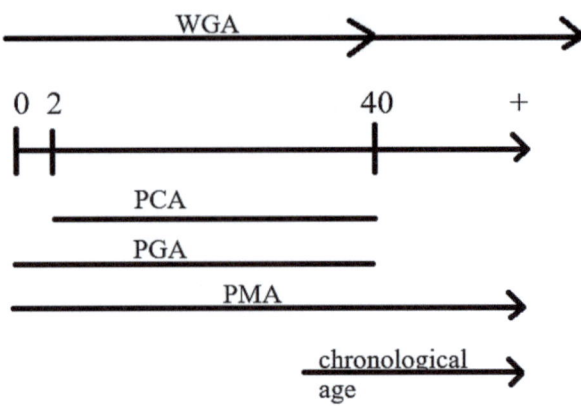

Fig. 2.1 Schematic of different terms related to ages of neonates. *0* represents the first day of last menstrual period and is time (week) zero. *Postgestational age* is the age of the neonate at birth, based on time zero being the first day of the last menstrual period. *2* represents the day of conception, so week 2 of gestation is based on the first day of last menstrual period or week (time) 0 of conceptional age. 40 is week 40 of gestation, based on time zero being the first day of the last menstrual period and is synonymous with week 38 if time zero is the time of conception. *Postconceptional age* is the week of the neonate at birth, based on time zero being the time of conception. *Postmenstrual age* is the age of the neonate in weeks, based on week 0 being the first day of the last menstrual period. *Chronological age* is the time since birth. Adjusted age (not shown in the diagram) factors in the prematurity of a baby and is defined as the age of the baby if they were born at 40 WGA

For this guidebook, the standard for representing the age of the neonate will be week gestational age (WGA), which is also the *postmenstrual age*

PCA postconceptual age, *PGA* postgestational age, *PMA* postmenstrual age, *WCA* weeks conceptional age, *WGA* weeks gestational age

Table 2.1 Comparison of different terminology for the same age neonate

	Born at 24 WGA, 6 months of age	Born at 40 WGA, 2 months of age
WCA	46 WCA	46 WCA
WGA	48 WGA	48 WGA
PMA	48 weeks	48 weeks
Chronological age	6 months	2 months
Adjusted/corrected age	2 months	2 months
Guide book standard	48 WGA	48 WGA

The following example is of two infants with different birth dates but with the same conceptional age. In other words, their mothers both had the same expected due date at the beginning of their pregnancies. These two patients will have similar appearing EEG studies, assuming all else is equal. This guidebook will use the standard of WGA to represent the age of the neonate

PMA postmenstrual age, *WCA* weeks conceptional age, *WGA* weeks gestational age

Corrected age: Adjusted age, calculates the age based on a 40 WGA birth date. Examples of how to calculate ages with different terminology are provided in Tables 2.1 and 2.2.

Table 2.2 Comparison of different terminology for different age neonates

	Born at 30 WGA, 1 month old	Born at 30 WGA, 3 months old
WCA	32 WCA	40 WCA
WGA	34 WGA	42 WGA
PMA	34 WGA	42 WGA
Chronological age	1 month	3 months
Adjusted/corrected age	34 WGA premature	2 weeks old
Guide book standard	34 WGA	42 WGA

The following example is of two infants with the same gestational age at birth but born on different days. These babies have different postconceptional ages and their mothers had different expected due dates. Their EEG studies will not be similar

PMA postmenstrual age, *WCA* weeks conceptional age, *WGA* weeks gestational age

Table 2.3 Criteria for active and quiet sleep in a term infant when the eyes are closed for more than 30 s

	Active sleep	Quiet sleep
Respiratory rate	Irregular	Regular
Limb movements	Yes	No
Eye movements	Yes	No
Chin movement	Minimal	Frequent
Indeterminate sleep, does not meet either criteria		

The column on the left represents the parameters that may be detected during an EEG study

2.3　State Changes/Mental Status

Similar to older children and adults, a normal mental status should correlate with a normal background EEG activity pattern. However, assessment of a neonate's mental status involves unique observations and criteria that are only seen in neonates. T. Berry Brazelton published *Neonatal Behavioral Assessment Scale* [3] to outline the objective criteria for assessing a full-term neonate's normal expected behavior. Brazelton uses the term "state" to represent the neonate's level of consciousness. He described neonatal behaviors that correlate with the three states of full-term neonates that are identified in EEG recordings (Table 2.3):

Awake: eyes open

>responds to sensory stimuli
>focuses
>fussy/crying
>irregular respirations

Active sleep: eyes closed and can appreciate rapid eye movements under closed lids, may open briefly.

>Low activity level, can have body movements
>Irregular respirations
>Sucking movements intermittent

Responds to external stimuli with arousal
Precursor to REM (rapid eye movement) sleep

Quiet sleep: eyes closed, no eye movements

Minimal spontaneous movements
Deep sleep with regular breathing
Responds to external stimulation with startle but no state change (returns to quiet sleep); this is a precursor to non-REM sleep

Within a 60-min period, the full-term neonate should cycle between wakefulness, active sleep, and quiet sleep on its own or with minimal intervention. Neonates are expected to arouse due to hunger cues or pain and self-soothe spontaneously or following feeds. Also, it is not atypical for a fussy infant to need rocking, patting, or swaddling to be calmed.

However, internal and external factors may affect these expected behaviors. If a neonate does not display these three states within a 60-min period, there is a concern. Being an inpatient with procedures, intravenous lines, feeding tubes, and environments of high stimulation can affect a neonate's ability to self-regulate. Experiencing withdrawals from in utero substance exposures may also affect the cycles as these infants have poor self-soothing and brief quiet sleep. Likewise, the use of sedative medications can limit wakefulness and active sleep. Underlying encephalopathy can also cause abnormal state changes corresponding to abnormal EEG background activity.

Premature infants may not display these state changes with EEG background correlation until at least 30 weeks of gestation. Even so, at the age of 30 WGA, the regulation and response of these states may be immature and not clearly defined.

Recall that routine neonatal EEG duration is 60 min so that these three states can be captured. Additional electrodes for eye movement, chin muscle movement, and respiratory belt are used to help define these three states.

2.4 Overall Background Patterns of Maturity

As the background activity matures, there are some overall patterns that are seen.
Background patterns (Fig. 2.2)

– As the neonate matures, the background becomes more continuous and more reactive (Figs. 2.3 and 2.4).

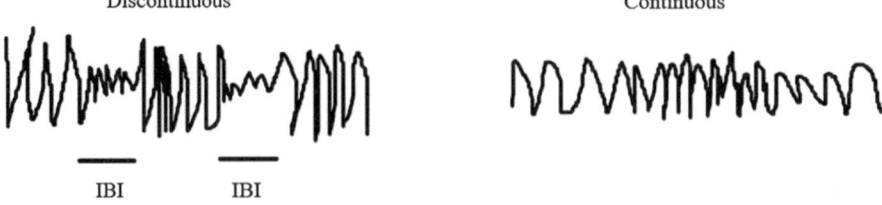

Fig. 2.2 Schematic showing the overall difference between a discontinuous background pattern and a continuous background pattern. The interburst interval is abbreviated IBI, which is the lower voltage period between the higher amplitude burst activity in a neonate. *IBI* interburst interval

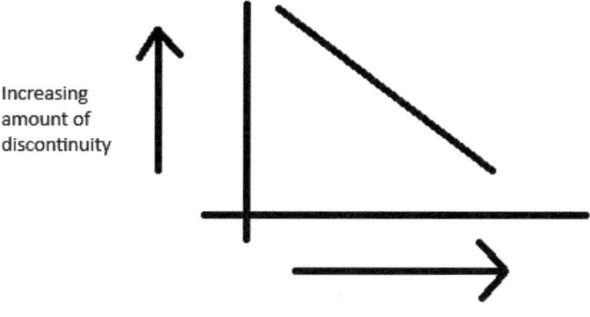

Fig. 2.3 Graph showing increase in gestational age correlates with less discontinuity. Likewise, there is an increase in continuity as the neonate matures

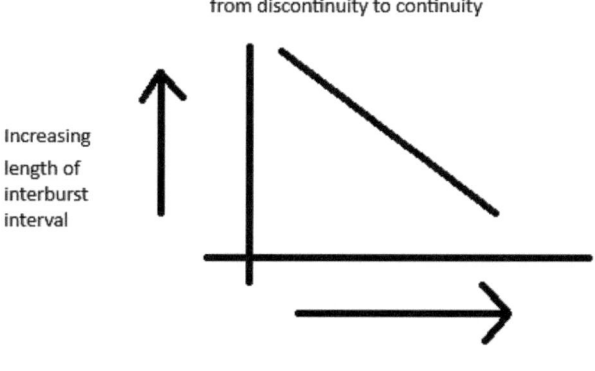

Fig. 2.4 Graph showing increase in length of bursts correlate with decreasing length of interburst interval. This also is a direct relation with increasing gestational age and translates to a more continuous background activity with maturity

- Younger age neonates tend to have a discontinuous background with higher amplitude and lower frequency activity within the bursts (Fig. 2.5).
- Mature neonates show lower amplitude activity with a mixture of low and higher frequencies (Fig. 2.5).
- Very premature and full-term neonates have a synchronous background. Asynchrony in quiet sleep begins around 28 WGA and abates about 32 WGA, with maximal asynchrony around 29–31 WGA (Fig. 2.6).

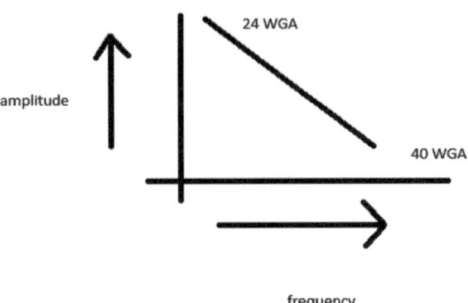

Fig. 2.5 Graph showing premature neonate activity consists of high-amplitude low-frequency activity, seen mostly in the burst activity. With maturity, amplitude lowers and frequencies are mixed of high and low on a continuous background

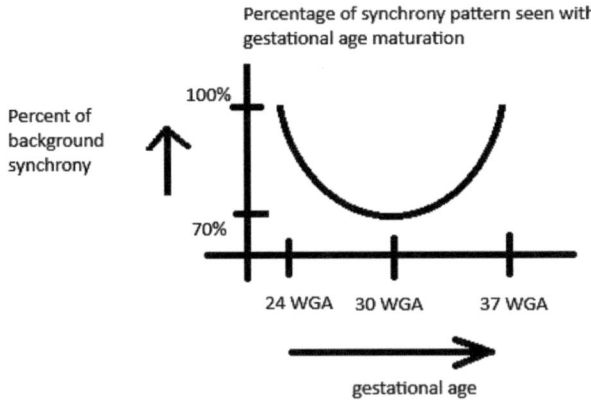

Fig. 2.6 The amount of synchronization varies during neonatal EEG maturation. Before 29–30 weeks CA, bursts are 100% synchronous. Synchrony decreases to approximately 70% between 29 and 31 weeks gestational age. Different sources vary on the exact age of maximal asynchrony. However, synchrony increases progressively thereafter until reaching 100% synchrony at age 37 weeks

2.5 EEG Tidbit

Regardless of gestational age, activity should be symmetric. If asymmetry is present, hemispheric dysfunction is suggested. Between 31 and 36 weeks of gestation, burst activity may be asynchronous. This means that the bursts may occur in each hemisphere at different times. In this case, it may be difficult to ascertain symmetry. Shortening the page to contain a longer duration of data or manually counting the

2 Developmental Maturation of the EEG in Neonates, from Preterm to Term...

Table 2.4 Chart demonstrating background parameters for a 21–22 WGA neonate

Burst length	3–5 s	Tracé discontinu
Burst amplitude	50–330 µV	
Burst frequencies	0.5–1 Hz	
IBI length	5–25 s	
IBI amplitude	5–25 µV	
Synchrony	Yes	
Discontinuous %	70%	
Continuous %	5%	
Sleep/wake	No	
Reactivity	No	

The discontinuous portion of the recording is called tracé discontinu. Only about 5% of the recording is continuous
IBI interburst interval, *WGA* weeks gestational age

left hemisphere activity and right hemisphere activity over a period of time may be necessary.

Below is a listing of developmental features per age. For purposes of convention for this chapter, age is listed as weeks gestational age (WGA). The following characteristics have been compiled based on multiple sources, and since maturation is a gradual process and continuum, ranges of gestational age are used as best fit [1, 2, 4–11]. Every infant will develop and mature at different rates and the range of normal can be broad with many overlaps in characteristics. When assessing the developmental appropriateness for any neonate, factors such as medical course, medications, surroundings, and other health problems need to be considered.

2.6   21–22 Weeks Gestational Age

This age group is challenging to determine normal or abnormal findings. Merely the birth of a baby with this early gestational age typically corresponds to a disrupted in utero environment and high risk of brain injury. Normal graphoelements (sharp waves and frequencies) are not well established for this age group. However, it is known and agreed upon that the background activity is discontinuous with long interburst intervals (Table 2.4).

2.7   EEG Tidbit

Q: If the pattern is not discontinuous and not continuous, then what is it?
A: This is called indeterminate background activity. In this case, the background may show a mixture of discontinuous and continuous patterns, with neither pattern occurring for a duration long enough to clearly state if it is discontinuous or continuous. As the baby matures, indeterminate background activity is considered to be a type of sleep, in which the baby has eyes closed but specific sleep criteria cannot be made. Amount of indeterminate sleep lessens as the baby matures.

2.8 23–24 Weeks Gestational Age

This age demonstrates certain background parameters (Table 2.5). The discontinuous portion of the recording is called tracé discontinu (Fig. 2.7). Only about 25% of the recording is continuous. Reactivity is not present, and there is no definable sleep and waking states. Sharp transients and certain frequencies are known to occur in specific regions (Table 2.6).

- Sharp transients can occur during the continuous activity, but they should mostly be seen in the discontinuous periods, and mostly in the bursts.
- Certain characteristic frequency activity mentioned above can occur during the discontinuous periods or continuous periods.

EEG Tidbit: What is a sharp transient? Sharp wave?

Sharp waves can be normal findings in neonates (unlike in older patients). The sharp wave is called a sharp transient, in that it is a temporary occurrence and is a normal phenomenon in this certain age group. The term "sharp transient" is only used in neonates. In addition, a sharp wave (or sharp transient) is usually an isolated waveform, which may occur in runs but is distinct from the background. Abnormal

Table 2.5 Chart demonstrating background parameters for a 23–24 WGA neonate

Burst length	3–5 s		Tracé discontinu
Burst amplitude	50–330 µV		
Burst frequencies	0.5–1 Hz		
IBI length	5–18 s		
IBI amplitude	5–25 µV		
Synchrony	Yes		
Discontinuous %	50%		
Continuous %	25%		
Sleep/wake	No		
Reactivity	No		

The discontinuous portion of the recording is called tracé discontinu. Only about 25% of the recording is continuous

IBI interburst interval, *WGA* weeks gestational age

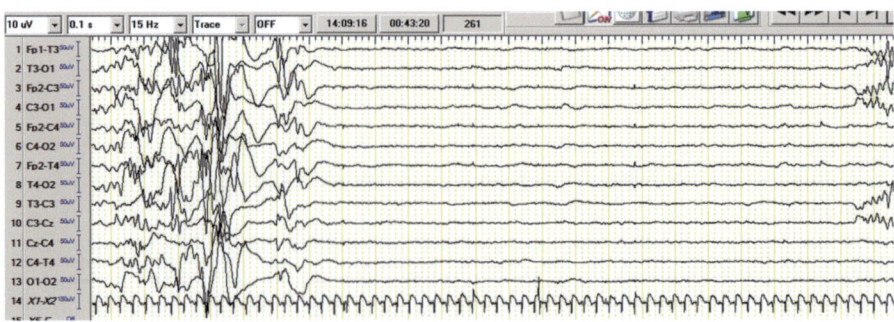

Fig. 2.7 Background pattern at a glance, setting is 30 s per page of a neonate between the gestational age of 23–24 weeks. This pattern is tracé discontinu

Table 2.6 Location of sharp transients and certain frequency patterns commonly seen in 23–24 weeks gestational age

	Sharp activity	Frequency activity
Bursts in DISCONTINUOUS periods		
Frontal	Sharp transients (unilateral or bilateral)	
Central	Sharp transients, rare	
Temporal	Sharp transients, rare	Theta, 200 µV, unilateral or bilateral but symmetric
Occipital	Negative sharps	
CONTINUOUS periods		
Diffuse		Theta, 200 µV, unilateral or bilateral, symmetric

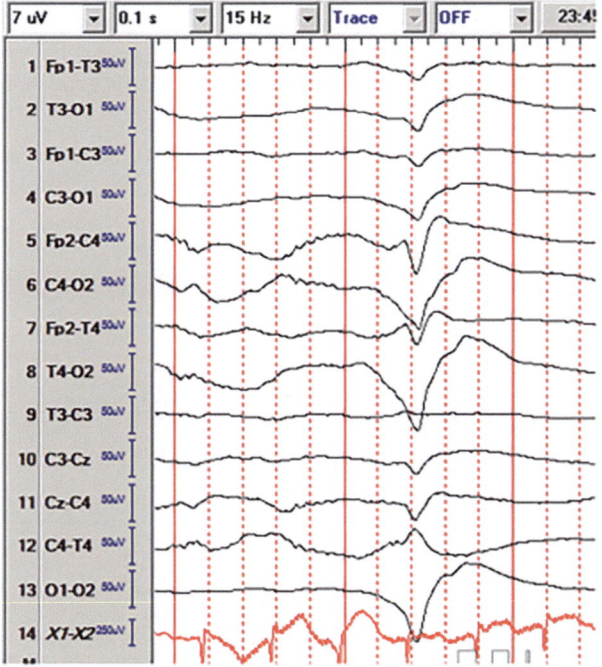

Fig. 2.8 Frontal sharp transients in a 23–24 WGA neonate

sharp waves or abnormal sharp transients in neonates suggest focal region of dysfunction and/or focal region of epileptogenicity. The connotation in older patient EEGs of a "sharp wave" is that of an epileptic waveform.

Frontal and occipital sharp transients are the most common regions of normal sharp activity in this age (Figs. 2.8, 2.9, 2.10 and 2.11).

Temporal theta is seen bilaterally or unilaterally but should be equal overall in occurrence between the two hemispheres (Figs. 2.12, 2.13 and 2.14).

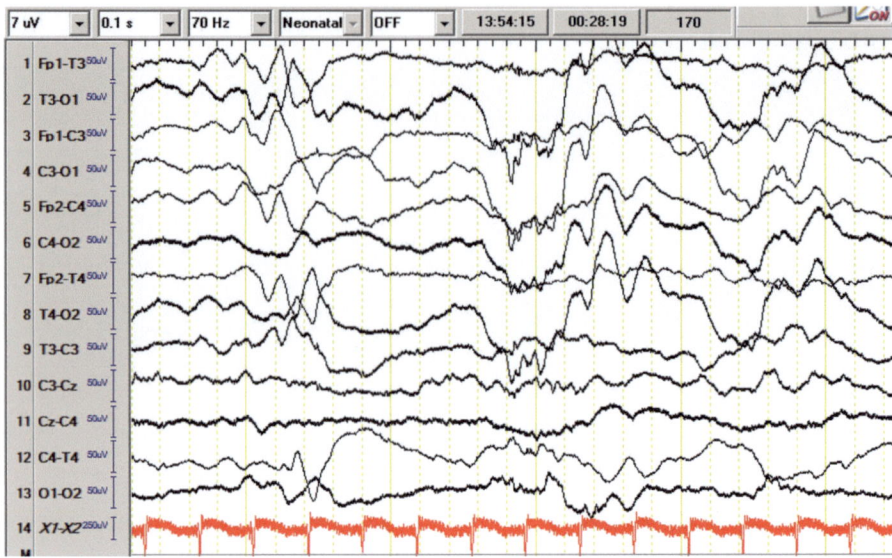

Fig. 2.9 Frontal sharp transients in a neonate of 23–24 WGA. Occipital sharp transients are also present

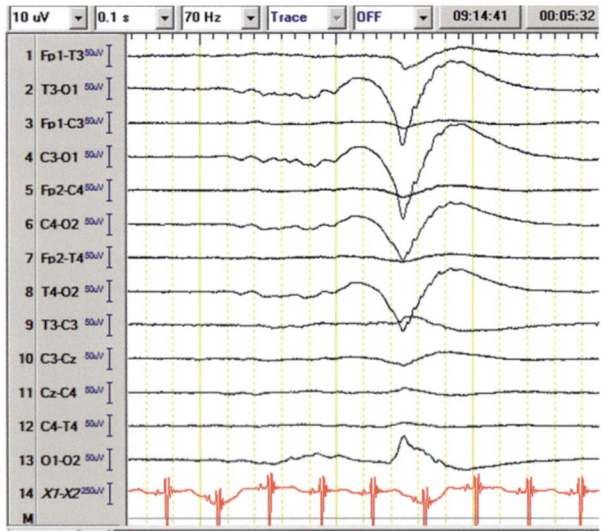

Fig. 2.10 Occipital sharp transients in a neonate of 23–24 WGA

Fig. 2.11 Occipital sharp transients in a neonate of 23–24 WGA

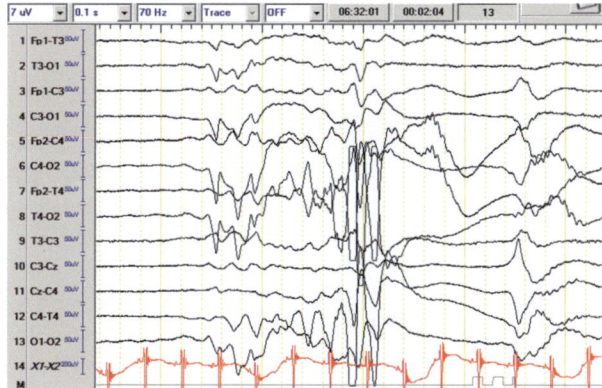

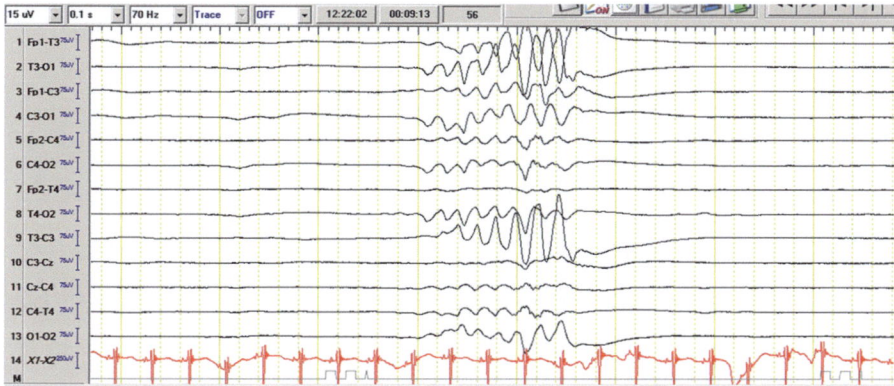

Fig. 2.12 Diffuse and temporal theta in a 23–24 WGA neonate. Diffuse (seen in all leads) theta frequencies in which the left temporal region shows highest amplitude. The theta activity is not often equal amplitude in all the leads. Temporal dominance is accepted since the temporal region shows its own independent theta frequencies

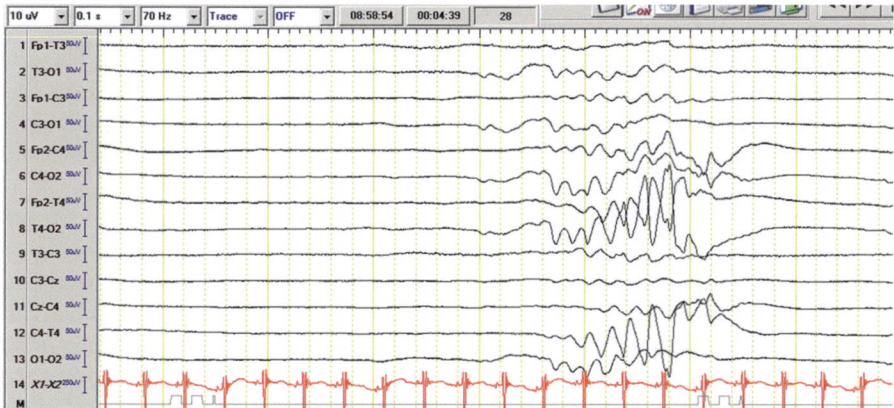

Fig. 2.13 Diffuse and temporal theta in a 23–24 WGA neonate. Diffuse theta, maximal in the right temporal region. This activity is seen mostly in bilateral temporal regions

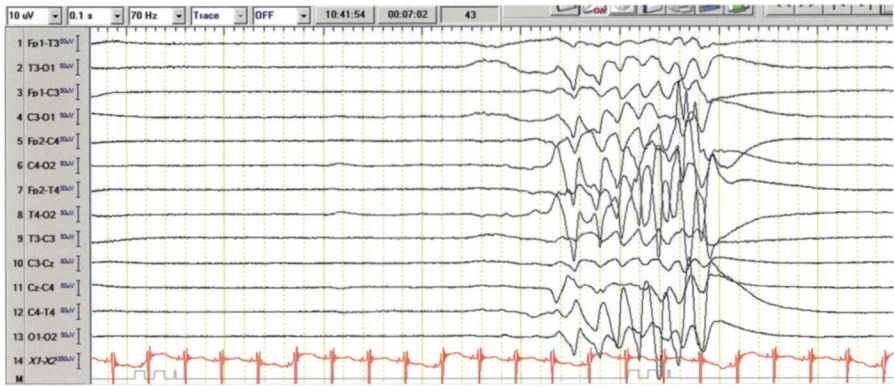

Fig. 2.14 Diffuse and temporal theta in a 23–24 WGA neonate. Example of diffuse theta, occurring in all leads. Right temporal region shows theta activity as highest in amplitude

Table 2.7 Background EEG parameters typical for 25–27 WGA

Burst length	3–6 s	Tracé discontinu
Burst amplitude	100–330 µV	
Burst frequency	0.5–1 Hz	
IBI length	3–12 s	
IBI amplitude	5–25 µV	
Synchrony	Yes	
Discontinuous %	50%	
Continuous %	50%, may see eye movements during continuous activity	Emerging continuous activity
Sleep/wake	No	
Reactivity	No	

IBI interburst interval, *WGA* weeks gestational age

2.9 25–27 Weeks Gestational Age

Below are background parameters for a 25–27 WGA neonate (Table 2.7). The discontinuous portion of the recording is called tracé discontinu (Fig. 2.15). At this age, continuous activity begins to occur up to 50% of the time. However, reactivity is not present and there is no definable sleep and waking states. Sharp transients and certain frequencies are known to occur in specific regions (Table 2.8).

Frontal and occipital sharp transients continue to be the most common normal transients (Figs. 2.16, 2.17 and 2.23).

Delta frequencies occur localized to the frontal, central, temporal, and occipital head regions (Figs. 2.17, 2.18, 2.19, 2.20 and 2.21). Frontal delta activity in particular can be sharp and short (rapid) (Fig. 2.17) or smooth and longer in duration (slow) (Fig. 2.18). In addition, delta waveforms can be seen in all the leads, or most of the leads, which is referred to as being *diffuse* (Figs. 2.20 and 2.28). Often, delta

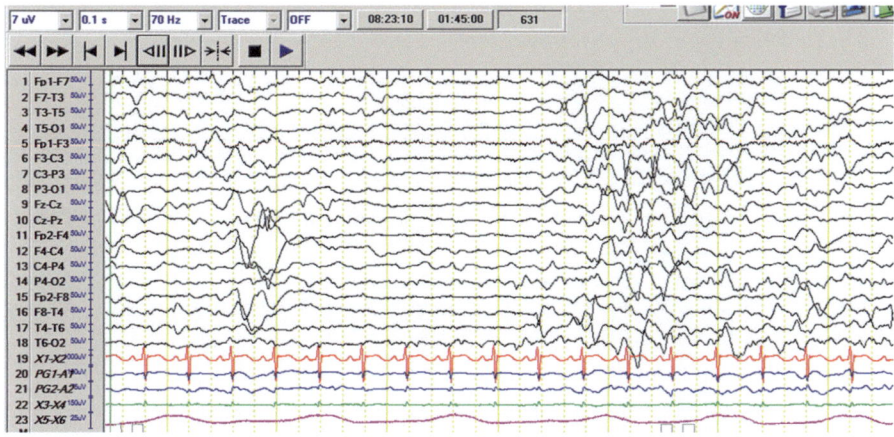

Fig. 2.15 Background pattern at a glance, setting is 30 s per page of a neonate between the gestational age of 25–27 weeks. This pattern is tracé discontinu. The interburst length is shortening compared to earlier gestational ages

Table 2.8 Location of sharp transients and certain frequency patterns commonly seen in 25–27 WGA

	Sharp activity	Frequency activity
Bursts in DISCONTINUOUS periods		
Frontal	Sharp transients (unilateral or bilateral)	Delta waves (sharp/rapid or smooth/slow)
Central	Rare	Smooth delta with superimposed alpha, beta
Temporal	Rare	Delta bilateral or unilateral Theta (25–120 µV, 1–2 s)—bilateral but may be independent
Occipital	Negative sharps	Smooth delta (synchronized, bilateral, unilateral) with superimposed theta or beta Theta lasting 2–10 s
CONTINUOUS activity		
Diffuse		Theta, delta

Note the term independent, which describes the occurrence of bilateral waveforms occurring asynchronously. Symmetry is implied

frequencies can have superimposed faster frequencies (usually alpha or beta) that give the appearance of the common household brush (Figs. 2.22, 2.23, 2.24 and 2.25). Identifying a certain frequency pattern implies ongoing activity, as opposed to a sharp wave, which may be monophasic. However, the distinction between a certain sharp wave that might repeat itself and a pattern of certain persistent frequency activity is very difficult at times and subject to individual reader interpretation. The examples below aim to demonstrate the correlation between terms and wave morphology.

Similar to delta frequencies occurring in one location or being diffuse, theta frequencies follow the same patterns (Figs. 2.17, 2.26, 2.27 and 2.28).

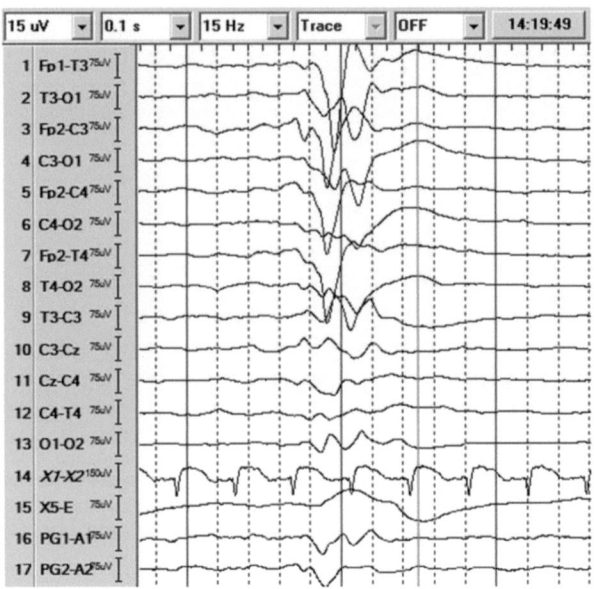

Fig. 2.16 Frontal sharp transients in a patient 25–27 WGA

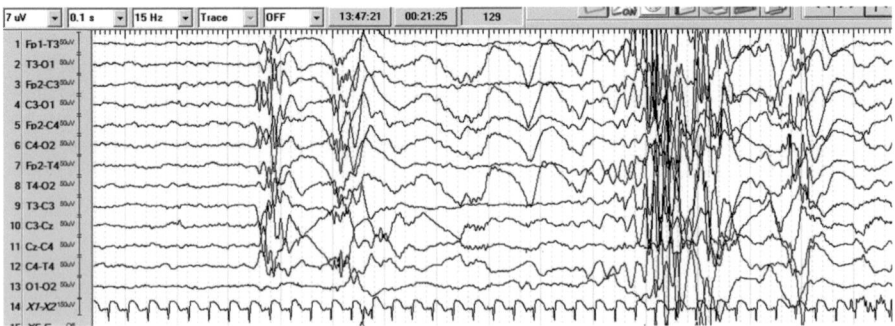

Fig. 2.17 Occipital negative sharps, frontal delta waveforms (sharp and rapid) and diffuse theta frequencies (temporal maximal and amplitude as high as 120 µV) in a neonate between 25 and 27 WGA

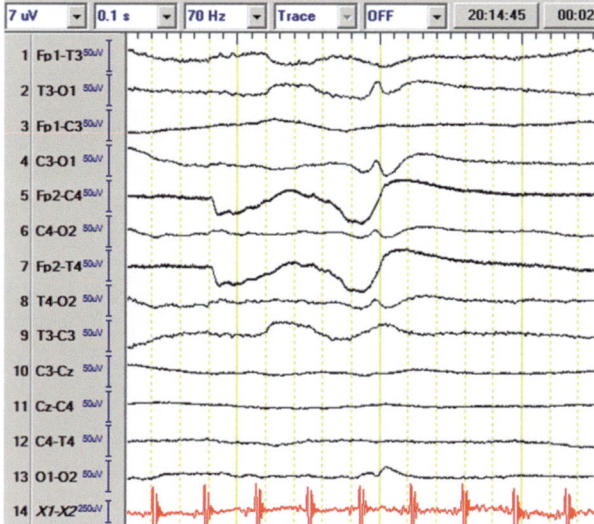

Fig. 2.18 Smooth and slow frontal delta waveforms in a neonate between 25 and 27 WGA. These waveforms are longer than the typical frontal sharp transient so would be considered a type of frequency pattern

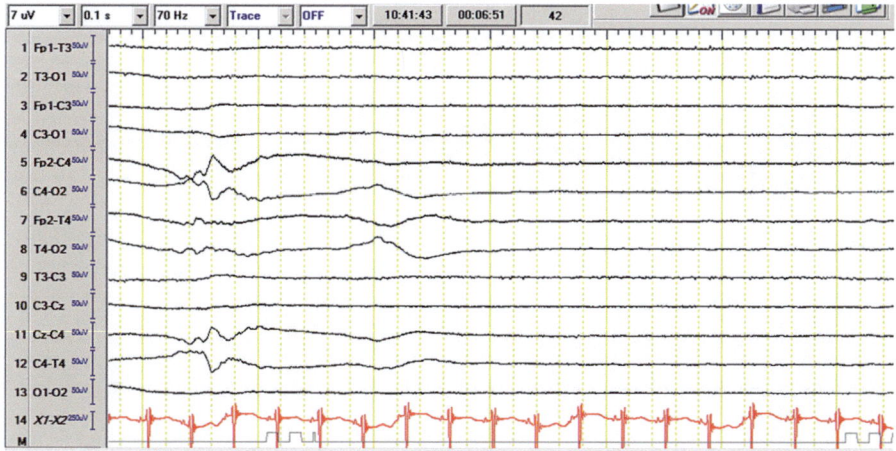

Fig. 2.19 Central delta frequencies in a neonate between 25 and 27 WGA. Note how this frequency fades into the background

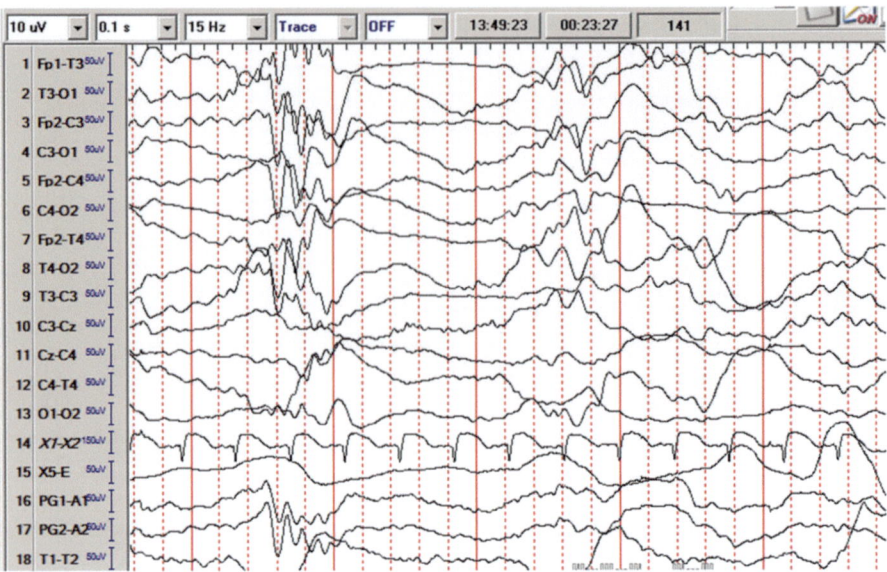

Fig. 2.20 Delta frequencies in temporal regions and diffusely (in all leads) in a neonate between 25 and 27 WGA

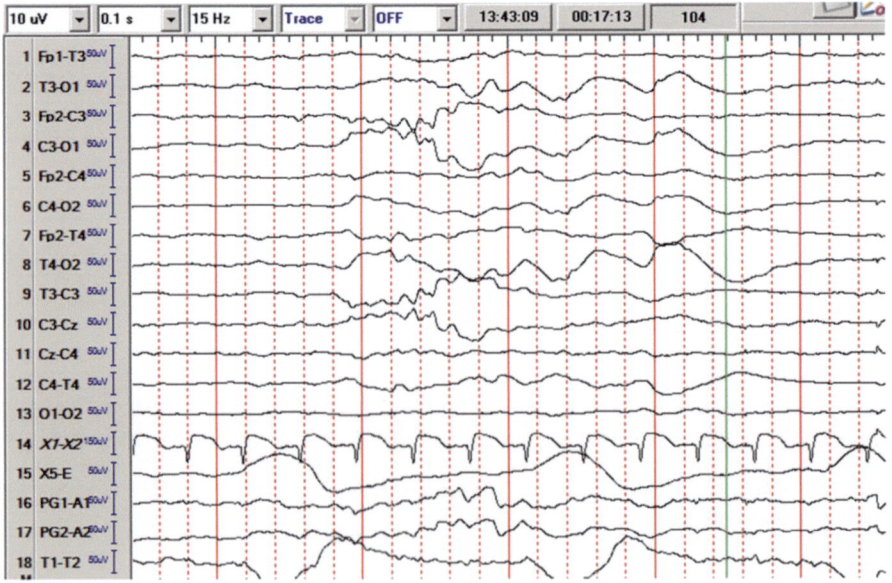

Fig. 2.21 Delta frequencies in occipital regions in a neonate between 25 and 27 WGA

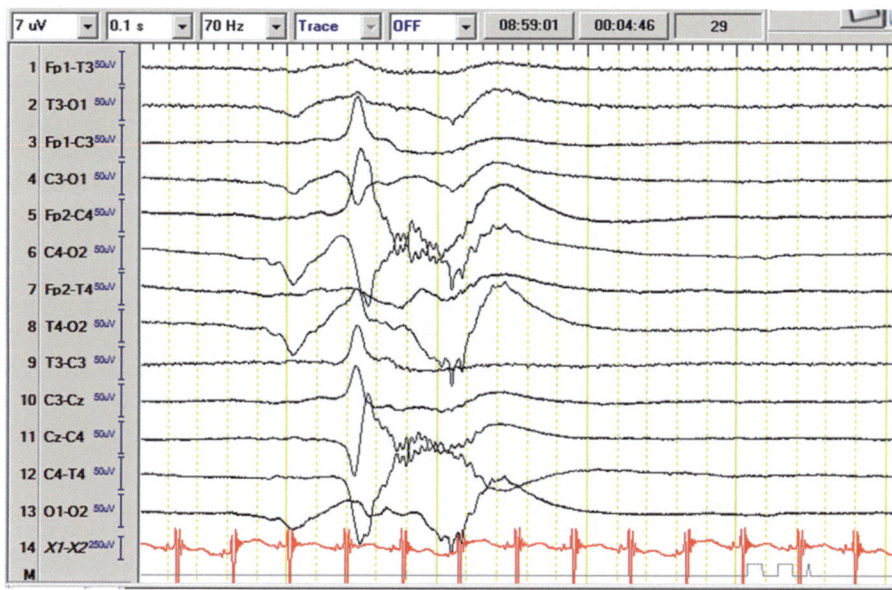

Fig. 2.22 Premature central delta brush and occipital delta in a neonate between 25 and 27 WGA. Central delta waveforms with superimposed beta frequencies constitute a premature delta brush. Note how the central delta brush has a beginning and an end; it can be traced from the start to finish. Occipital delta frequency has a sharp wave phase at onset, then blends into the background

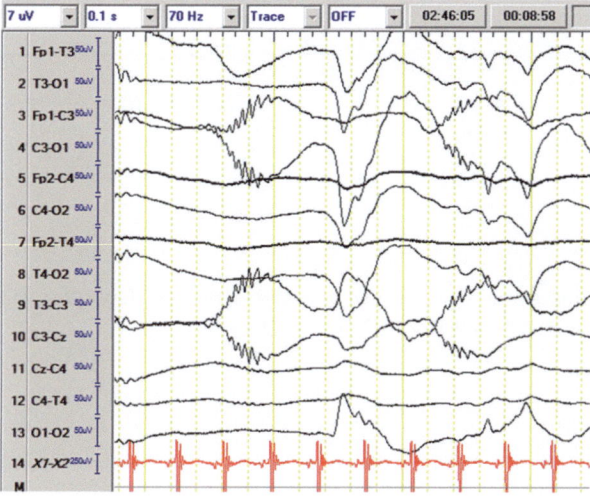

Fig. 2.23 Premature (central) delta brush and frontal sharp transients in a neonate between 25 and 27 WGA. Central delta activity with superimposed beta frequencies, considered the premature delta brush. Frontal sharp transients are also present in this figure

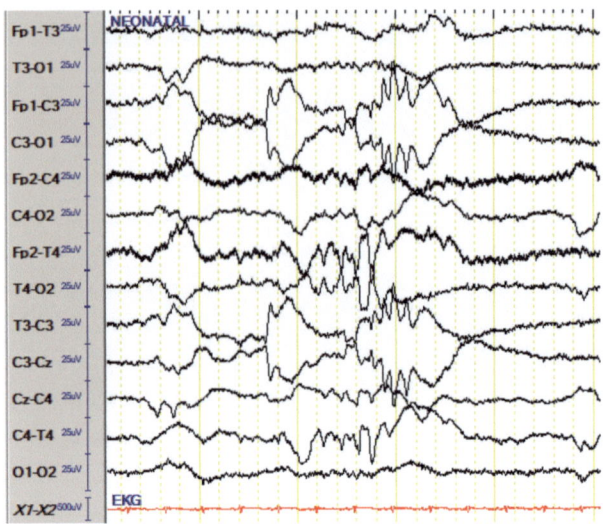

Fig. 2.24 Central delta waveforms with superimposed alpha frequencies in a neonate between 25 and 27 WGA

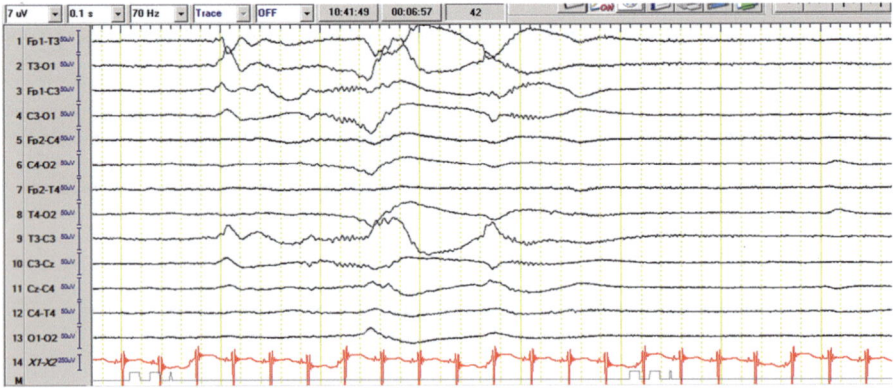

Fig. 2.25 Beta frequencies superimposed on central delta waveforms and delta frequencies in temporal regions in a neonate between 25 and 27 WGA

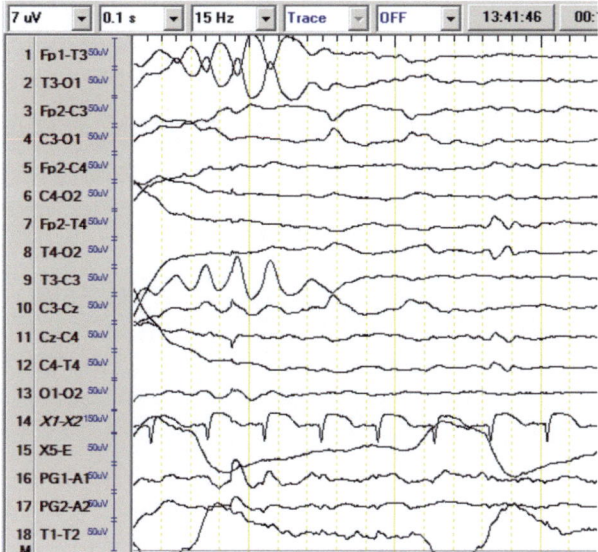

Fig. 2.26 Theta frequencies in temporal regions in a neonate between 25 and 27 WGA

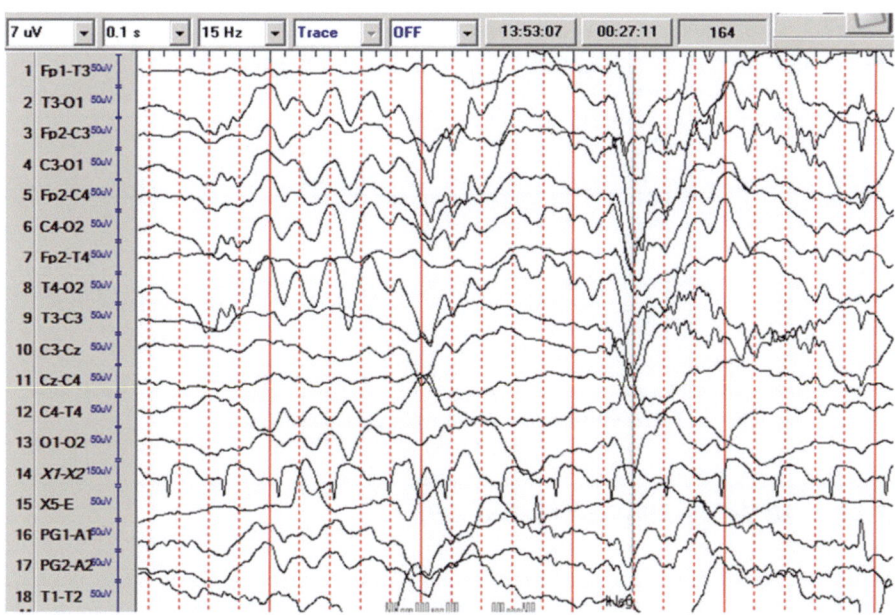

Fig. 2.27 Theta frequencies occurring diffusely and in occipital regions in a neonate between 25 and 27 WGA

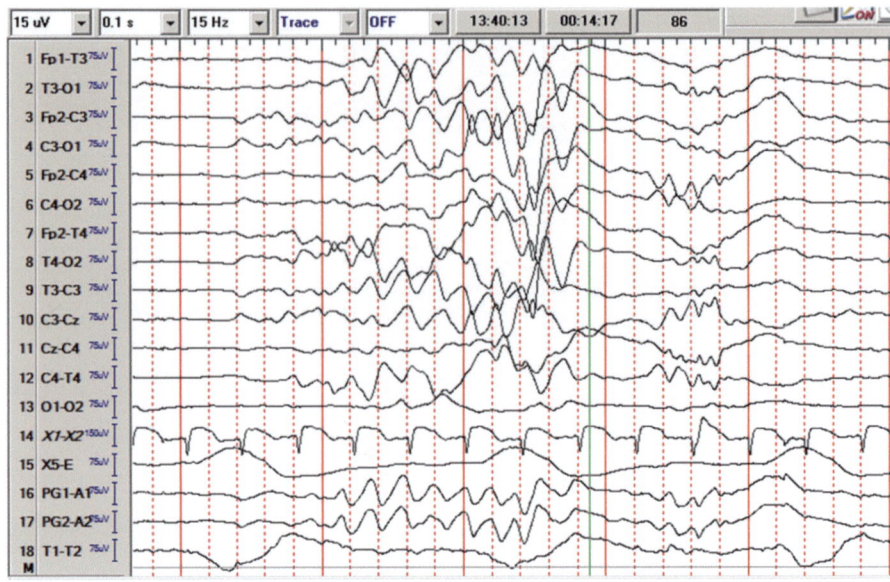

Fig. 2.28 Diffuse theta and delta frequencies in a neonate between 25 and 27 WGA

Table 2.9 Background EEG parameters typical for 28–29 WGA

Burst length	3–6 s	Tracé discontinu (TD)
Burst amplitude	30–300 µV	
Burst frequency	0.5–2 Hz	
IBI length	3–12 s	
IBI amplitude	5–25 µV	
Synchrony	In TD, some asynchrony is present/continuous activity is synchronous	
Discontinuous %	50%	
Continuous %	50%—may see eye movements during continuous activity	Continuous activity but no clear identifiers yet of awake or active sleep
Sleep/wake	No	
Reactivity	No	

IBI interburst interval, *TD* tracé discontinu, *WGA* week gestational age

2.10 28 WGA–29 WGA (Table 2.9)

Below is a chart demonstrating background parameters for a 28–29 WGA neonate (Table 2.9). The discontinuous portion of the recording is called tracé discontinu. At this age, discontinuous and continuous activity occurs about the same amount and eye movements are noted in the continuous segment (Figs. 2.29 and 2.30). However, reactivity is not present and there is no definable sleep and waking states. Sharp transients and certain frequency patterns are unique to this age (Table 2.10).

Frontal and occipital sharp transients continue to be a common finding in the normal background of neonates between 28 and 29 WGA (Figs. 2.31 and 2.32). Rolandic dips

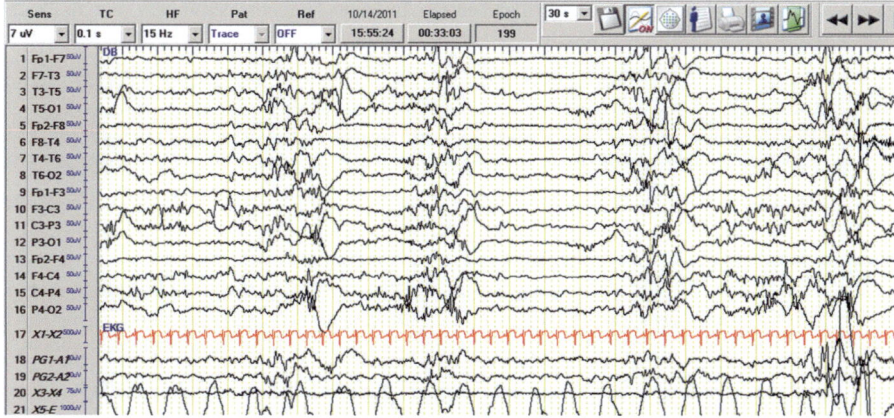

Fig. 2.29 Background pattern at a glance of a neonate between the gestational age of 28–29 weeks, setting is 30 s per page in this. This pattern is tracé discontinu. The interburst length continues to shorten compared to earlier gestational ages

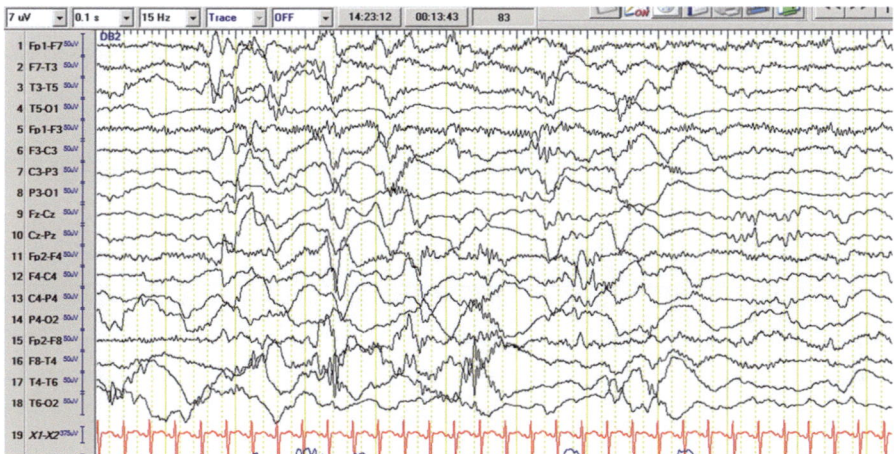

Fig. 2.30 Continuous background activity in a 28 WGA neonate. Monorhythmic delta activity is present

may begin at this age (Fig. 2.33). These are centrally located positive waveforms seen as part of normal maturational background activity. The Rolandic fissure is where the primary sensory and motor cortices meet in the developed cortex. In preterm babies, the term Rolandic refers to the parasagittal central regions, where cortical activity is displayed in the central EEG scalp electrodes (C3 or C4). Temporal saw tooth waveforms may also appear at this age (Fig. 2.34), which are seen in the left or right temporal regions. Frequency is between 6 and 10 Hz and morphology is oscillatory, in that the upward and downward deflections are equal in shape and frequency.

Diffuse delta and theta frequencies occur in this age group. Superimposed alpha activity can display a spindle-like picture (Figs. 2.35, 2.36, and 2.37).

Table 2.10 Location of sharp transients and certain frequency patterns commonly seen in 28–29 WGA neonates

	Sharp activity	Frequency activity
Bursts in DISCONTINUOUS periods, which is now considered quiet sleep		
Frontal	Sharp transients (unilateral or bilateral)	
Central	May see Rolandic dip	Delta low amplitude <1 s, superimposed alpha (10–75 μV) giving spindle-like picture), or superimposed beta (5–35 μV)
Temporal	Sawtooth	Delta moderate amplitude Theta burst (25–120 μV), bilateral but may be independent
Occipital	Negative sharps	Delta high amplitude, synchronized or isolated, superimposed alpha (10–75 μV) giving spindle[a]-like picture Theta burst (20–260 μV) 2–10 s
CONTINUOUS		
Diffuse		Theta, delta (monorhythmic)

[a]Spindle is a particular type of waveform, is not a defined frequency but is mentioned in this chart for concept introduction. At 2 months of age (48 WGA) in sleep, sleep spindles begin to occur. These waveforms are low amplitude and are centrally located at a frequency of 11–16 Hz. Some premature neonatal background waveforms are described as having a "spindle-like" appearance, in which superimposed alpha frequencies are present on slower waveforms. This appearance may remind the reader of a sleep spindle, although not having any other similarities to a sleep spindle besides the frequency of 11–16 Hz. Using this term in neonatal EEGs can be very confusing and misleading

QS quiet sleep, *WGA* weeks gestational age

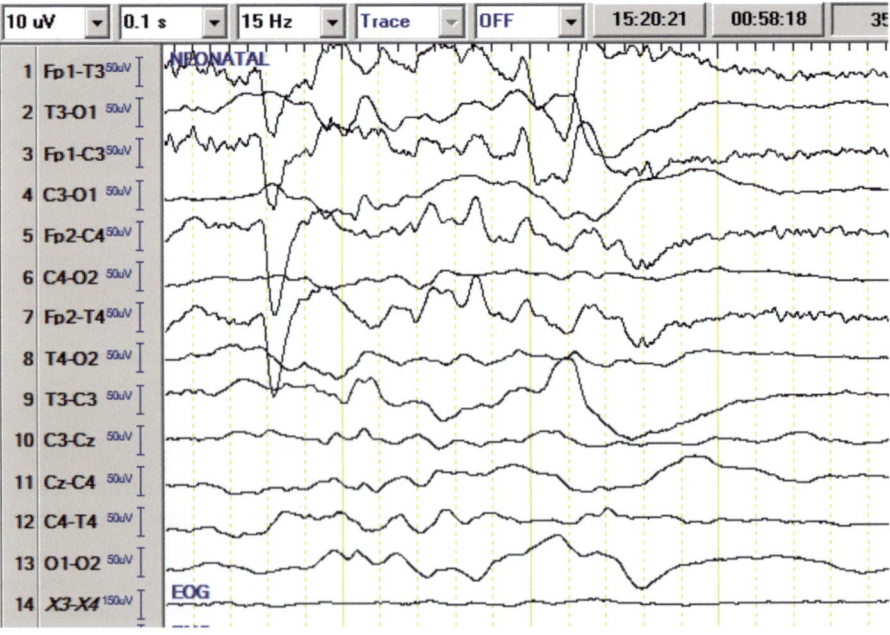

Fig. 2.31 Frontal sharp transients and temporal theta frequencies in a neonate between 28 and 29 WGA

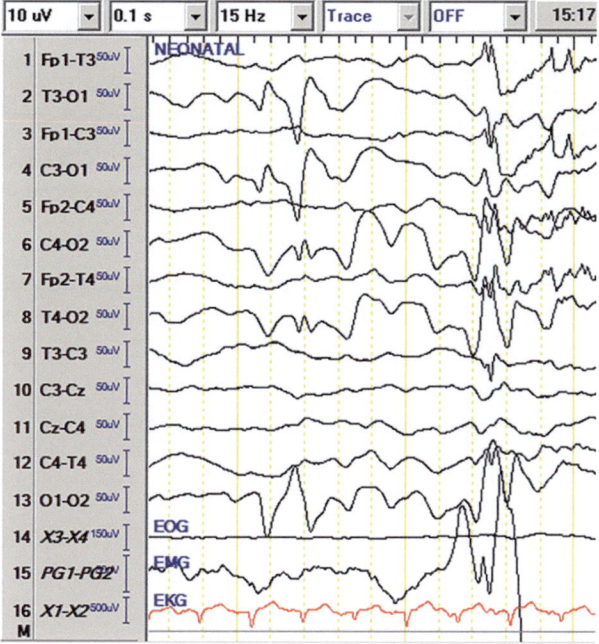

Fig. 2.32 Occipital negative sharp transient in a neonate between 28 and 29 WGA

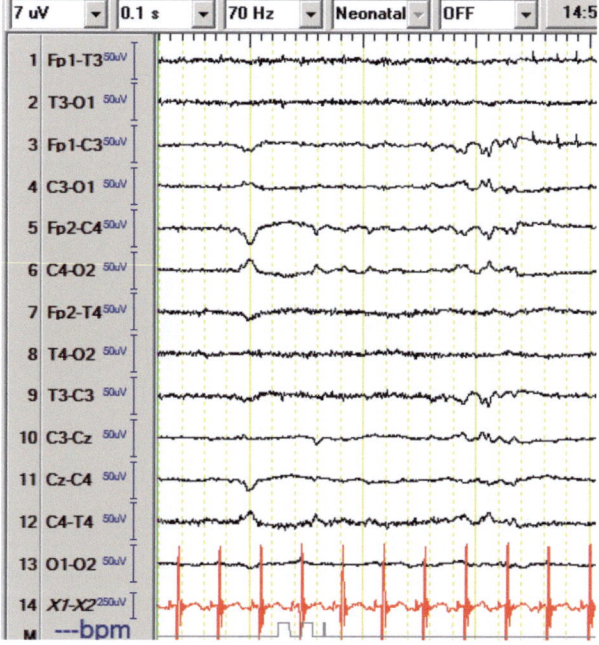

Fig. 2.33 Rolandic dip in a neonate between 28 and 29 WGA in the C4 electrode. This waveform is negative, small, and in central regions

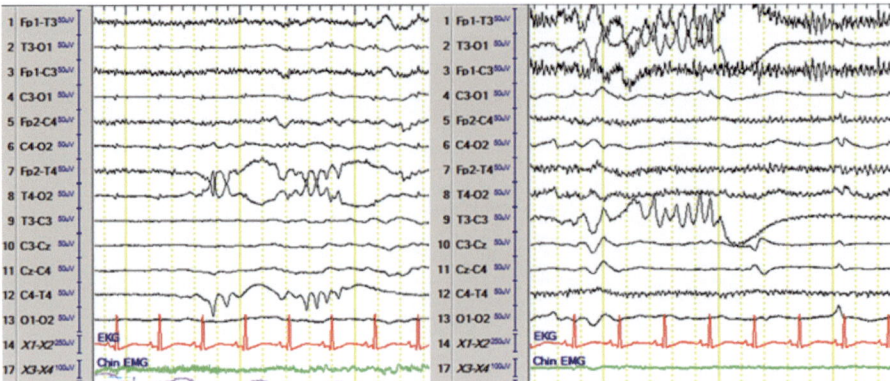

Fig. 2.34 Temporal saw tooth waveforms in a neonate between 28 and 29 WGA. Left image, right temporal location (T4 electrode); right image, left temporal (T3 electrode) location. Frequency is between 6 and 10 Hz and morphology is oscillatory, in that the upward and downward deflections are equal in shape and frequency

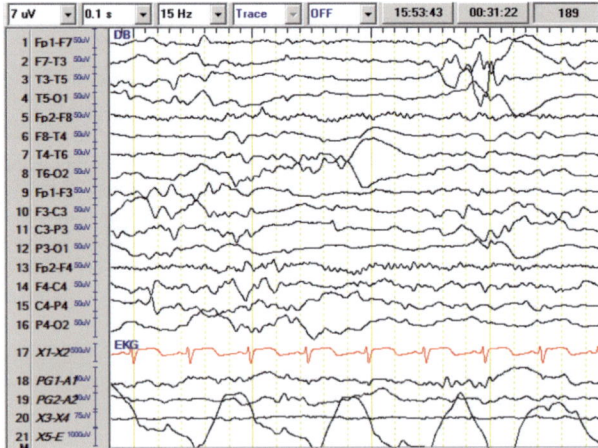

Fig. 2.35 Temporal and occipital delta frequencies in a neonate between 28 and 29 WGA

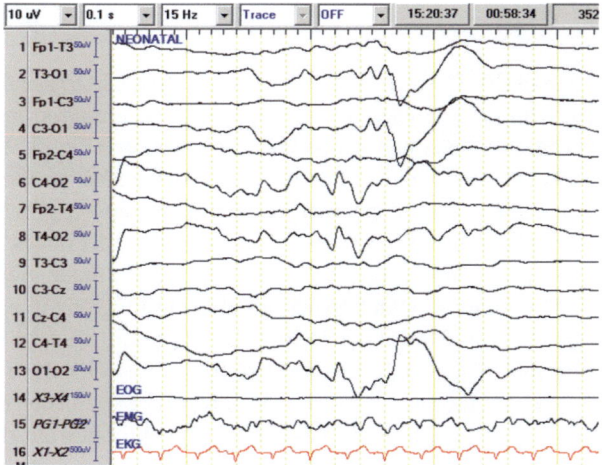

Fig. 2.36 Occipital theta frequencies with an amplitude of 20–260 µV and duration of 3 s in a neonate between 28 and 29 WGA

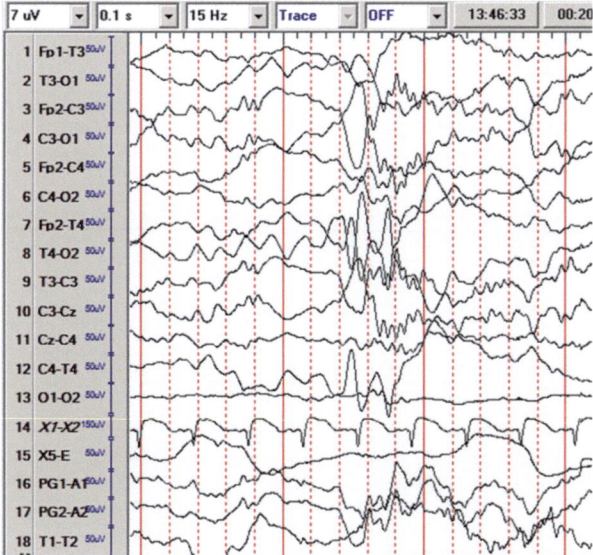

Fig. 2.37 Low-amplitude delta frequencies with superimposed alpha frequencies in the central region in a neonate between 28 and 29 WGA. This may look "spindle-like"

2.11 30–31 WGA

The gestational age of 30–31 weeks is the time when we begin to see reactivity and a fair amount of continuous activity, which represent wakefulness and active sleep (Fig. 2.38). The discontinuous periods represent quiet sleep (Fig. 2.39). Also, asynchrony peaks around this time, most often during the discontinuous segment. In addition, the premature delta brush (maximal in central regions) begins to shift to the temporal and occipital regions to create the full-term delta brush (Tables 2.11 and 2.12).

Below is a chart describing the change in delta brushes from the premature to term neonate (Table 2.13). Preterm delta brushes are in central regions in active sleep and term delta brushes occur in quiet sleep. Delta brushes present after 44 WGA are considered to be abnormal. The actual waveform consists of a delta wave of 0.3–1.5 Hz with a peak-to-peak amplitude of 50–250 µV. Superimposed faster beta activity is 8–20 Hz and is low voltage. Delta brushes can be asynchronous but should be symmetric. Delta brush synonyms are beta-delta complexes, spindle-delta bursts, spindle-like fast waves, ripples of prematurity or spindle/delta bursts. Spindles are typically low-amplitude frequencies between 11 and 16 Hz, and ripples are typically low-amplitude frequencies between 16 and 20 Hz. All of the above synonyms describe low-amplitude fast activity superimposed on high-amplitude slow activity (Fig. 2.40).

As this neonatal age demonstrates reactivity, the background activity often correlates with diffuse theta frequencies (Fig. 2.41).

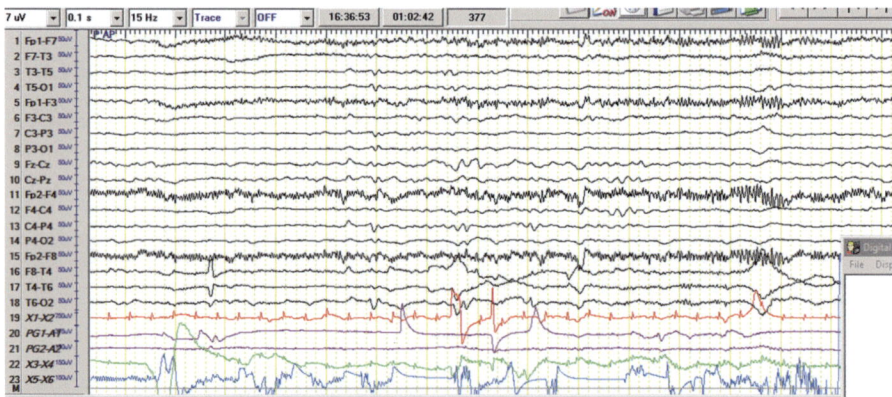

Fig. 2.38 Continuous background in a neonate between 30 and 31 WGA. The lower leads (purple is eye movement, green is chin movement, and blue is respiratory movement) show that the neonate is very active. Difference between wakefulness (open eyes with eye movements) and active sleep (closed eyes with eye movements) may be difficult to discern based on EEG alone

2 Developmental Maturation of the EEG in Neonates, from Preterm to Term... 51

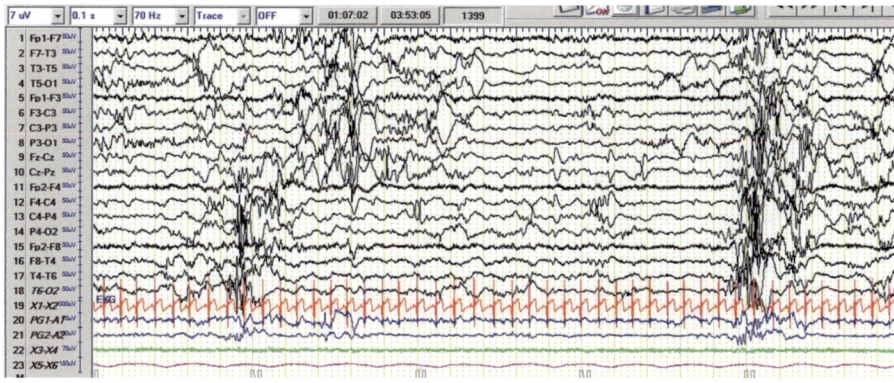

Fig. 2.39 Discontinuous background at a glance of a neonate between 30 and 31 WGA. In quiet sleep, synchronous and asynchronous bursts may both occur

Table 2.11 Chart demonstrating background parameters for a 30–31 WGA neonate

Burst length	3–6 s	Tracé discontinu is the pattern equitable to quiet sleep
Burst amplitude	100–200 μV	
Burst frequency	0.7–2 Hz	
IBI length	3–12 s	
IBI amplitude	5–25 μV	
Synchrony	Quiet sleep more asynchronous than active sleep	
Discontinuous %	50%	
Continuous %	50%	Active sleep/waking[a]
Continuous activity	Delta frequency	
Sleep/wake	Yes beginning: quiet sleep may be differentiated from active sleep/awake but active sleep/awake may look the same, eye movement may be helpful, and clinical exam may be helpful	Quiet sleep tracé discontinu/active sleep and waking look the same—continuous
Reactivity	Yes beginning	

The discontinuous portion of the recording is called tracé discontinu and is quiet sleep. Discontinuous and continuous activity occurs about the same amount. Eye movements become frequent and can help define active sleep from wakefulness. Reactivity is beginning to occur
[a]Difference is whether eyes are open or closed (waking and active sleep)
IBI interburst interval, *WGA* weeks gestational age

Table 2.12 Location of sharp transients and certain frequency patterns commonly seen in 30–31 WGA neonates

	Sharp activity	Frequency activity
Bursts in DISCONTINUOUS periods, which is quiet sleep		
Frontal	Sharp transients (unilateral or bilateral)	
Central	Rolandic dip (central phase reversal, bilateral or unilateral)	Beta delta complex
Temporal	Small positive, sharp transients, saw tooth	Most of theta is in temporal region (25–120 µV, 1–2 s) and theta mostly in QS, delta (3 Hz) rhythmic low amp
Occipital	Negative sharps	Theta (less than temporal), most delta beta complexes (brushes), Delta rhythmic lasting 2–60 s
CONTINUOUS		
Diffuse		Delta, theta

Amp amplitude, *Hz* Hertz, *QS* quiet sleep, *WGA* weeks gestational age

Table 2.13 The evolution of delta brushes in neonates as seen in EEG recordings

	24–32 WGA	32–42 WGA	44 WGA+
Location	Central	Temporal/occipital	Not present
State	Active sleep	Quiet sleep	

WGA weeks gestational age

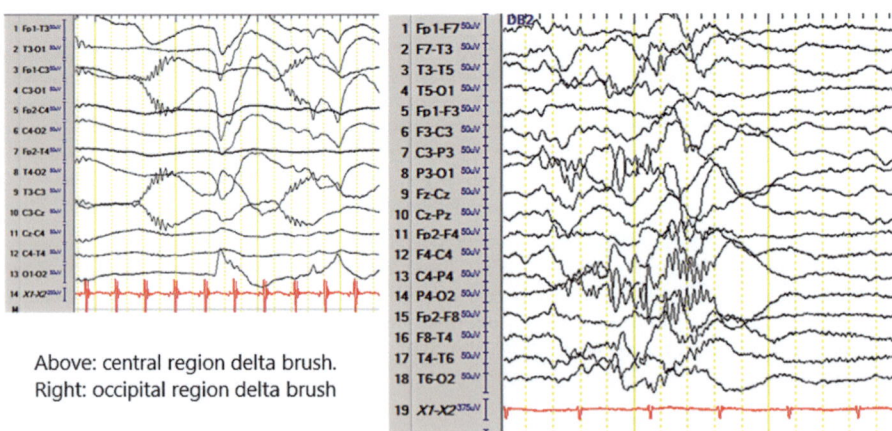

Above: central region delta brush.
Right: occipital region delta brush

Fig. 2.40 Comparison of premature and term delta brush location. Left image is premature delta brush with superimposed fast activity on delta frequencies in the central head regions. Right image is the term delta brush, in which superimposed fast activity on delta frequencies in the occipital regions

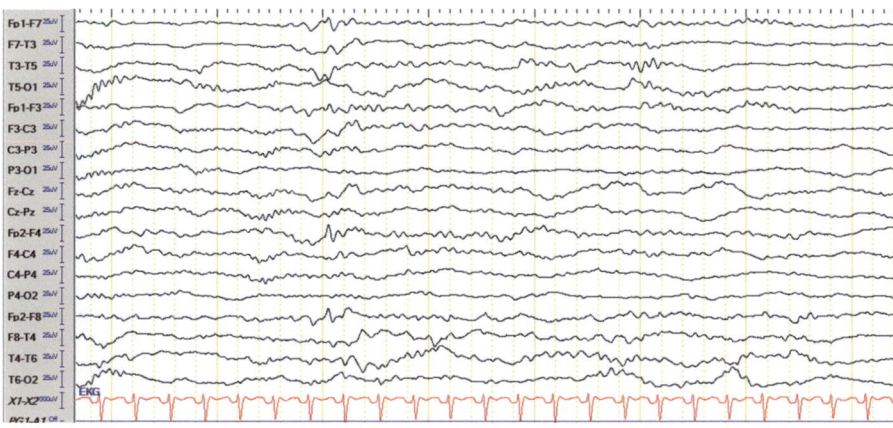

Fig. 2.41 Diffuse theta frequencies in a neonate between 30 and 31 WGA

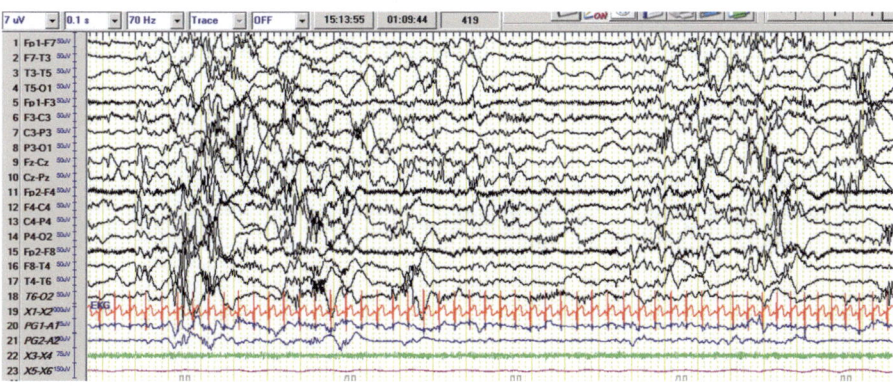

Fig. 2.42 Background at a glance of a neonate between 32 and 33 WGA. The bursts are longer in duration, and the IBI amplitude is higher compared to earlier ages. This overall pattern change during quiet sleep causes the disappearing of tracé discontinu and emerging of tracé alternant

2.12 32–33 WGA

At 32 WGA, the interburst interval amplitude changes to be consistently around 25 μV, which causes an evolution of the background pattern from tracé discontinu to tracé alternant (Fig. 2.42). Reactivity occurs and the continuous portion of the recording represents wakefulness or active sleep (Fig. 2.43). Presence of eye opening can help distinguish the two. Attenuation occurred with reactivity (Fig. 2.44 and Table 2.14).

Between 32 and 33 WGA, frontal, temporal, and occipital sharp transients continue to occur (Fig. 2.45). In particular, frontal sharp transients may begin to take on a form known as encoches frontales (see Table 2.18). Central (Rolandic) sharp waves are also present (Fig. 2.46). Delta activity is less frequent and is replaced by theta and alpha frequencies (Figs. 2.47 and 2.48, and Table 2.15).

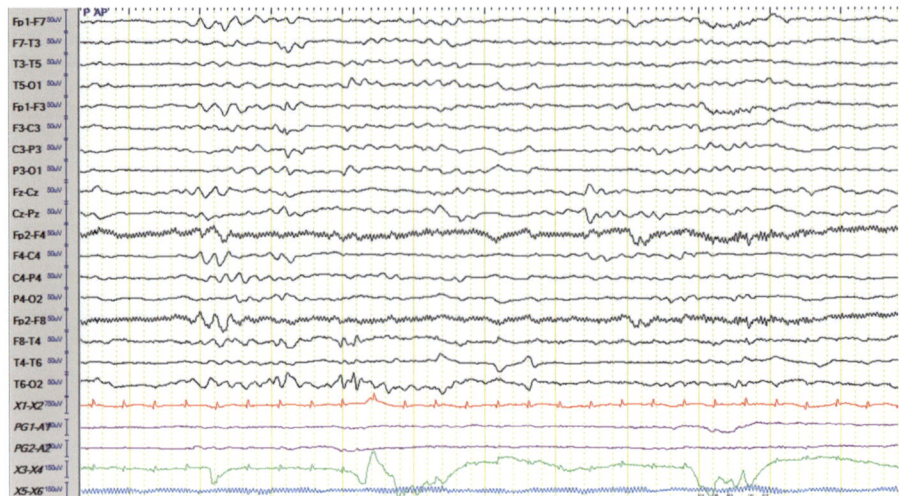

Fig. 2.43 Background at a glance of a neonate between 32 and 33 WGA. Continuous activity shows a pattern of continuous delta frequencies with intermixed theta frequencies. A broad range of amplitudes can be seen

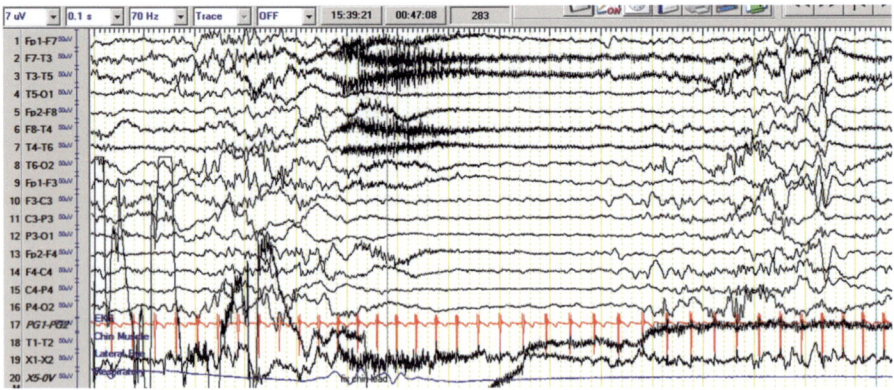

Fig. 2.44 Background at a glance of a neonate between 32 and 33 WGA. Present is an arousal during which the patient awakens from quiet sleep. A brief 5 s period of attenuation occurs with the arousal

2 Developmental Maturation of the EEG in Neonates, from Preterm to Term...

Table 2.14 Chart demonstrating background parameters for a 32–33 WGA neonate

Burst length	3–7 s	Tracé discontinu evolves to tracé alternant in quiet sleep
Burst amplitude	100–200 µV	
Burst frequency	1–4 Hz	
IBI length	3–10 s	
IBI amplitude	May be around or above 25 µV[a]	
Discontinuous %	50%	
Synchrony	Asynchrony in quiet sleep but not as often as in earlier ages	
Continuous %	50%	Active sleep with eye movements (eyes closed).
Continuous activity asleep	Irregular occipital delta	Awake with eye movements (eyes open)
Continuous activity awake	Diffuse regular delta, occipital maximum	Starting to see the difference
Sleep/awake	Yes	QS/AS/awake
Reactivity	Yes	Attenuation up to 12 s

The discontinuous quiet sleep portion of the recording changes from tracé discontinu to tracé alternant. Discontinuous and continuous activity occurs about the same amount. Eye movements become frequent, and presence of eyes being open can help define active sleep from wakefulness. Reactivity occurs

[a]IBI amplitude around 25 µV leads the way from tracé discontinu to tracé alternant where the burst and interburst interval are not as distinct

AS active sleep, *IBI* interburst interval, *QS* quiet sleep

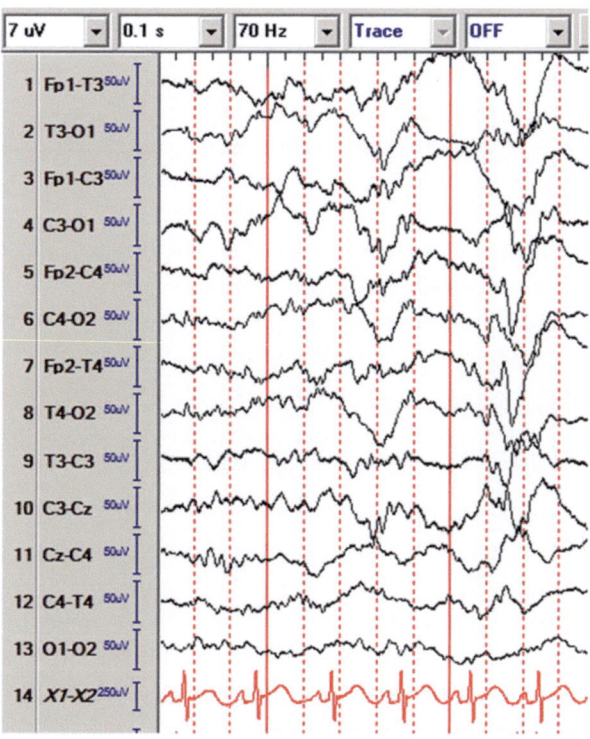

Fig. 2.45 Frontal, temporal, and occipital sharp transients in a neonate between 32 and 33 WGA

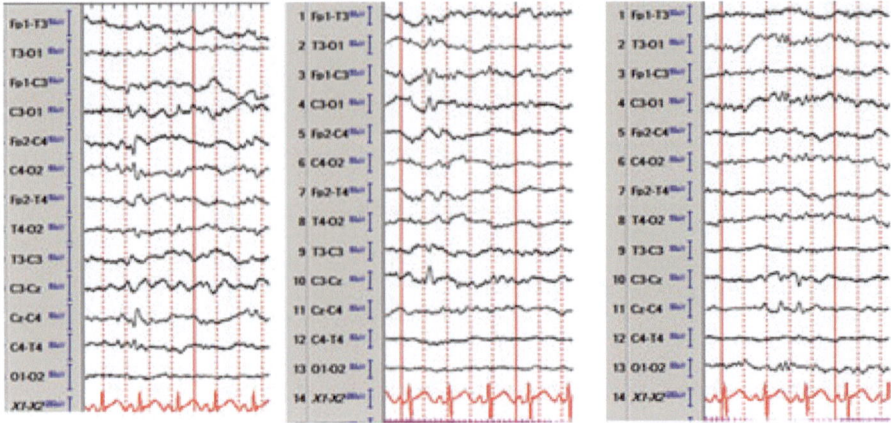

Fig. 2.46 Rolandic sharp waves in a neonate between 32 and 33 WGA. Rolandic sharp waves are in the central head regions. The Rolandic region is anatomically the central sulcus

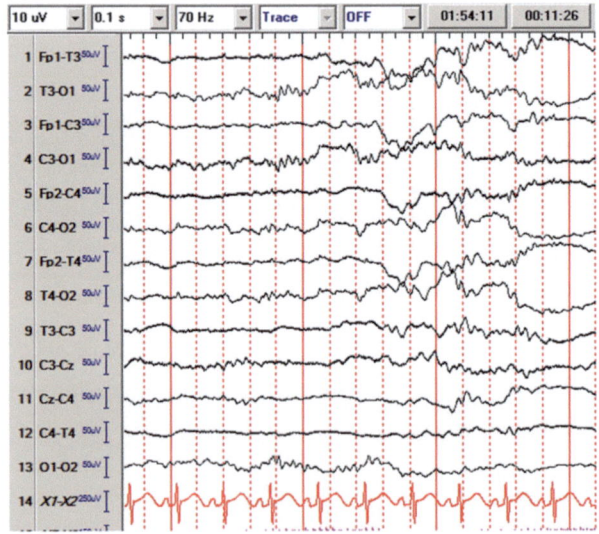

Fig. 2.47 Temporal alpha in a neonate between 32 and 33 WGA

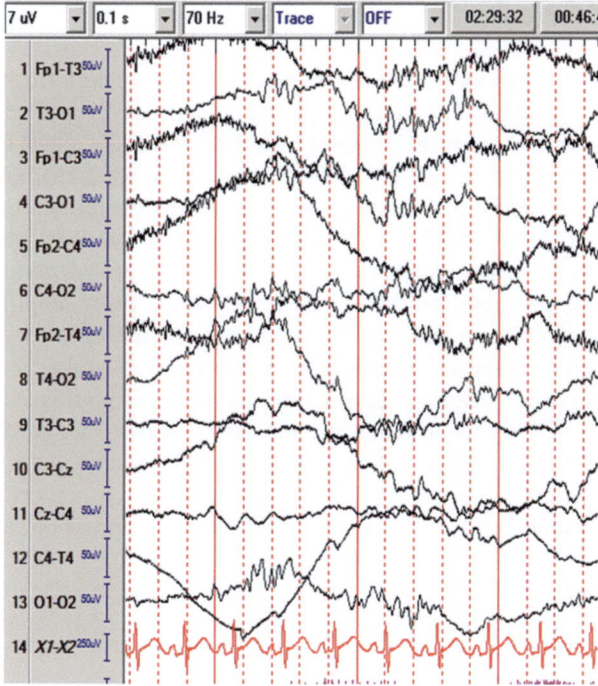

Fig. 2.48 Temporal alpha and ripple (16–20 Hz) activity in a neonate between 32 and 33 WGA

Table 2.15 Location of sharp transients and certain frequency patterns commonly seen in 32–33 WGA neonates

	Sharp activity	Frequency activity
Bursts in DISCONTINUOUS periods of quiet sleep		
Frontal	Sharp transients (unilateral or bilateral) May see emerging encoche frontales	
Central	Rolandic sharp unilateral or bilateral sharps	Fewer delta brushes
Temporal	Negative sharp	Bursts of theta (decreasing), alpha frequency—new beta delta complex
Occipital	Negative sharps	Theta (increasing), beta delta complex increasing monorhythmic delta
CONTINUOUS AWAKE		
Diffuse		Frequent ripples[a] or brushes (16–20 Hz) when awake

Additional reference: Hayakawa et al. [6]

[a]The term ripple may be confusing. It is an older term describing 16–20 Hz (beta) activity, which is often superimposed on slow delta activity. This fast activity may be seen during continuous periods. The term ripple may also be described in older textbooks as a "ripple of prematurity" when describing the more modern term *delta brush*

Hz Hertz, *QS* quiet sleep

2.13   34–35 Weeks Gestational Age

This age demonstrates an important transition from the preterm patterns to the term patterns. Typical term patterns may not be fully developed but background activity may show some of their characteristics. Below is a chart demonstrating background parameters for a 34–35 WGA neonate (Table 2.16). The discontinuous portion of the recording is now a well-defined tracé alternant pattern in quiet sleep (Fig. 2.49) in which the IBI amplitude increases and the burst amplitude decreases, so that the overall appearance of the discontinuous pattern is less pronounced. In other words, the difference between the burst amplitudes and IBI amplitudes is less pronounced and bursts and IBI "alternate" between 25 µV and 50–150 µV. Active sleep and wakefulness, the continuous segments, are showing a variety of amplitudes and frequencies. Some sources cite this increasing varying continuous activity as an emerging pattern of activité moyenne (Fig. 2.50). Activite moyenne is considered the waking background seen in term neonates. In addition, the difference between waking and active sleep is more apparent and reactivity is present. With reactivity, low-amplitude (suppression) activity occurs (Fig. 2.51).

During 34 and 35 WGA, frontal sharp waves become encoches frontales (EF), continuing to shape into the typical EF morphology (Fig. 2.52). Anterior dysrhythmia arises as a frontal frequency pattern and is similar to the EF morphology (Fig. 2.53 and Tables 2.17 and 2.18). Background frequencies are in the delta and theta ranges.

Table 2.16 Chart showing parameters of the background activity of neonates between 34 and 35 WGA

Burst length	3–7 s	Tracé alternant is quiet sleep pattern
Burst amplitude	50–150 µV	
Burst frequency	1–4 Hz	
IBI length	3–10 s	
IBI amplitude	25 µV	
Synchrony	No/yes Asynchrony in quiet sleep and very rare	
Discontinuous %	50%	
Continuous %	50%	Continuous delta changing to activité moyenne
Continuous activity asleep	Irregular occipital delta	Active sleep with eye movements and eyes closed
Continuous activity awake	Diffuse regular delta, occipital maximum	Awake with eye movements and eyes open
Sleep/wake	Yes	QS/AS/awake all 3 different
Reactivity	Yes	Attenuation up to 10 s

AS active sleep, *IBI* interburst interval, *Hz* Hertz, *QS* quiet sleep

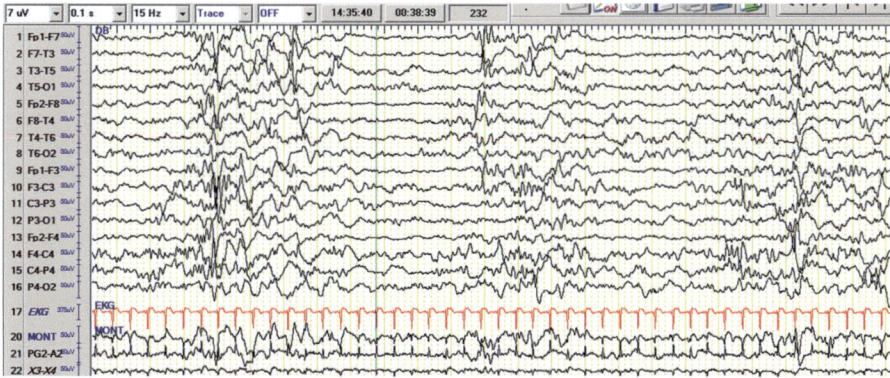

Fig. 2.49 Background at a glance of a neonate between 34 and 35 WGA. Quiet sleep is termed tracé alternant. The IBI length and burst length are both about 4–5 s in this depiction

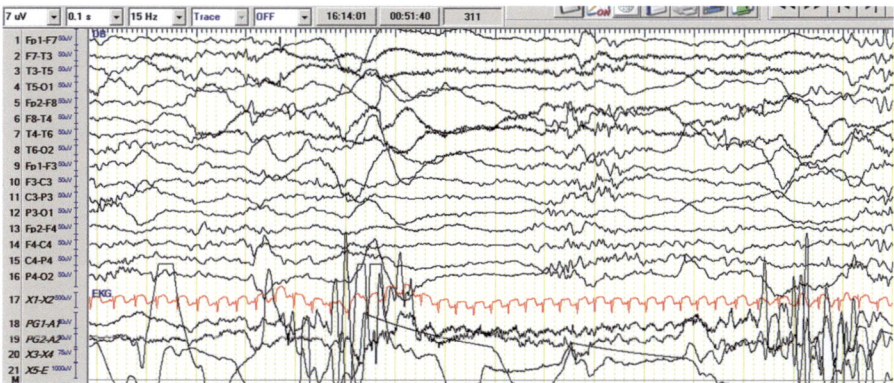

Fig. 2.50 Background at a glance of a neonate between 34 and 35 WGA. This segment captures continuous activity and can be considered to be activité moyenne. Waking and active sleep can be differentiated by eyes being open or closed. Note the artifacts occurring in the accessory leads, indicating patient movement

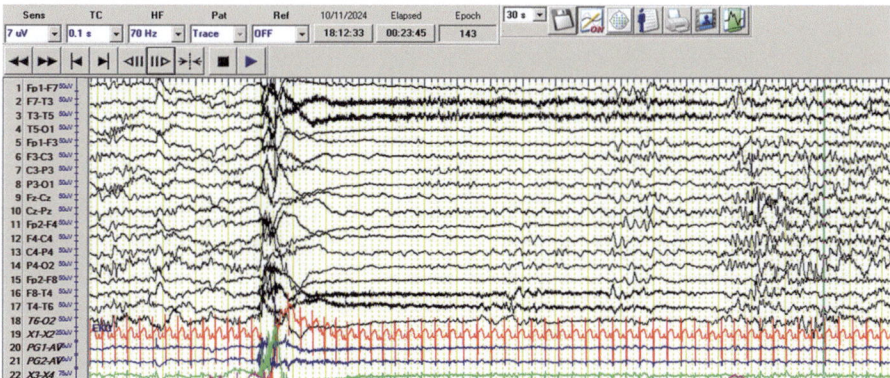

Fig. 2.51 Background at a glance of a neonate between 34 and 35 WGA. This figure shows an attenuation of approximately 5 s with an arousal. The patient likely had a startle or jerking movement that produced the high-amplitude artifactual waveforms

Fig. 2.52 Encoches frontales in a neonate between 34 and 35 WGA. These waveforms are frontal located with a broad waveform. They are synchronous and symmetric. If frontal sharp waves are not synchronous and symmetric, they may be epileptiform

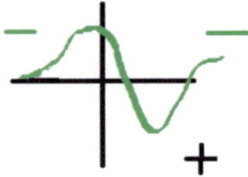

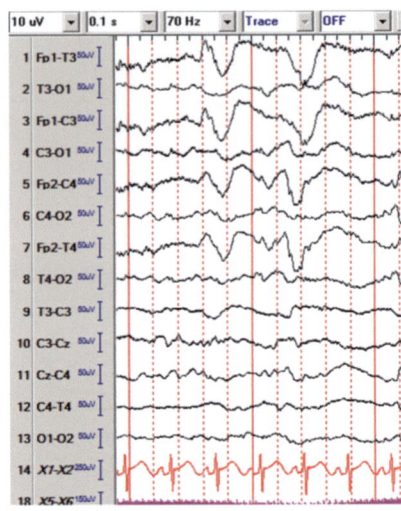

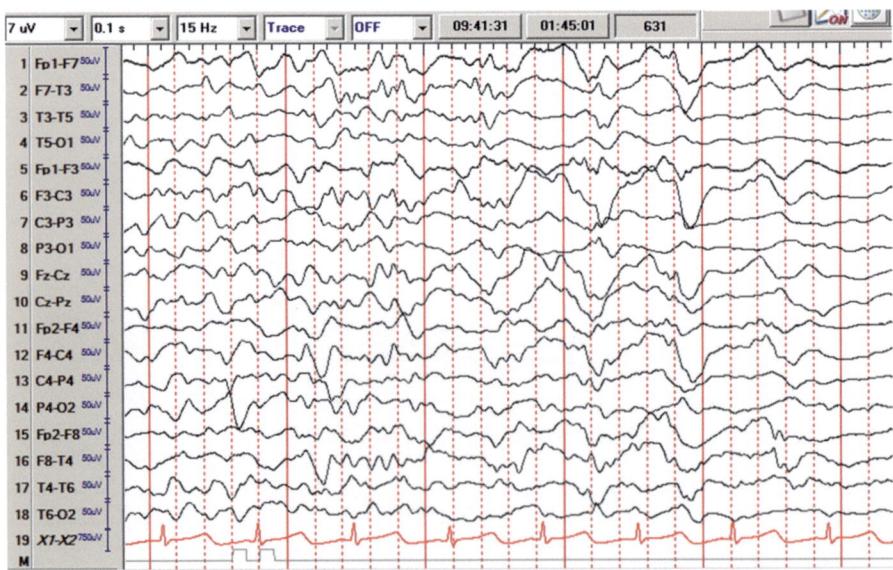

Fig. 2.53 Symmetric anterior dysrhythmia in a neonate between 34 and 35 WGA

Table 2.17 Location of sharp transients and certain frequency patterns commonly seen in 34–35 WGA neonates

	Sharp activity	Frequency activity
Bursts in DISCONTINUOUS QS		
Frontal	Sharp transients synchronous now EF: 50–100 μV, diphasic (small initial negative then larger positive), each wave duration 0.5–0.75 s Synchronous and symmetric and occur during active to quiet sleep transition	Anterior dysrhythmia: delta: 50–100 μV, runs last a few seconds, synchronous, symmetrical
Central		
Temporal		No temporal alpha bursts Beta delta complexes Rare theta
Occipital		Beta delta complex
CONTINUOUS		
Diffuse		Delta, theta

EF encoches frontales, *QS* quiet sleep, *WGA* weeks gestational age

Table 2.18 Chart showing the differences between normal encoches frontales, normal anterior dysrhythmia, and abnormal frontal sharp waves

	Normal—EF	Normal—AD	Abnormal
Symmetry	Symmetric	Symmetric	Asymmetric
Synchrony	Yes	Yes	No
Frequency of waveform	2–4 Hz	1.5–2 Hz	10 Hz
Duration of waveform	<2 s	2–5 s	5 s
Amplitude	<200 μV	50–150 μV	200 μV
State	Transitional/quiet sleep	Transitional/quiet sleep	Any
Age	<42/44 WGA	38–44 WGA	42/44 WGA

Hayakawa et al. [6] and Mizrahi and Hrachovy [8].
AD anterior dysrhythmia, *EF* enoches frontales, *WGA* weeks gestational age

2.14 36–37 Weeks Gestational Age

Below is a chart demonstrating background parameters for a 36–37 WGA neonate (Table 2.19). The discontinuous portion of the recording is a tracé alternant pattern in quiet sleep (Fig. 2.54). Continuous activity is activité moyenne, and the difference between waking and active sleep is apparent (Figs. 2.55 and 2.56). Activité moyenne is considered to be the pattern of continuous activity that is moderate voltage (25–50 μV) with a mixture of frequencies in the delta, theta, and beta ranges. Reactivity is present (Fig. 2.57). Transitional sleep is present and is when the baby's eyes are closed but clear criteria for a certain sleep stage are not met. This can be considered to be a brief period of indeterminate sleep. Below is a chart showing normal expected sharp activity and frequencies present in neonates between 36 and 37 WGA (Table 2.20).

Table 2.19 Chart showing background patterns for a 36–37 WGA neonate

Burst length	3–8 s	Tracé alternant is quiet sleep pattern
Burst amplitude	100–200 µV	
Burst frequency	0.5–4 Hz	
IBI length	3–8 s	
IBI amplitude	Over 25 µV	
Synchrony	No asynchrony	
Discontinuous %	50%	
Continuous %	50%	Activité moyenne is pattern in active sleep and awake
Continuous activity—active sleep	1–8 Hz 20–30 µV amplitude	
Continuous activity—awake	Moderate voltage, typically higher than 25 µV 1–8 Hz, mostly delta range	
Sleep/wake	Yes	Can differentiate all 3 states
Reactivity	Yes	Attenuation up to 10 s

Hz Hertz, *IBI* interburst interval

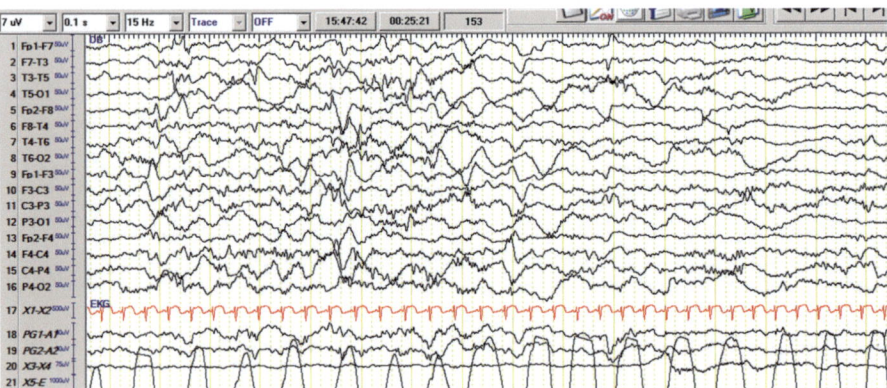

Fig. 2.54 Background activity at a glance in a neonate between 36 and 37 WGA. This figure shows quiet sleep and the IBI amplitudes are at this age are greater than 25 µV

2 Developmental Maturation of the EEG in Neonates, from Preterm to Term... 63

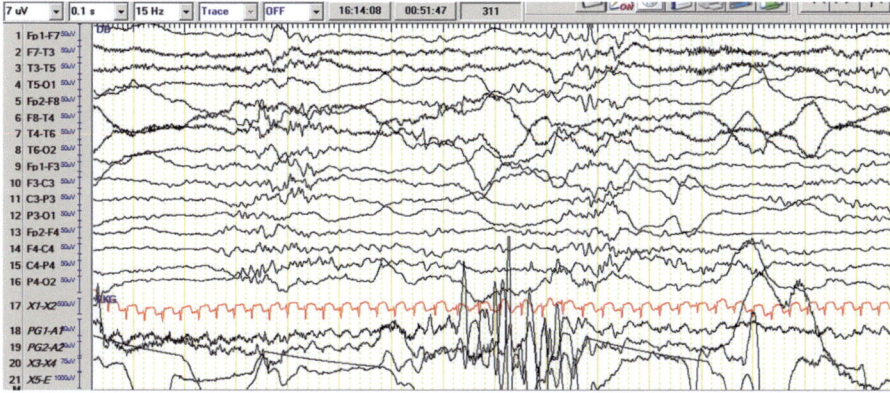

Fig. 2.55 Background activity at a glance in a neonate between 36 and 37 WGA. This figure shows active sleep. The background activity is continuous, and the respiratory belt lead shows irregular respirations. Some movement artifact is noted in the accessory leads, but lack of movement artifact in the head leads suggests the baby's body is relatively still, a constellation of findings typical of active sleep

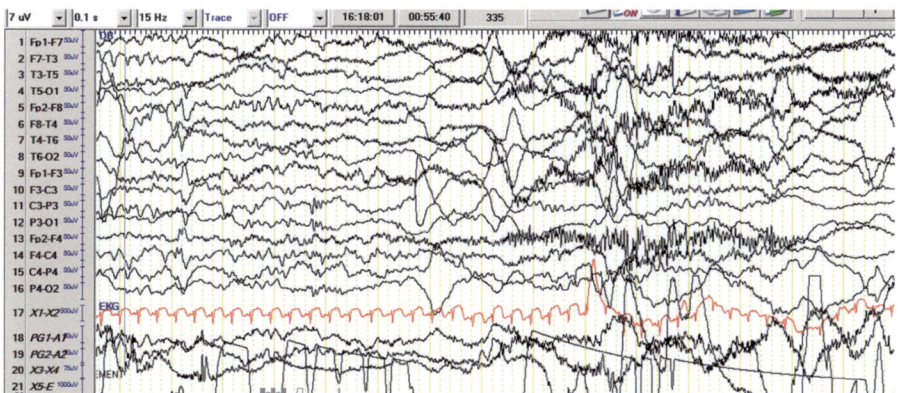

Fig. 2.56 Background activity at a glance in a neonate between 36 and 37 WGA. This figure shows wakefulness. In the right side of the picture, there is muscle artifact in all the leads that represents the baby being active and interacting with its environment

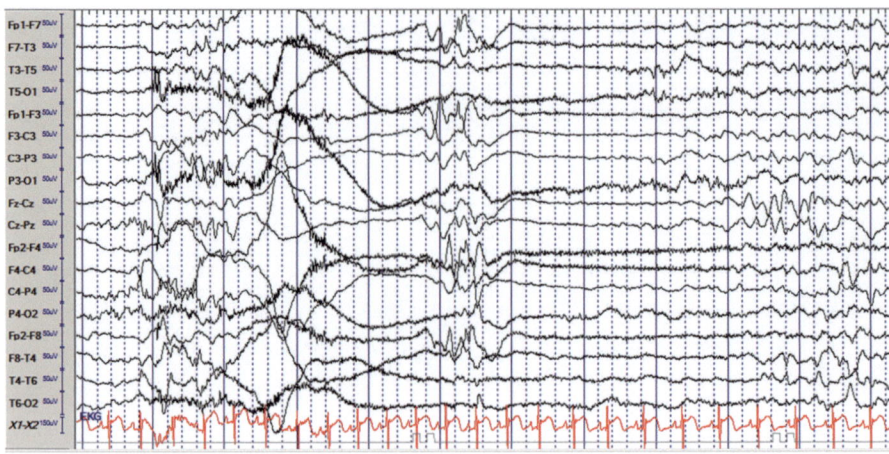

Fig. 2.57 Background at a glance in a neonate between 36 and 37 WGA. In this picture, an arousal occurs with a 2 s period of attenuation following

Table 2.20 Location of sharp transients and certain frequency patterns commonly seen in 36–37 WGA neonates

	Sharp activity	Frequency activity
Bursts in DISCONTINUOUS periods		
Frontal	Encoches frontales: 50–100 µV, diphasic (small initial negative then larger positive), each wave duration 0.5–0.75 s Synchronous and symmetric Active to quiet sleep transition	Anterior dysrhythmia: Delta, 50–100 µV, runs last a few seconds, synchronous, symmetric
Central	Sharp transients	Mixed frequencies
Temporal	Sharp transients	Fewer beta delta Decreasing temporal theta
Occipital	Sharp transients	Theta, fewer beta delta
CONTINUOUS periods		
Diffuse		Delta, theta, fast activity (ripples)

WGA weeks gestational age

2.15　38–40 Weeks Gestational Age

Below is a chart demonstrating background parameters for a 38–40 WGA neonate (Table 2.21). The discontinuous portion of the recording is a tracé alternant pattern in quiet sleep (Fig. 2.58). Continuous activity is activité moyenne, and the difference between waking and active sleep is apparent (Figs. 2.59 and 2.60). Reactivity

Table 2.21 Background parameters for a 38–40 WGA neonate EEG

Burst length	3–8 s	Tracé alternant is quiet sleep pattern
Burst amplitude	100–200 µV	
Burst frequency	0.5–4 Hz	
IBI length	3–8 s	
IBI amplitude	Over 25 µV	
Synchrony	Yes No asynchrony	
Discontinuous %	50%	
Continuous %	50%	Activité moyenne is pattern in active sleep and awake
Continuous activity—Active sleep	1–8 Hz 20–30 µV amplitude	
Continuous activity—Awake	Moderate voltage, typically higher than 25 µV 1–8 Hz, mostly delta range	
Sleep/wake	Yes	Can differentiate all 3 states
Reactivity	Yes	Attenuation up to 6 s

IBI interburst interval, *Hz* Hertz

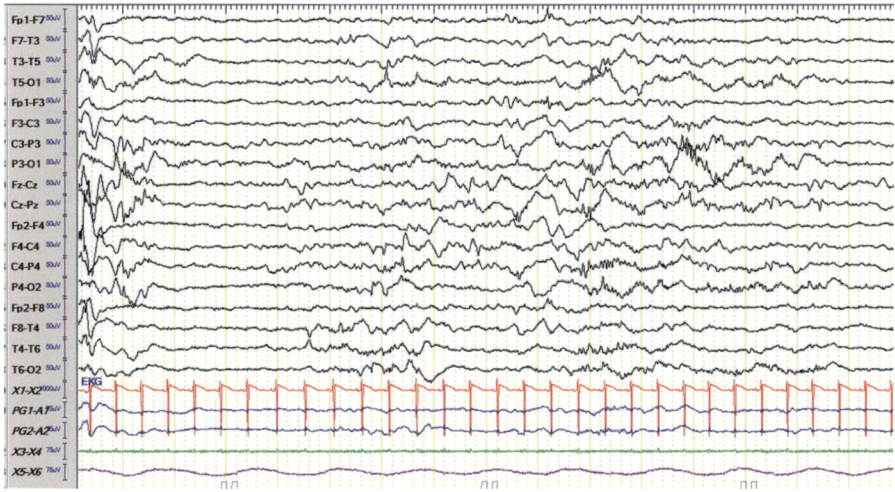

Fig. 2.58 Background at a glance. Quiet sleep, showing a tracé alternant pattern in a neonate between 38 and 40 WGA. Blue eye leads—quiet, so minimal eye movements, green chin lead—calm chin, purple respiratory lead—regular respirations

is present. Transitional sleep is present and occurs between active and quiet sleep when there may be a mixture of active sleep and quiet sleep criteria met (Fig. 2.61). The three sleep stages can be identified using simple criteria (Table 2.22). Sharp transients can be seen in any region; however, they should be symmetric and follow certain criteria to be considered normal (Fig. 2.62 and Table 2.23).

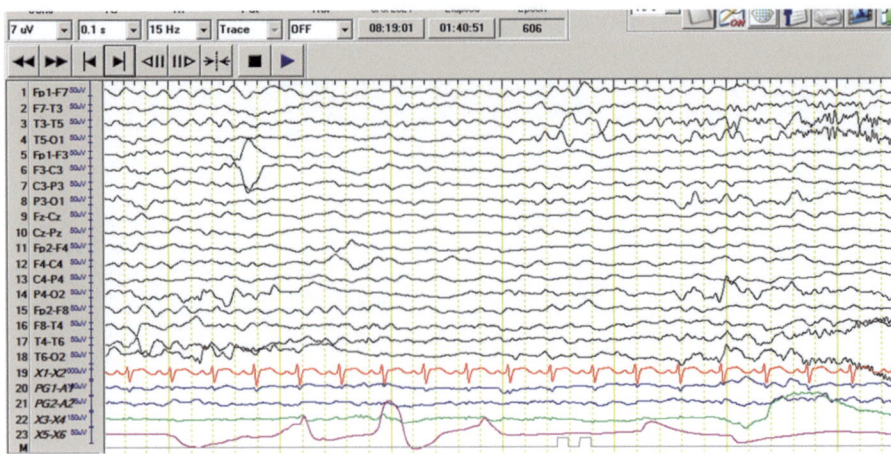

Fig. 2.59 Background at a glance. Active sleep, showing continuous pattern in a neonate between 38 and 40 WGA. Blue eye leads—active eye movements, green chin lead—calm chin, Purple respiratory lead—irregular respirations

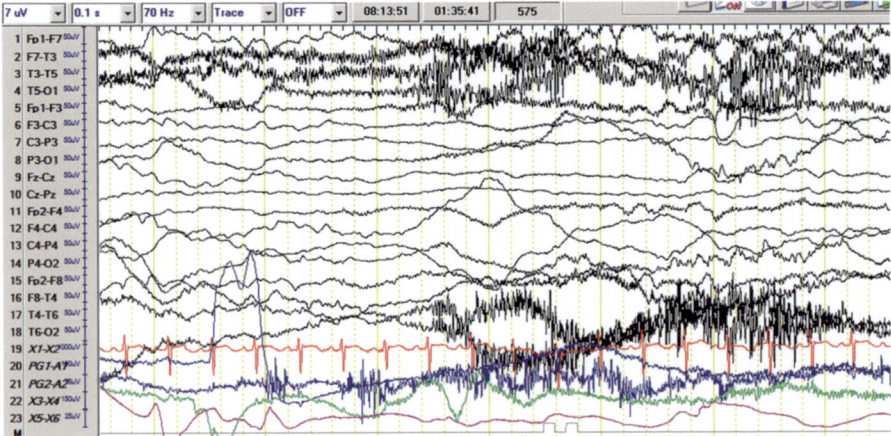

Fig. 2.60 Background at a glance. Wakefulness, showing continuous pattern with abundant muscle and movement artifact in a neonate between 38 and 40 WGA. Blue eye leads—active eye movements, green chin lead—active chin movements, purple respiratory lead—irregular respirations

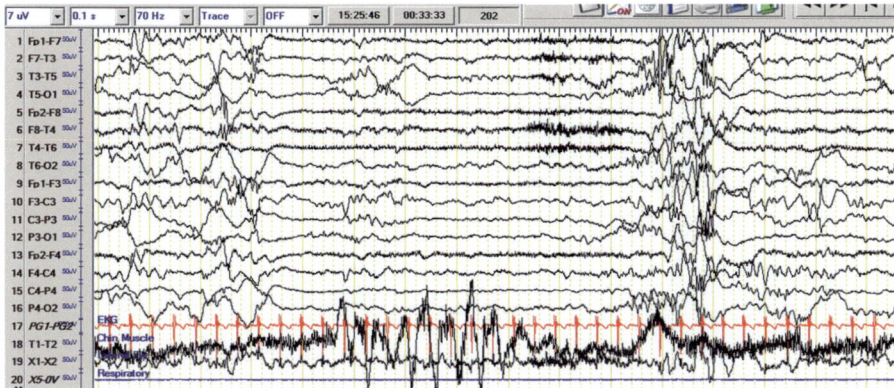

Fig. 2.61 Background at a glance. Indeterminate sleep in a neonate between 38 and 40 WGA. The pattern looks like tracé alternant; however, chin movement is occurring

Table 2.22 Sleep criteria in term neonates based on accessory EEG lead findings

	Awake	Active sleep	Quiet sleep
Eyes	Open	Closed	Closed
Eye leads	Active	Active (REM)	None
Chin EMG	Active	Calm	Calm
Respiratory belt	Irregular	Irregular	Regular
Body movements	Yes	Yes	Minimal

EMG electromyogram, *REM* rapid eye movement

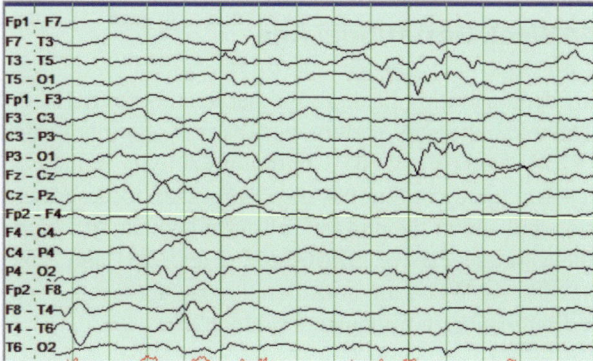

Fig. 2.62 Term sharp transients in the central, temporal, and occipital regions

Table 2.23 Location of sharp transients and certain frequency patterns in neonates between 38 and 40 WGA

	Sharp activity	Frequency activity
Bursts of DISCONTINUOUS periods		
Frontal	Encoches frontales: 50–100 µV, diphasic (small initial negative then larger positive), each wave duration 0.5–0.75 s Synchronous and symmetric Active to quiet sleep transition	Anterior dysrhythmia: delta, 50–100 µV, runs last a few seconds, synchronous, symmetric Theta (50–200 µV—May be sharp, bursts less than 1.5 s)
Central	Sharp transients, max here	Mixed frequencies Theta (50–200 µV)
Temporal	Sharp transients, max here	Fewer beta delta No temporal theta
Occipital	Sharp transients	Theta, fewer beta delta Rhythmic theta (4–6 Hz, 50–100 µV, less than 1 s, wake or sleep, bilateral asynchronous or unilateral)
CONTINUOUS periods		
Diffuse		Decreasing ripples, delta, theta

Hz Hertz, *µV* microvolt

Signs of <u>abnormal</u> sharp transient:

- Different location than deemed to be a normal graphoelement
- Focality (persistent in one region)
- Long runs, more than approximately three in a row (anterior dysrhythmia is an exception).

2.16 41–44 Week Gestational Age

Below is a chart demonstrating background parameters for a 41–44 WGA neonate (Table 2.24). The tracé alternant pattern evolves into continuous delta activity representing non-REM sleep (Fig. 2.63). Continuous activity remains as activité moyenne. An older term, tracé continu has also been used to describe this continuous pattern of waking and active sleep in the full-term neonate in which there is irregular delta and theta frequencies of 50–100 µV (Figs. 2.64 and 2.65). Any isolated sharp transients after 42 WGA are considered to be abnormal. Encoches frontales are present but diminishing in frequency (Table 2.25).

2 Developmental Maturation of the EEG in Neonates, from Preterm to Term...

Table 2.24 Background parameters for a neonate between the gestational age of 41–44 weeks

Burst length	Quiet sleep:	Tracé alternant is quiet sleep
Burst amplitude	tracé alternant evolves to continuous delta by 44 WGA	pattern
Burst frequency		Abates by 44 WGA and
IBI length		transitions to continuous delta
IBI amplitude		activity
Synchrony	Yes	
Continuous %	100%	Activité moyenne is pattern in
Continuous activity—active sleep	1–8 Hz 25–50 µV amplitude Delta and some theta	active sleep and awake
Continuous activity—awake	Moderate voltage (25–50 µV), delta and theta range, some alpha	

IBI interburst interval, *Hz* Hertz, *WGA* weeks gestational age, *REM* rapid eye movement

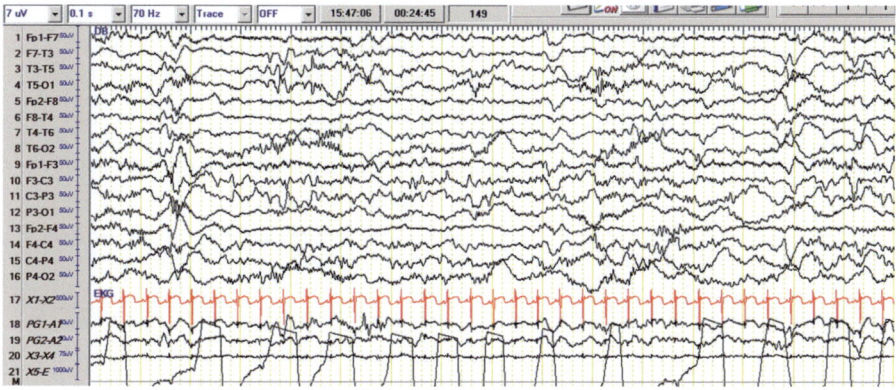

Fig. 2.63 Background at a glance. Quiet sleep, showing a tracé alternant pattern in a neonate between 41 and 44 WGA. Eye leads (PG1-A1, PG2-A2)—calm so minimal eye movements, chin (X3-X4)—calm chin, respiratory (X5-E)—regular respirations

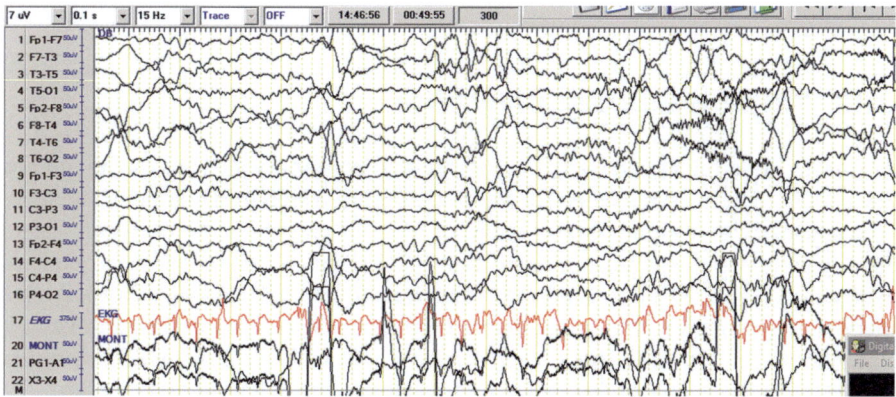

Fig. 2.64 Background at a glance. Active sleep, showing a continuous pattern in a neonate between 41 and 44 WGA. Eye lead left (PG1-A1)—active eye movement, chin (X3-X4)—calm chin movement, respiratory (X5-E)—irregular respirations. Lead marking is not shown in this picture but high-amplitude waveforms are present representing this lead activity

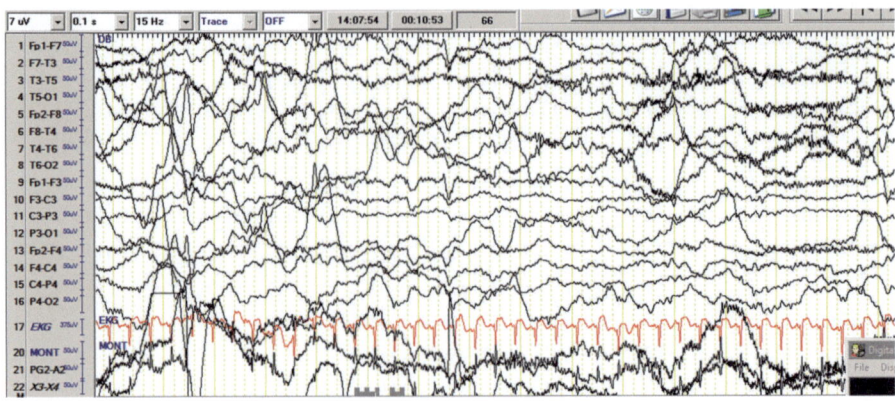

Fig. 2.65 Background at a glance. Wakefulness, showing a continuous pattern in a neonate between 41 and 44 WGA. Right eye lead (PG2-A2)—active eye movement, chin (X3-X4)—active chin movements, respiratory (X5-E)—irregular respirations. Lead marking is not shown in this picture but high-amplitude waveforms are present representing this lead activity

Table 2.25 Location of sharp transients and certain frequency patterns in neonates between 41 and 44 WGA

	Sharp activity	Frequency activity
Bursts of DISCONTINUOUS periods		
Frontal	Encoches frontales: 50–100 µV, diphasic (small initial negative then larger positive), each wave duration 0.5–0.75 s Synchronous and symmetric Active to quiet sleep transition	Anterior dysrhythmia: Delta: 50–100 µV, runs last a few seconds, synchronous, symmetric
Central		Delta, theta
Temporal		Delta
Occipital		Less delta, theta
CONTINUOUS periods		
Diffuse		Delta, theta

2.17 45–48 Weeks Gestational Age

Post term, wakefulness and active sleep begin to appear distinct. Waking maintains the pattern of activité moyenne (or tracé continu) in which irregular delta and theta frequencies within an amplitude range of 50–100 µV occur. Active sleep shows mostly delta with some theta frequencies. Quiet sleep consists of delta frequencies with the presence of primordial sleep spindles (Table 2.26 and Fig. 2.66). Active sleep may require a study longer than a 60-min study to capture. Sharp waves are not normal in this age group, and encoches frontales should not be present (Table 2.27). Background frequencies are mostly in the delta and theta ranges.

Table 2.26 Chart demonstrating background parameters for a 45–48 WGA neonate. Active sleep may require overnight study to capture

Burst length	Quiet sleep	Rudimentary sleep spindles, may not be synchronous but should be symmetric (12–14 Hz) Continuous delta
Burst amplitude	continuous delta	
Burst frequency	higher voltage (50–150 μV)	
IBI length	stimulation causes continuous activity	
IBI amplitude		
Synchrony	Yes	
Continuous %	100%	
Continuous activity—active sleep	1–8 Hz 20–50 μV amplitude Stimulation causes attenuation	Continuous slow, delta and theta
Continuous activity—awake Tracé continu	Moderate voltage (25–50 μV, some say 100–200 μV), irregular delta and theta range, some alpha Stimulation causes attenuation	Activité moyenne is pattern in wakefulness See mixed frequencies

IBI interburst interval, *Hz* Hertz

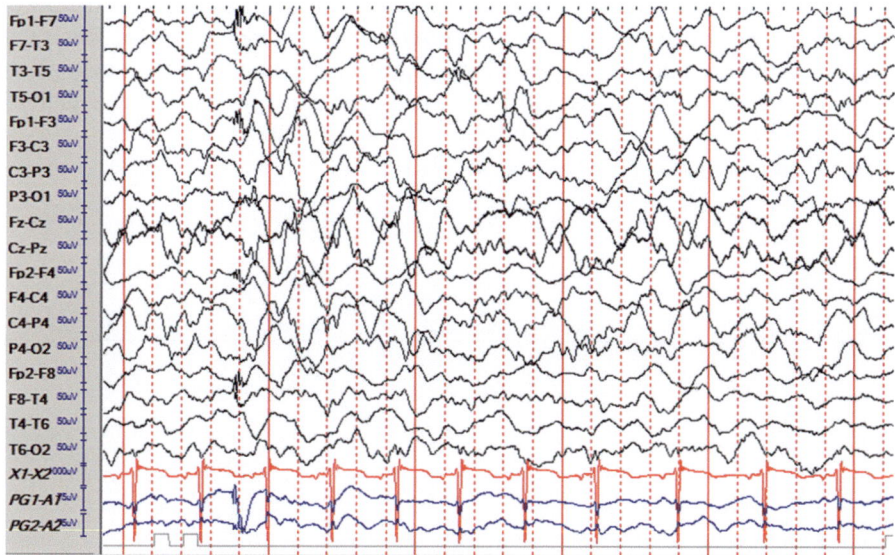

Fig. 2.66 Primordial sleep spindles in a neonate between 45 and 48 WGA. Sleep spindles are central in location with frequency of 16–20 Hz and begin around 48 WGA. They may not be synchronous but should be symmetric when first identified

Table 2.27 Location of sharp transients and certain frequency patterns in neonates 45–48 weeks

NO SHARP TRANSIENTS ARE NORMAL		
Bursts of DISCONTINUOUS periods	No discontinuous activity	
CONTINUOUS periods		
Diffuse		Delta, theta

Below is a table, followed by a schematic, depicting the transition of background patterns in the preterm to term neonate. Discontinuity predominates the early ages and by full term, three stages are identified. Awake, active, and quiet sleep then lead to normal wakefulness, stage II sleep, and REM sleep (Table 2.28 and Fig. 2.67).

Below is a pinwheel chart showing a layout of the maturational characteristics in the neonatal EEG recording from 24 WGA to 46 WGA (Fig. 2.68). The center of the wheel is 24 WGA, and the wheel expansion correlates with advancing developmental age. Sharp transients and frequencies are mentioned for each region as depicted in the wedges representing the frontal, central, temporal, and occipital regions. In addition, a fifth wedge is present, which represents the overall background pattern development. The inner circle marks 30 WGA, when the distinction between active sleep/waking and quiet sleep begins. This is also when many of the sharp transients and frequencies change. The background pattern wedge further divides around 40 WGA, when the distinction between awake, active sleep, and quiet sleep may be observed.

2 Developmental Maturation of the EEG in Neonates, from Preterm to Term…

Table 2.28 Transition of these developmental progressions. Exact gestational age may vary among patients

	24–29 WGA	28–35 WGA	32–38 WGA	36–41 WGA	40–48		48+	4 months +
	TD 50–300 µV Then <25 µV	Delta continuous, reactive	Delta and theta	Activité moyenne 25–50 µV Theta delta, beta	Activité moyenne/ tracé continu Mixed frequencies 50–100 µV	Awake	Continuous and mixed frequencies	Continuous PDR
	TD 50–300 µV Then <25 µV	Delta continuous	Delta	Activité moyenne 25–50 µV Theta delta, beta	Activité moyenne/ tracé continu Delta, some theta, 50–100 µV	Active sleep	REM Continuous delta and theta	REM Alpha
	TD 50–300 µV Then <25 µV	TD 50–300 µV Then <25 µV	TA 50–150 µV Delta 4 s/brief theta delta 25–50 µV	TA 50–150 µV Delta 4 s/brief theta delta 25–50	Continuous delta	Quiet sleep	Sleep spindles Also slow waves	Stage 2 sleep Spindles, vertex wave Stage 3 sleep Slow waves

µV microvolt, *PDR* posterior dominant rhythm, *TA* tracé alternant, *TD* tracé discontinu, *REM* rapid eye movement, *WGA* weeks gestational age

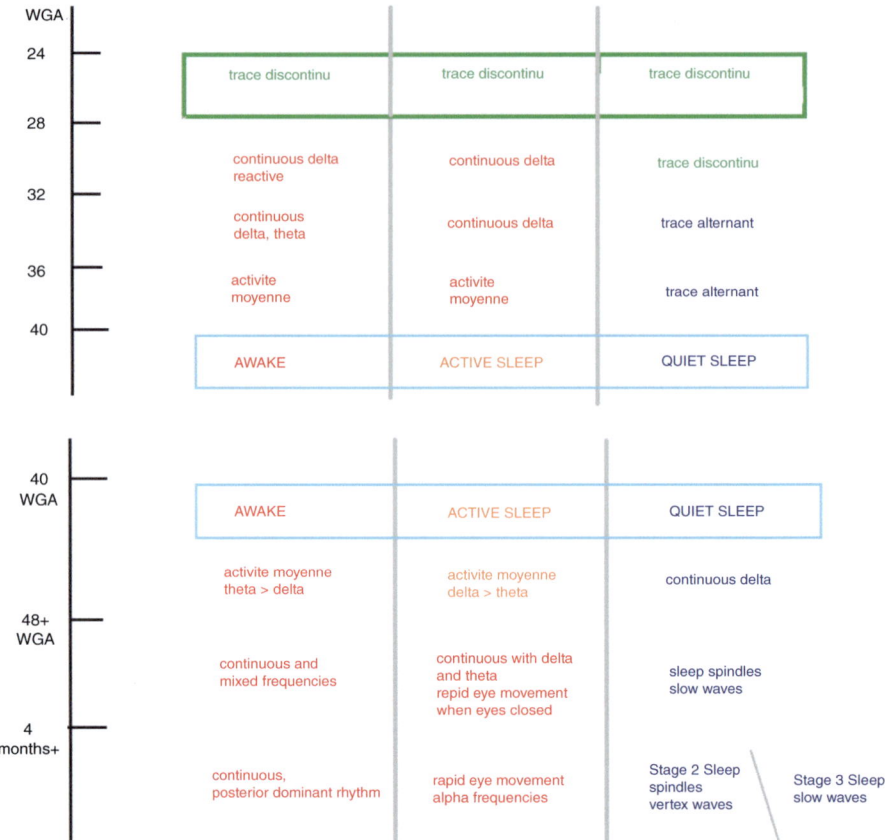

Fig. 2.67 Schematic representing Table 2.28, showing the maturation and development of background patterns from premature trace discontinu to term wakefulness, active sleep, and quiet sleep. By 4 months of age, wakefulness shows presence of regional differentiation, active sleep is consistent with REM sleep and quiet sleep is either stage 2 or 3 sleep

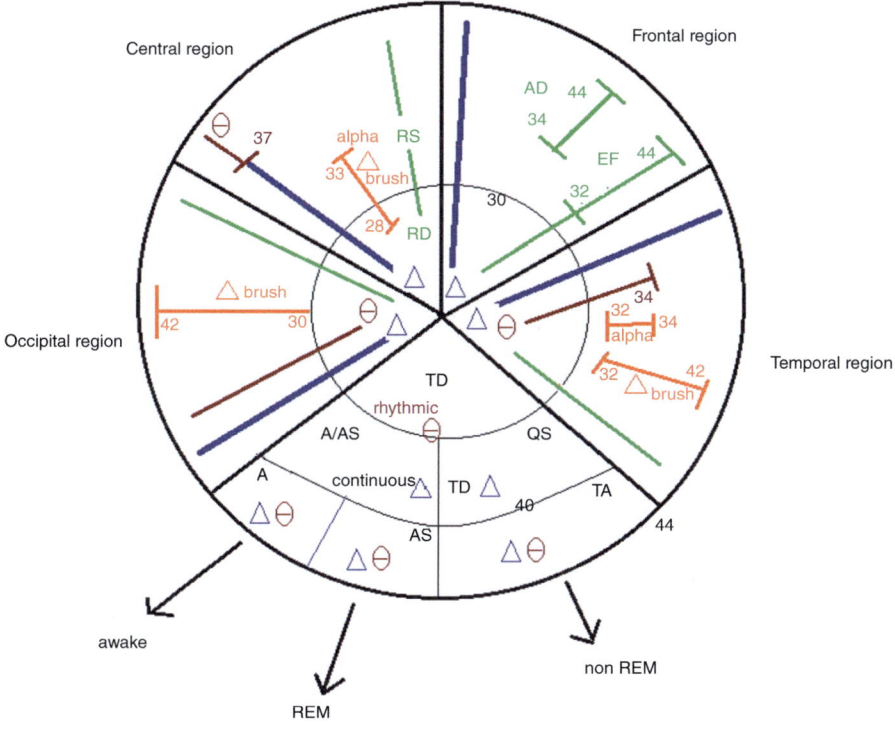

Fig. 2.68 Pinwheel chart depicting the EEG pattern transitions and evolutions from preterm to term neonatal ages. Key: Numbers correspond to WGA, Delta ▲, Theta ⬤. *A* awake, *AS* active sleep, *QS* quiet sleep, *TD* tracé discontinu, *TA* tracé alternant, *REM* rapid eye movement

References

1. Blume W, Kaibara M. Atlas of pediatric electroencephalopagraphy. 2nd ed. New York: Lippincott-Raven; 1998.
2. Bourel-Ponchel E, Gueden S, Hasaerts D, et al. Normal EEG during the neonatal period: maturational aspects from premature to full-term newborns. Neurophysiol Clin. 2021;51(1):61–88. https://doi.org/10.1016/j.neucli.2020.10.004. Epub 2020 Nov 22
3. Brazelton TB. Neonatal behavioral assessment scale. Philadelphia: J.B. Lippincott Co; 1984.
4. Britton J, Frey L, Hopp J, et al. Electroencephalography: an introductory text and atlas of Normal and abnormal findings in adults, children and Infants. Chicago: American Epilepsy Society; 2016.
5. Hahn JS, Monyer H, Tharp BR. Interburst interval measurements in the EEGs of premature infants with normal neurological outcome. Electrocencephalogr Clin Neurophysiol. 1989;73(5):410–8. https://doi.org/10.1016/0013-4694(89)90090-4.

6. Hayakawa F, Watanabe K, Hakamada S, et al. FZ theta/alpha bursts: a transient EEG pattern in healthy newborns. Electroencephalogr Clin Neurophysiol. 1987;67:27–31.
7. Hrachovy RA, Mizrahi EM, Kellway P. Electroencephalography of the newborn. In: Daly D, Pedley TA, editors. Current practice of clinical electroencephalography. 2nd ed. New York: Raven Press; 1990. p. 201–41.
8. Mizrahi E, Hrachovy R. Atlas of neonatal electroencephalography. 4th ed. New York: Demos Medical; 2016.
9. Selton D, Andre M, Hascoet JM. Normal EEG in very premature infants: reference criteria. Clin Neurophysiol. 2000;111(12):2116–24. https://doi.org/10.1016/s1388-2457(00)00440-5.
10. Tsuchida T, Wusthoff C, Shellhaas R, et al. ACNS standardized EEG terminology and categorization for the description of continuous EEG monitoring in neonates. Report of the American Clinical Neurophysiology Society, Critical Care Monitoring Committee. J Clin Neurophysiol. 2013;2:161–73. https://doi.org/10.1097/WNP.0b013e3182872b24.
11. Vecchierini MF, d'Allest AM, Verpillat P. EEG patterns in 10 extreme premature neonates with normal neurological outcome: qualitative and quantitative data. Brain Dev. 2002;25:330–7.

Abnormal Background Activity in Neonatal EEGs: Encephalopathy and Abnormal Frequency and Amplitude Findings

Mary Payne

3.1 Introduction

Presence of encephalopathy or focal dysfunction is demonstrated by electroencephalograms (EEGs). The reasons for such abnormalities may be broad; however, the EEG can help identify the degree of dysfunction and the regions involved. At the bedside, these electrographic findings can be especially helpful as radiographs do not always show abnormalities in a patient who is clearly altered. The EEG is a very sensitive test to evaluate actual neuronal functioning. This chapter will discuss different patterns identified in abnormal cortical functioning and their clinical implications.

3.2 Part 1: Abnormal Background Patterns: Encephalopathy

An encephalopathic full-term infant clinically may show absence of or decreased state changes, as in poor self-arousing for feeding, overall lethargy, or minimal response to stimulation [10]. The EEG background activity will correlate with these bedside findings, showing an encephalopathic background activity. However, observational signs of encephalopathy of a preterm infant can be more difficult to discern. Prior to 30 weeks gestational age (WGA), neonates do not typically arouse for feeds or have a significant identifiable waking state. Fortunately, the EEG background can be helpful in identifying encephalopathy in all gestational ages as encephalopathy manifests with the same overall background activity pattern across all gestational ages [2, 3, 6, 7].

M. Payne (✉)
Department of Pediatrics, Division of Pediatric Neurology, Joan C. Edwards School of Medicine, Hoops Family Children's Hospital, Marshall University, Huntington, WV, USA
e-mail: paynem@marshall.edu

3.2.1 Neuro Tidbit

Encephalopathy is a nonspecific finding and can occur from certain medications, therapeutic hypothermia, infection, metabolic errors, or hypoxic-ischemic encephalopathy. It can also be transient or intermittent. In older children and adults, encephalopathy corresponds to a patient having an altered mental status.

A. Mild encephalopathic findings manifest as excessive discontinuity, which can mimic a maturational abnormality.

Mild encephalopathy causes longer interburst intervals (IBI) and lower amplitudes overall, a term called *excessive discontinuity*. Sometimes the frequencies within the bursts and interbursts are also slower than would be expected. This pattern change can sometimes mimic the background activity of a younger gestational age infant. For example, a 32 WGA infant who is encephalopathic may show a background pattern that would be typical for a 28 WGA infant. This rewinding in age can be seen in any cause of encephalopathy, including use of sedative medications, infection, metabolic disorders, or hypoxic-ischemic encephalopathy.

In addition to immature background patterns, other findings may occur in mild encephalopathy:

– Minimal to no state change
– Amplitude and/or frequency abnormalities
– Unstimulated generalized and regional voltage attenuation
– Multifocal sharp waves

When assessing the degree of mild encephalopathy, there are two distinct patterns:

Internal Dyschronism
- Waking background is normal for gestational age
- Quiet sleep is abnormal
  – Excessive discontinuity (immature background)
  – Burst and interburst interval activity may be low amplitude.
  – Reactivity may still be present
- Suggests brain dysfunction but not as severe as external dyschronism
- Applicable term when neonate is at least 30 WGA, when all 3 state changes are often present at baseline

External Dyschronism
- All states (awake, active sleep, quiet sleep) are immature for gestational age.
  – Burst and interburst interval activity may be low amplitude.
- Reactivity may still be present.
- Suggests brain dysfunction, more severe compared to internal dyschronism.
- Applicable term when neonate is at least 30 WGA, when all 3 state changes may be present at baseline [9].

3.2.2 EEG Tidbit

Distinction between internal and external dyschronism can only be determined in certain gestational age infants (approximately greater than 30 WGA) who are expected to have state changes of waking and sleep at baseline. Identification of internal versus external dyschronism is typically made in infants who have minimal encephalopathy, such as in mild hypoxic-ischemic encephalopathy or those patients administered low-dose sedative medications.

Excessive discontinuity alone implies a mild degree of encephalopathy in which the background pattern becomes less mature based on the lengthening of the interburst interval duration. As encephalopathy worsens, there can be a progression of this excessive discontinuity so that the interburst interval durations are longer than would be seen in any gestational age (Figs. 3.1 and 3.2).

Below is a table (Table 3.1) outlining approximate ranges for a normal interburst interval (IBI) and abnormal IBI based on gestational age. The column on the right is the longest acceptable interburst length that has been documented in infants with normal neurological outcome. An interburst interval less than what is listed below in the far-right column may still indicate encephalopathy; however, the clinical scenario and other EEG findings need to be incorporated into the declaration of encephalopathy.

A. Moderate to severe encephalopathy manifests as a burst suppression pattern and ultimately electrocerebral silence.

As encephalopathy worsens, the pattern of excessive discontinuity changes to a burst suppression pattern, followed by diffuse low-amplitude activity and ultimately an extreme voltage-suppressed pattern.

1. Burst suppression pattern is part of a continuum with further progression of excessive discontinuity (Figs. 3.3, 3.4 and 3.5).

   Features of burst suppression:
   - The activity in the bursts is higher amplitude than the activity during the interburst interval and has the following characteristics:
     – Duration of bursts can vary.
     – Voltages may vary but are higher than 5 µV.
     – Frequencies can be delta, theta, or beta.
     – Sharp waves often intermixed.
     – Asymmetric activity within the bursts suggests focal dysfunction.
     – BURSTS DO NOT CONTAIN NORMAL GRAPHOELEMENTS.
   - IBI activity is low amplitude, <5 µV.
   - No state change (no change from waking to sleep).
   - No reactivity (no change with stimulation).

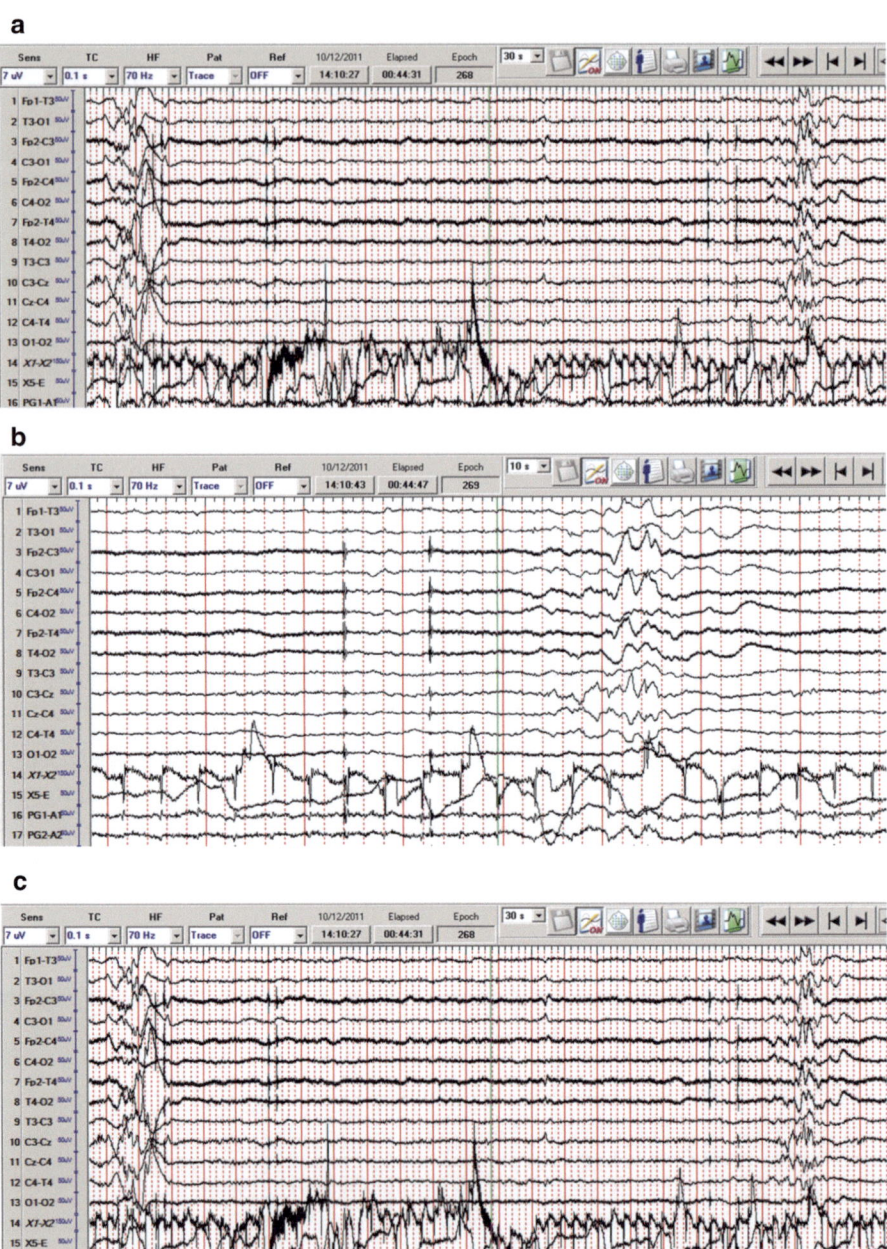

Fig. 3.1 Examples of discontinuous backgrounds in a neonate. *IBI* interburst interval. (**a**) This pattern could be normal for a very premature infant or abnormal for a term infant. Picture is of 25 s. IBI is 20 s. IBI amplitude is greater than 5 μV. (**b**) Burst activity with IBI at least 5 s, according to this picture. (**c**) Changing the setting so longer period of time is viewed on the screen shows the IBI period to last 18 s. This is an example of excessive discontinuity

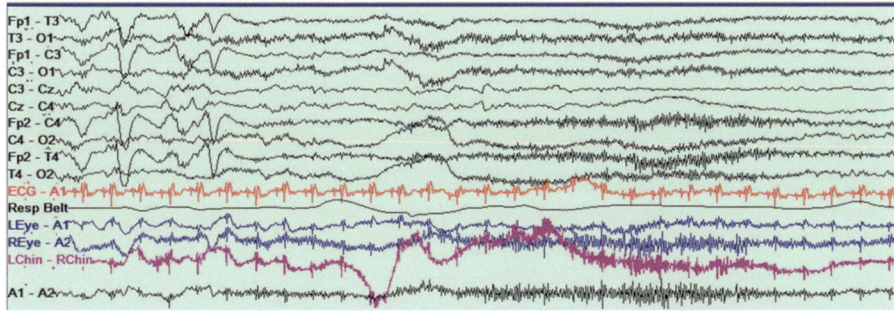

Fig. 3.2 Example of prolonged abnormal attenuation in a neonate. Abnormal prolonged attenuation, which is not triggered by stimulation, is shown in this segment and suggests encephalopathy. Also note that this baby has normal anterior dysrhythmia, reminding that in mild encephalopathy preservation of some normal graphoelements can occur

Table 3.1 Gestational ages and comparison of normal and abnormal interburst intervals

WGA	IBI average normal	Longest acceptable interval
24	5–25 s	60 s
26	3–12 s	46 s
27	3–12 s	36 s
28–30	3-12 s	30–35 s
31–33	2-10 s	20 s
34–36	2–8 s	10 s
37–40	2–6 s	10 s

Grigg-Damberger et al. [4], Hahn et al. [5], Holmes and Lombroso [6], Selton et al. [11], and Vecchierini et al. [13]
IBI interburst interval, *WGA* weeks gestational age

Medically induced burst suppression, such as in case of refractory seizure treatment, can show very clearly the progression from excessive discontinuity to burst suppression pattern. With continued administration of medications, the burst lengths become shorter and the IBI intervals become lower in voltage. Likewise, if medications are being lowered to bring a patient out of burst suppression, we see a similar reverse change of bursts become longer in duration, IBI amplitude becomes higher (Fig. 3.6).

2. Myoclonic jerks in the setting of burst suppression background pattern
    (a) Myoclonic jerks occurring time-locked with electrographic epileptic bursts suggest that the clinical jerk is epileptic myoclonus and the burst activity is thus epileptic. Electrographic epileptic bursts may occur without a clinical accompaniment, especially following anti-epileptic treatment. Most of the time, the clinical and electrographic epileptic activity is bilateral with minor asymmetries. However, the presence of unilateral clinical jerk-like movements and/or unilateral electrographic epileptic activity suggests a structural abnormality in the associated electrographic epileptic region. Epileptic myoclonus indicates a poor prognosis and in the setting of anoxic injury is termed post-anoxic myoclonus.

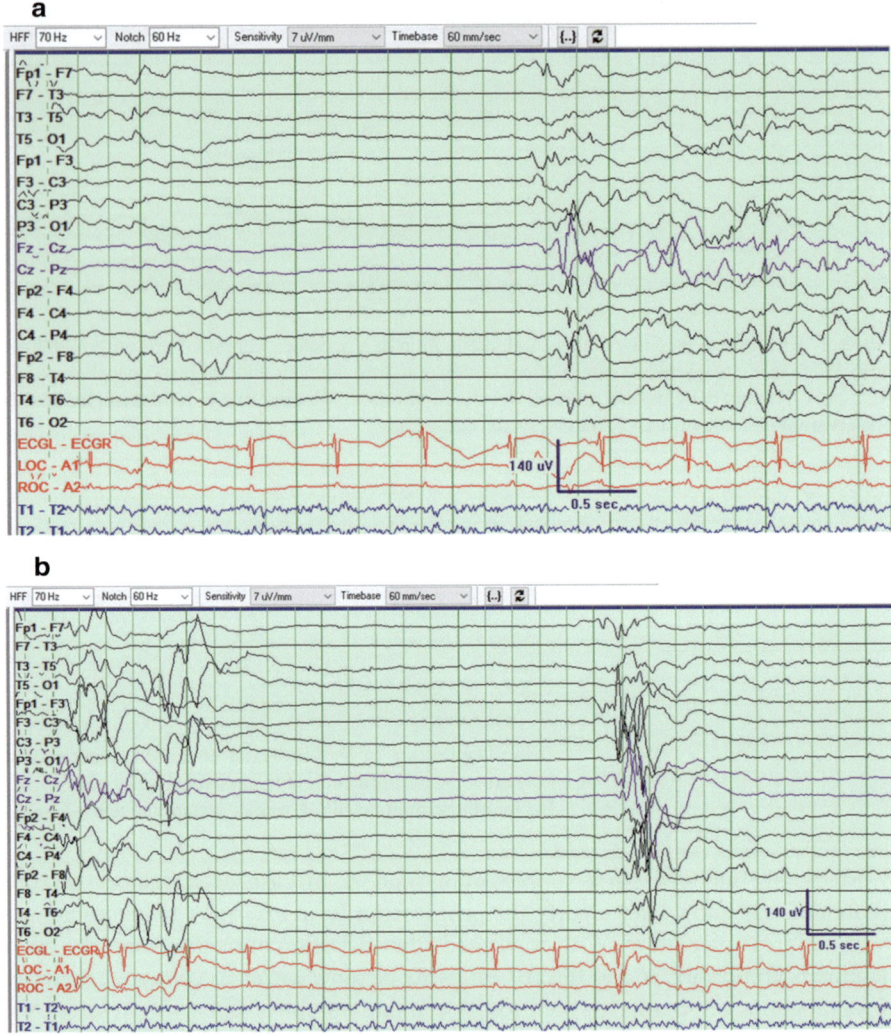

Fig. 3.3 (**a, b**) Burst suppression activity in a neonate. In this example, the burst activity is greater than 150 μV and consists of a mixture of delta and theta frequencies lasting 1–3 s. The period of suppression is about 2 s in duration and consists of low-amplitude (less than 5 μV) activity. Asymmetry is also present with higher amplitude activity in the right hemisphere, suggesting additional abnormality in one of the hemispheres. Patient is full term with severe hypoxic-ischemic encephalopathy. (**b**) Burst suppression activity in a neonate. This burst consists of a mixture of delta and theta frequencies. This patient has high-amplitude (greater than 200 μV) burst activity, The period of suppression is about 3 s in duration and consists of low-amplitude (less than 5 μV) activity

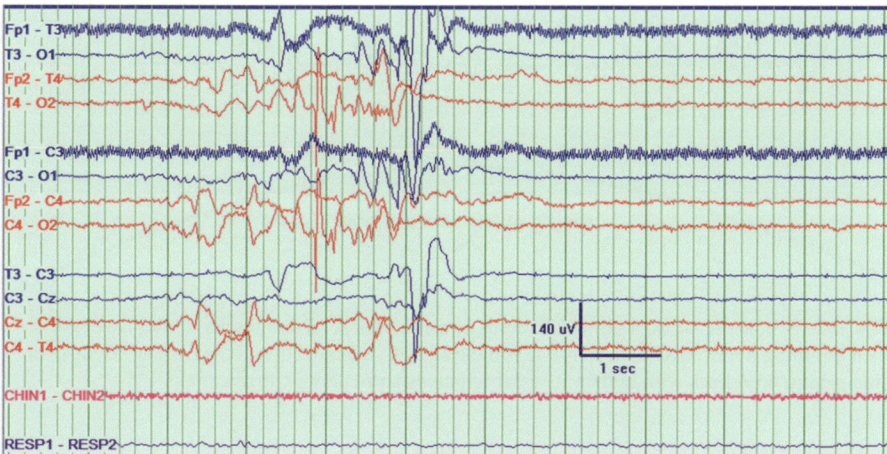

Fig. 3.4 Burst suppression activity in a neonate. Note the burst consists of a mixture of delta and theta frequencies lasting approximately 3 s. The period of suppression is greater than 5 s in duration and consists of low-amplitude (less than 5 µV) activity

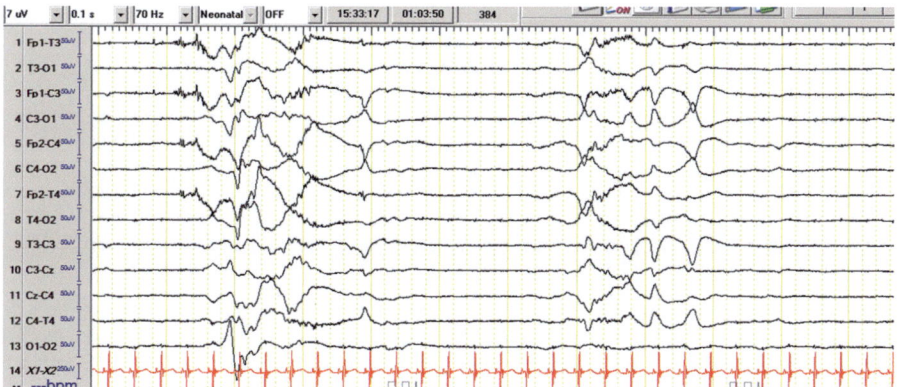

Fig. 3.5 Burst suppression activity in a neonate. These bursts consist of a mixture of delta, theta, and alpha frequencies with a duration of 2–3 s. The period of suppression is about 3 s in duration and consists of low-amplitude (less than 5 µV) activity. This patient's age is 27 WGA

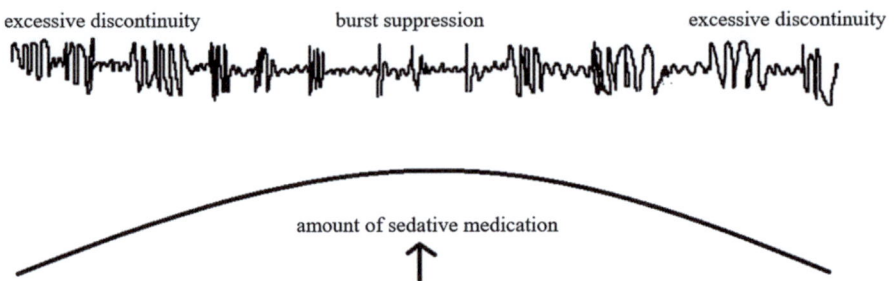

Fig. 3.6 Schematic of background patterns from excessive discontinuity to burst suppression, then returning the excessive discontinuity in the setting of medication changes. The burst suppression pattern correlates with higher doses of sedatives/anti-epileptic medications

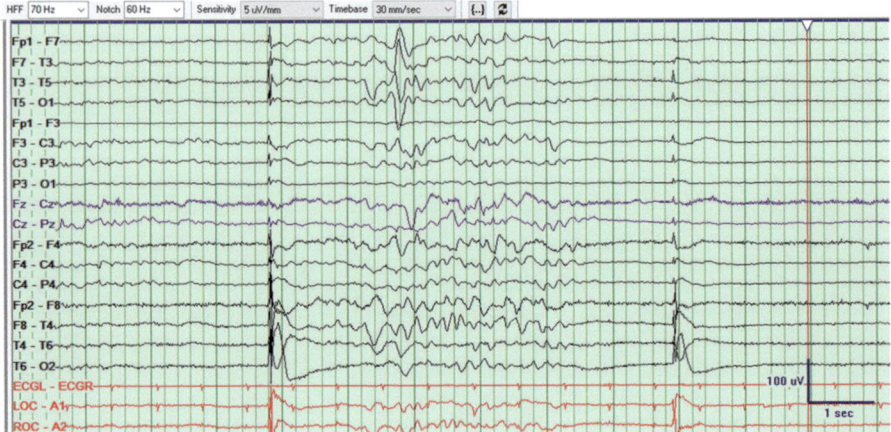

Fig. 3.7 Post-anoxic myoclonus with a burst suppression pattern in a neonate. High-amplitude brief bursts correlate with clinical myoclonus. The background pattern is burst suppression. Not all bursts are associated with a clinical myoclonus event of the patient; however, all clinical events are associated with an electrographic epileptic discharge

  (b) Myoclonic jerks that do not correlate in a time-locked manner with the high-amplitude electrographic burst activity are not considered to be epileptic myoclonus. Their etiology is likely due to subcortical or spinal circuitry. This scenario is also seen in severe encephalopathy and indicates a poor prognosis [1].
  (c) Myoclonic jerks occurring in the setting of a burst suppression background pattern is also a constellation seen with the developmental epileptic encephalopathies. In this case, myoclonic jerks are the ictal (seizure) signature and not necessarily associated with post-anoxic injury.

Post-anoxic Myoclonus Examples
In the examples below (Figs. 3.7 and 3.8), the patient was noted to have myoclonic jerks at the same time as the high-amplitude epileptiform spike

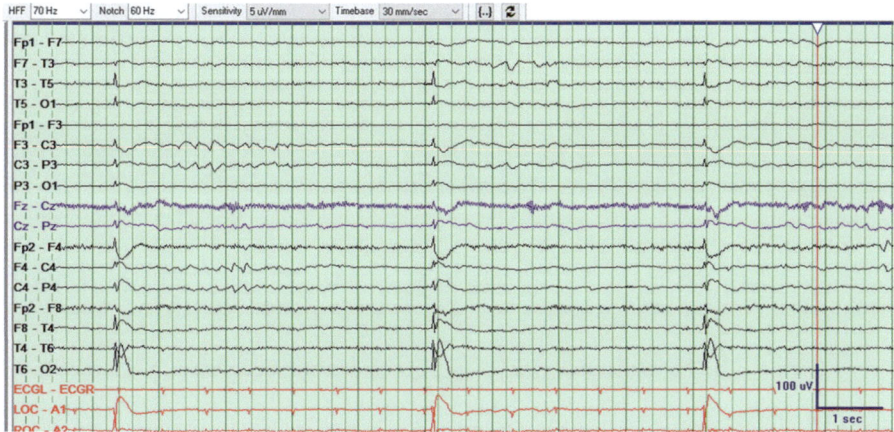

Fig. 3.8 Post-anoxic myoclonus with a burst suppression pattern in a neonate. High-amplitude brief bursts correlate with clinical myoclonus. The background pattern is burst suppression

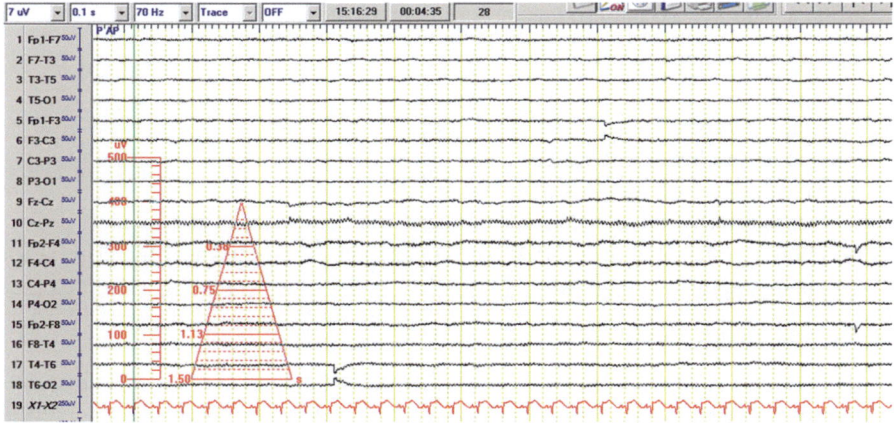

Fig. 3.9 Low voltage suppressed pattern in a neonate

discharges. The eye leads (LOC, ROC) are actually detecting cortical activity, not eye movement activity. When the overall EEG background is very low amplitude, the eye leads will often display high-amplitude activity from the cortex as no other contributing waveforms are present to be computed into the integrated signal output.

3. Low-voltage-suppressed pattern

The American Clinical Neurophysiology Society (ACNS) guidelines [12] define this pattern as being beyond burst suppression but not quite meeting the criteria for electrocerebral inactivity (Fig. 3.9). Presence of electrocerebral inactivity may be

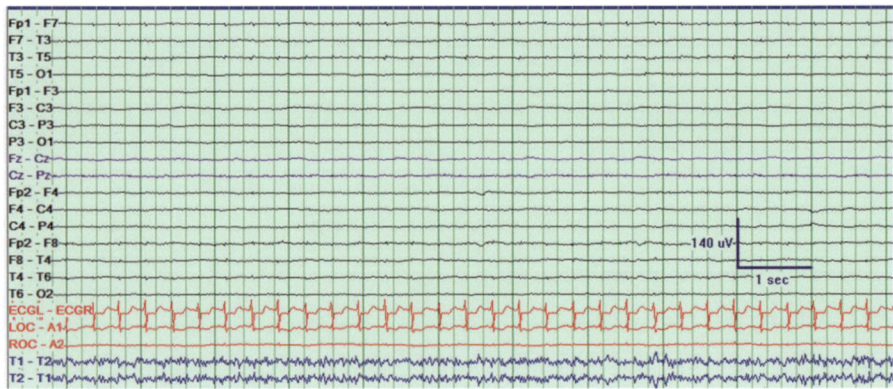

Fig. 3.10 Electrocerebral inactivity in a neonate. Background activity is suppressed and there is no cortical activity above 2 μV in amplitude

part of a brain death determination, so the occurrence of a less severe, low-voltage-suppressed pattern is important to discern for clinical implications.

Voltage-suppressed pattern has the following features:

- No normal graphoelements
- No reactivity
- No state changes
- Frequency is slow (delta range)
- Activity is low voltage, less than 10 μV
  - Occasionally higher voltages can occur, but not longer than 2 s
  - Higher voltages above 10 μV for longer than 2 s would meet the criteria for burst suppression pattern

4. Electrocerebral Inactivity

This pattern is beyond the low-voltage-suppressed pattern and indicates irreversible severe cortical dysfunction (Figs. 3.10 and 3.11). Prior terms are electrocerebral silence or isoelectric. A specific EEG protocol is used in this setting to minimize the possibilities of false signals or inaccurate recordings. The results of this EEG study may be criteria or a factor when making a decision about brain death determination. Features include

- No state change
- No reactivity
- No apparent cortical activity above 2 μV

C. Clarification of Terms: Excessive Discontinuity and Burst Suppression

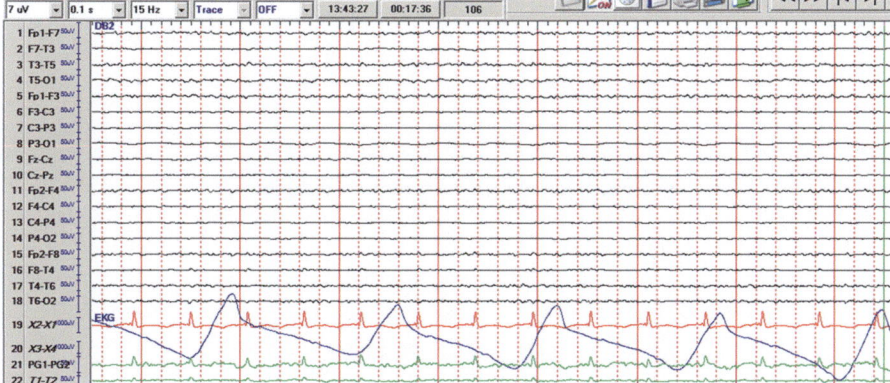

Fig. 3.11 Electrocerebral inactivity in a neonate. Background activity is suppressed and there is no cortical activity above 2 μV in amplitude. The blue line pattern is the respiratory belt movement, showing the patient's chest movements with a mechanical ventilator

The difference in these two terms can be confusing and may have some overlap and different interpretations by different readers. Below are some main differences:

Excessive Discontinuity
This term implies the presence of an immature background as seen in mild encephalopathy. This is the "rewind" of the background pattern. IBI duration may be longer than what would be normal for the patient's gestational age or longer than what would be expected for any neonate. Periods of lower amplitude activity (the IBI) may be attenuated but should remain in the range of normal background voltage. Reactivity and state change may be present. If these criteria are met, one could report the pattern as "excessive discontinuity for gestational age."

Burst Suppression
This term describes a pattern in which IBI amplitudes are extremely low voltage (less than 5 μV) and alternate with higher amplitude bursts. In addition, the duration of low-amplitude periods may be longer than what would be expected for the patient's gestational age (but not necessarily). There is no reactivity or state change. This pattern implies more severe encephalopathy than that seen with excessive discontinuity.

EEG Tidbit
Infants younger than 30 WGA are not expected to have reactivity or state change at baseline. Thus, the presence or absence of these changes cannot always be used to evaluate for encephalopathy. However, this younger premature infant cortical activity still follows the progression in overall background patterns as cortical function worsens.

D. Summary of Progression of Encephalopathic Findings Seen in EEG Background Activity:

Normal Maturation Background

Internal Dyschronism / Excessive Discontinuity

External Dyschronism / Excessive Discontinuity

Burst suppression

Low voltage Suppressed

Electrocerebral Inactivity

3.3 Part 2: Abnormal Background Patterns: Abnormal Amplitude

A. Low voltage in all leads
   1. Can be called diffuse low amplitude, implying low-amplitude activity is present in all leads (Fig. 3.12).
   2. Term does not imply a certain voltage criteria, but denotes that the overall background activity is lower voltage than would be expected for age.
   3. Nonspecific etiology, seen in, for example,
      (a) Encephalopathy
      (b) Medication use
            Opiates, barbiturates, benzodiazepines, anti-epileptic medications
      (c) Therapeutic hypothermia
   4. May be intermittent.
   5. Persistent amplitudes less than 10 µV without variation (no reactivity or state change) suggest poor prognosis. In this case, the term low-voltage-suppressed pattern can be used.

B. High voltage in all leads (Fig. 3.13)
   1. Can be called diffuse high amplitude (present in all leads).
   2. Unusual in neonates but can be seen in encephalopathy.
   3. High-amplitude background activity can be seen in patients with hypsarrhythmia, a background pattern seen in patients with a type of epileptic encephalopathy. This usually presents beyond the neonatal age.

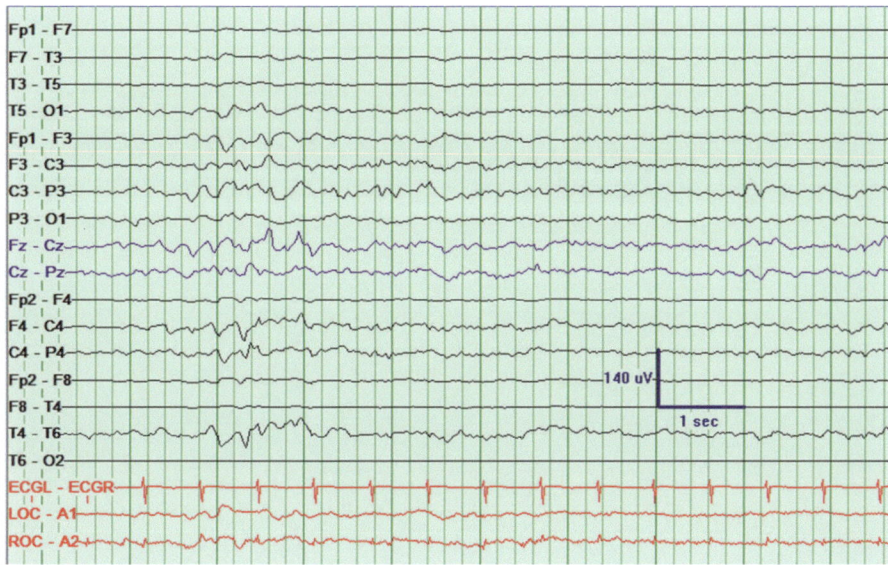

Fig. 3.12 Diffuse low-amplitude activity in a neonate. Low-amplitude activity is diffuse, meaning present in all leads. However, some leads (regions) show lower amplitude than others. In this patient, bilateral frontal and temporal regions demonstrate the largest degree of amplitude attenuation

C. Focal (in one region) abnormality of low or high amplitude (Figs. 3.14 and 3.15)
   1. May be constant or intermittent
   2. Suggests focal lesion
   3. May occur with normal background patterns
      (a) Structural lesion—may be low- or high-amplitude focal abnormality and is usually constant or near continuous
      (b) Extra-axial hemorrhage—causes low amplitude based on impedance of signal through the hemorrhage and is usually constant or near continuous
      (c) Post-ictal—low or high amplitude and transient
      (d) Artifact—low- or high-amplitude abnormality
D. Diffuse amplitude abnormality with additional focal amplitude abnormalities (Fig. 3.16)
   1. Diffuse amplitude abnormalities indicate global cortical dysfunction. When additional areas of focal amplitude abnormality occur, this suggests a focal area of dysfunction, in addition to the global (overall) cortical impairment.
   2. Usually seen in patients with a background abnormality of excessive discontinuity, low-voltage-suppressed or burst suppression.
   3. Also can be seen with diffuse cortical dysfunction with external factors affecting the scalp EEG signal, causing a false focal abnormality.

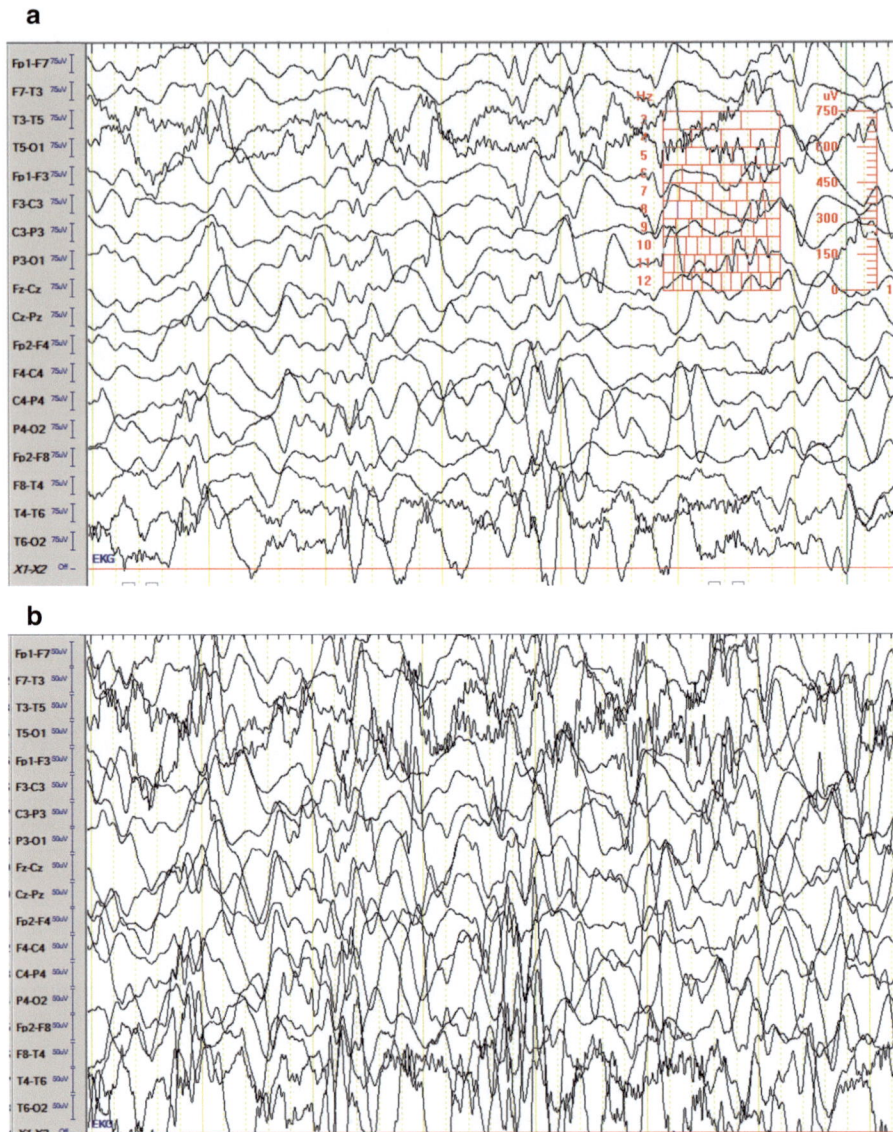

Fig. 3.13 (**a**, **b**) High-voltage activity in all leads in an infant EEG recording. (**a**) Sensitivity is set at 7 μV. (**b**) Sensitivity is set at 15 μV

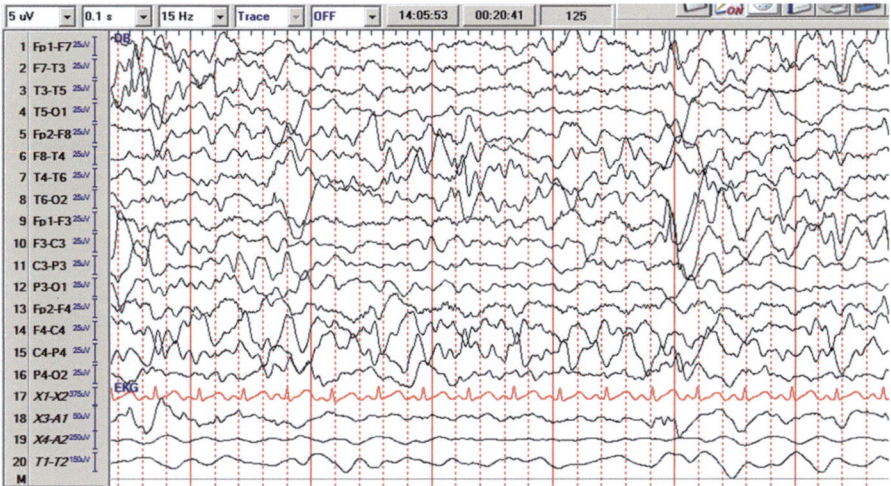

Fig. 3.14 Lower amplitude activity present in the left hemisphere of a neonate. This patient has a porencephalic cyst in the left hemisphere, which creates low-amplitude scalp-recorded EEG activity

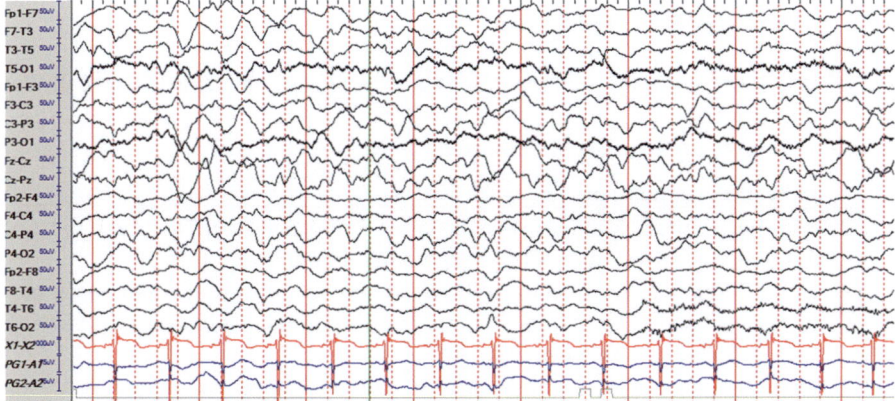

Fig. 3.15 Focal low-amplitude activity in the right hemisphere of a neonate. This patient has a subdural hematoma in the right hemisphere, which blunts the cortical activity perceived by the scalp electrodes over the right hemisphere

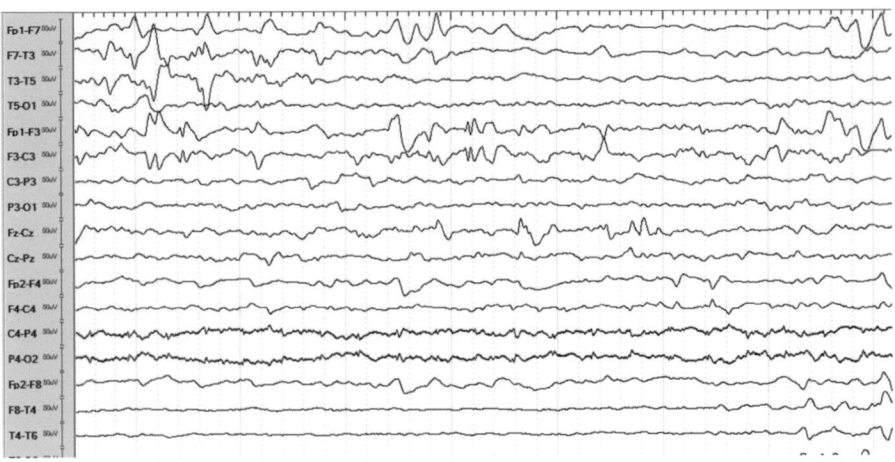

Fig. 3.16 Diffuse low-amplitude activity with additional regions of focal low-amplitude activity in bilateral temporal regions in a neonate with encephalitis. Also present are epileptiform sharp waves and low-frequency activity

3.4 Part 3: Abnormal Background Patterns: Abnormal Frequency

A. Diffuse low frequency—This is referred to as slowing in all leads. Recall that delta frequency is the slowest frequency (less than 4 Hz) and in neonates diffuse slowing typically consists of delta frequencies (Fig. 3.17).

1. Indicates encephalopathy.
2. May be seen in a continuous or discontinuous background in which most of the frequencies are in the delta range without much variation.
3. Delta frequencies can occur in the burst activity of a burst suppression pattern. Periods of suppression (IBI) are low amplitude, but if able to be viewed, will be noted to have delta frequencies.
4. Delta frequencies occur in the pattern of low-voltage-suppressed, in which the activity present is delta activity. Voltages are very low, so frequency may be difficult to clearly identify without artifacts. If the sensitivity is increased to view these waveforms, artifact waveforms will also be increased and may obscure the view of cortical activity.

B. Focal slowing, low frequency in one area (Figs. 3.18 and 3.19).

1. Indicates focal dysfunction in that area.
2. May be transient after a seizure.
3. Can also correlate with presence of soft tissue edema, blood, extra- or intra-axial; this would be considered secondary and not cortical in origin because the alteration of the waveforms is due to a noncortical structural reason.
4. Can be seen with normal background pattern activity.

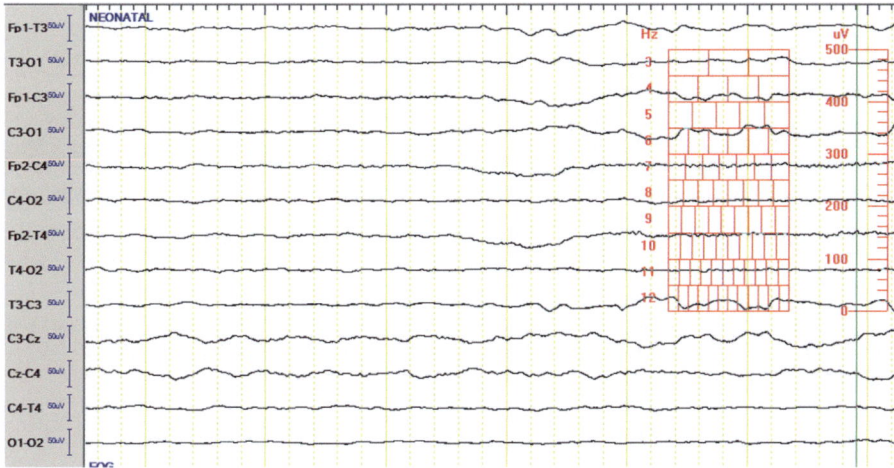

Fig. 3.17 Background activity showing diffusely low-amplitude and low-frequency activity in a neonatal EEG. Most amplitudes are between 10 and 20 μV

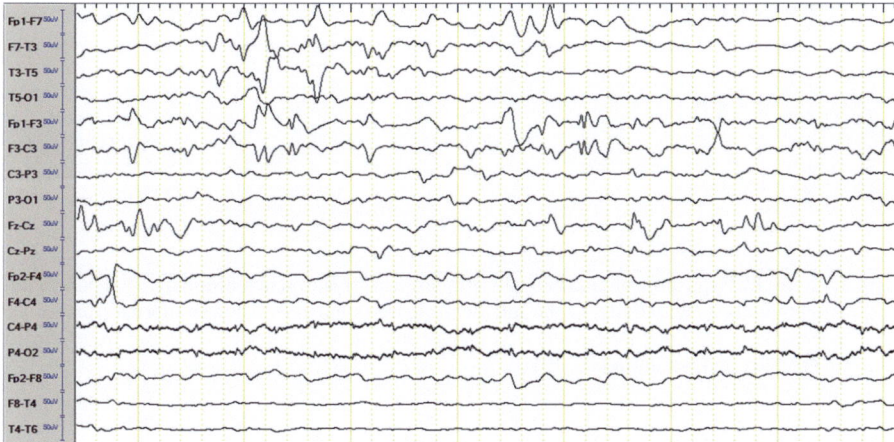

Fig. 3.18 Left frontal focal slowing with right temporal amplitude suppression in a neonatal EEG recording. The Fp1-F7 lead shows 1–2 Hz activity, which corresponds to a region of focal infarction

C. Abnormal rhythmic frequencies or abnormal runs of waveforms at a certain frequency; focal or generalized (Figs. 3.18, 3.19, 3.20, 3.21, and 3.22)

1. The term rhythmic implies a repeating waveform in a repeating pattern.
    (a) Rhythmic activity may consist of otherwise normal waveforms that occur in a repeated pattern.
    (b) Rhythmic activity may also consist of sharp waveforms that occur in a repeated pattern.

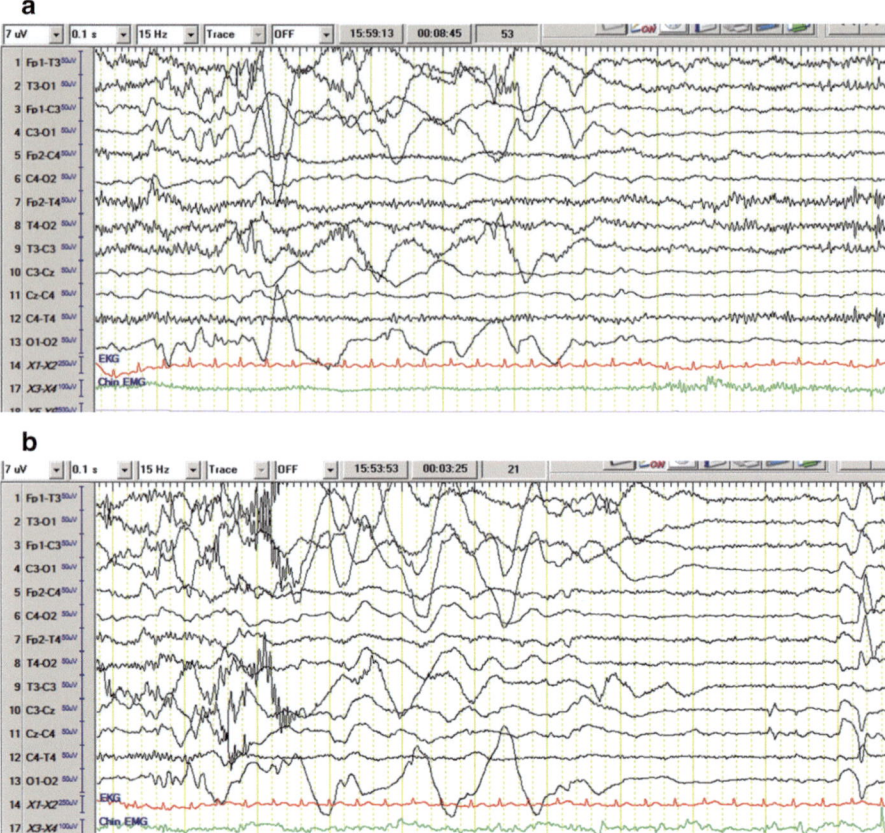

Fig. 3.19 (**a**, **b**) Focal slowing in a neonate with left hemisphere schizencephaly. This patient has high-amplitude 1–2 Hz activity in the left hemisphere compared to lower (normal) amplitude 2–3 Hz activity in the right hemisphere. Also notice that the focal slowing is demonstrated during the burst activity and not during the IBI.

    2. Semi-rhythmic may also be used to describe runs of activity that may not be completely repetitive but overtime are concerning and show a consistent pattern with being repeated.
    3. Usually seen with other abnormalities of the background pattern such as abnormal amplitudes, presence of sharp waves, or excessive discontinuity.
    4. When generalized, may be an indication of encephalopathy.
    5. When focal may be an indication of a corresponding focal area of dysfunction.
       Common abnormal rhythmic frequencies occurring in patients with encephalopathy, depicted in Table 3.2.
D. Diffuse cortical dysfunction with additional region of focal dysfunction
    1. Abnormal background pattern AND focal slowing AND/OR abnormal frequencies.

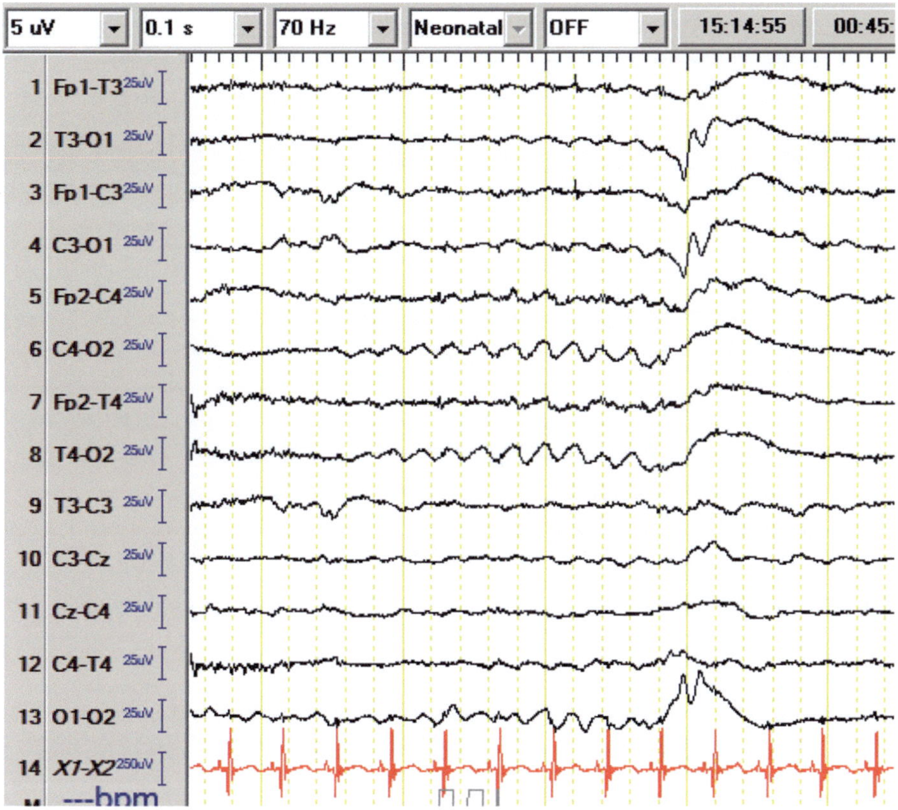

3 Abnormal Background Activity in Neonatal EEGs: Encephalopathy and Abnormal... 95

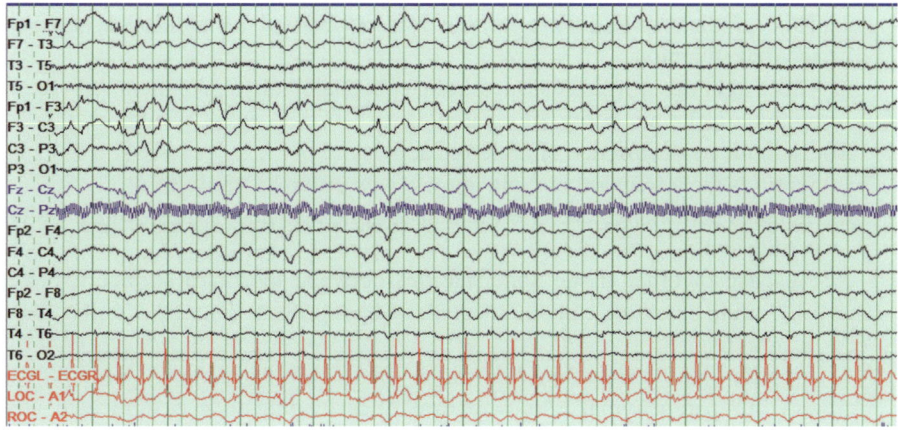

Fig. 3.20 Example of runs of 4–5 Hz occipital activity, right more than left hemisphere in a neonate with encephalopathy

Fig. 3.21 Runs of bifrontal sharply contoured delta activity in a neonate with seizures and bilateral frontal infarctions

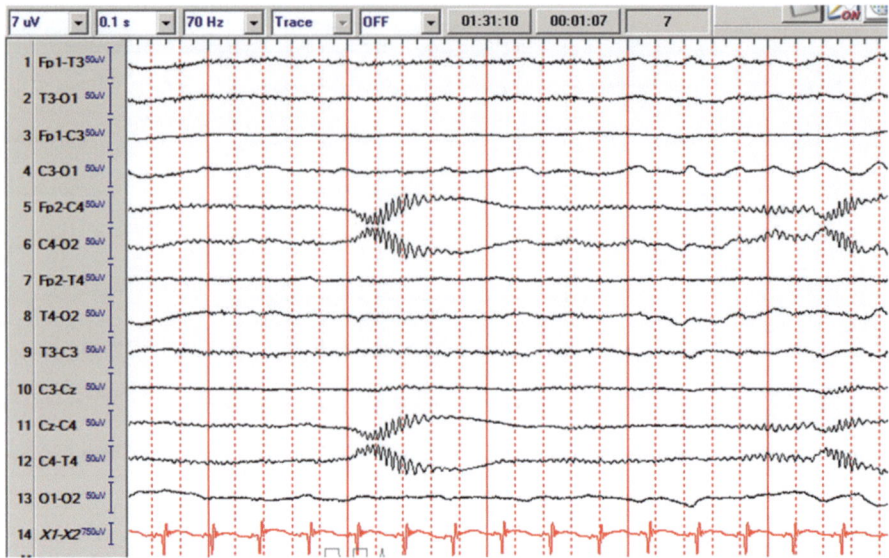

Fig. 3.22 Intermittent low-amplitude delta activity with superimposed fast activity in the right central lead in a neonate with ischemic encephalopathy

Table 3.2 Chart showing abnormal frequencies seen in neonates with cortical dysfunction

Frequency	Delta (0.5–4 Hz)	Theta (4–7 Hz)	Alpha (8–10 Hz)	Beta
Amplitude		40–100 µV	40–100 µV	
Location	Frontal or occipital	Focal or generalized	Focal or generalized	Focal or generalized

Holmes and Lombroso [6] and Mizrahi and Hrachovy [8]
Hz Hertz

   2. This is indicative of diffuse cortical dysfunction with an additional region of focal dysfunction.
   3. This might occur in case of metabolic encephalopathy in a patient with focal hypoxic-ischemic injury, for example.
 E. Notes about co-occurrence of epileptic activity
   1. Seizures are a frequent complication of any cranial pathology.
   2. Seizures can change background activity to cause post-ictal slowing, which is transient.
   3. Presence of other tissue abnormalities between the brain surface and the EEG scalp electrode can blunt signals of epileptiform discharges and epileptic activity.
   4. A patient with a traumatic brain injury may have extracranial, intracranial, and intraparenchymal tissue abnormalities leading to a complicated and often confusing picture of slowing, amplitude abnormalities, encephalopathy, and seizures.

3.5 Part 4: Combined Amplitude, Frequency, and Background Pattern Abnormalities Based on Abnormal Structure

A. Extracranial abnormalities (Fig. 3.23)
    1. Can cause low-amplitude and/or low-frequency activity due to interruption of the scalp signal. In the case of scalp swelling, cephalohematomas, and caput succedaneum, the electrical signals must pass through this abnormal tissue and fluid matter.
    2. The resultant signal seen on the surface EEG may become lower in amplitude and/or frequency, thus causing confusion for an area of possible cortical neuronal dysfunction.
B. Intracranial abnormalities can also cause blunting of the scalp signal, showing a low-amplitude and/or -frequency finding (Figs. 3.23 and 3.24).
    1. Presence of subdural hemorrhage or epidural hemorrhage may cause the EEG neuronal activity to appear asymmetric with apparent focal abnormalities.

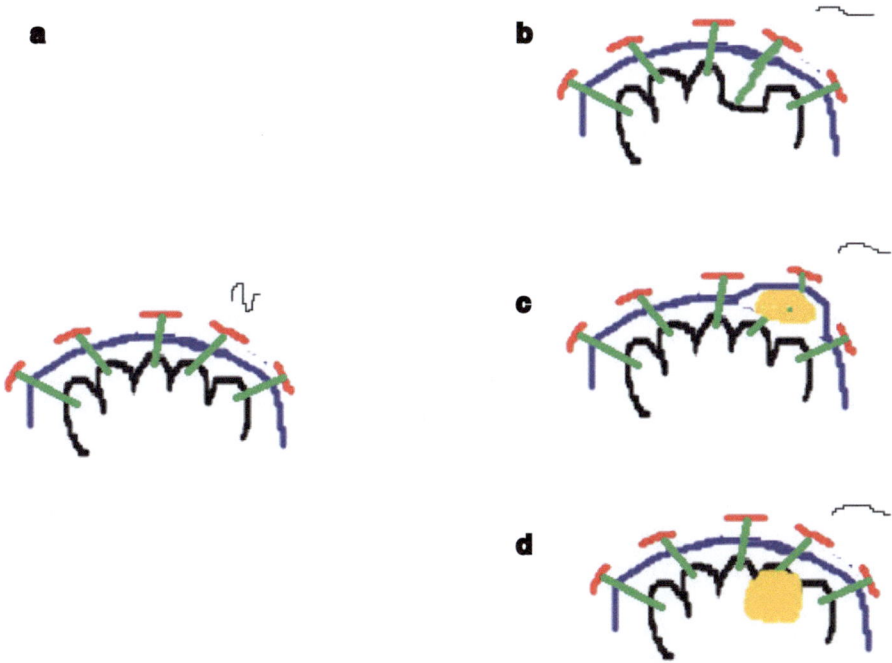

Fig. 3.23 Schematic showing how a focal abnormality can cause blunting of the amplitude as seen on the scalp EEG of a neonate. (**a**) Represents a normal anatomic distribution of cortical signals to the EEG electrodes. (**b**) Represents a focal dysplasia or gliosis causing absence of cortical tissue, thus leading to a CSF-filled space. Signals may traverse this space differently than otherwise. (**c**) Represents an extra-axial abnormality that leads to signal interruption from the cortex to the electrode. (**d**) Represents an intra-axial abnormality leading to disruption of the signal to the electrode. In this case, there is likely abnormal cortical functioning, in addition to the abnormal mass

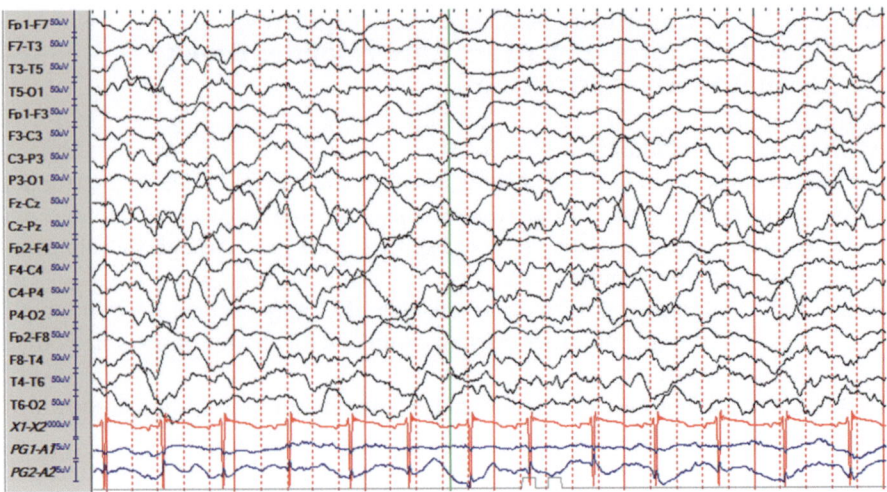

Fig. 3.24 Low-amplitude and low-frequency activity in the left hemisphere in a neonate with a left subdural hematoma

2. Presence of abnormal cerebrospinal fluid (CSF) collection (whether as a cyst or secondary to structural brain dysplasia) can also lead to abnormal focal EEG signals.
3. Intraparenchymal hemorrhage or infarction will also cause abnormal focal signals, correlating with the region of cellular injury.

EEG Tidbit
Complicating the issue, however, these focal extracranial and intracranial structural abnormalities may correlate with underlying neuronal dysfunction and epileptiform potential. Intraparenchymal hemorrhage can lead to neuronal irritability and abnormal CSF collections often correlate with abnormal cortex, which both have a high chance of yielding epileptic potential. Often these regions have the presence of epileptic activity or abnormal sharp waves. Effect of focal space occupying blood or CSF collection may blunt signal of these epileptic events or abnormal sharp waves and may be difficult to detect electrographic seizure activity.

3.6 Part 5: Abnormal Background Patterns: Symmetry and Synchrony

A. Any asymmetric background activity suggests focal dysfunction. Based only on the EEG, it may be difficult to determine which hemisphere is abnormal, but one can deduce that there is at least one abnormal hemisphere (Fig. 3.25). It is not unusual for both hemispheres to demonstrate abnormal findings but in different ways. Asymmetry can be present within the setting of excessive

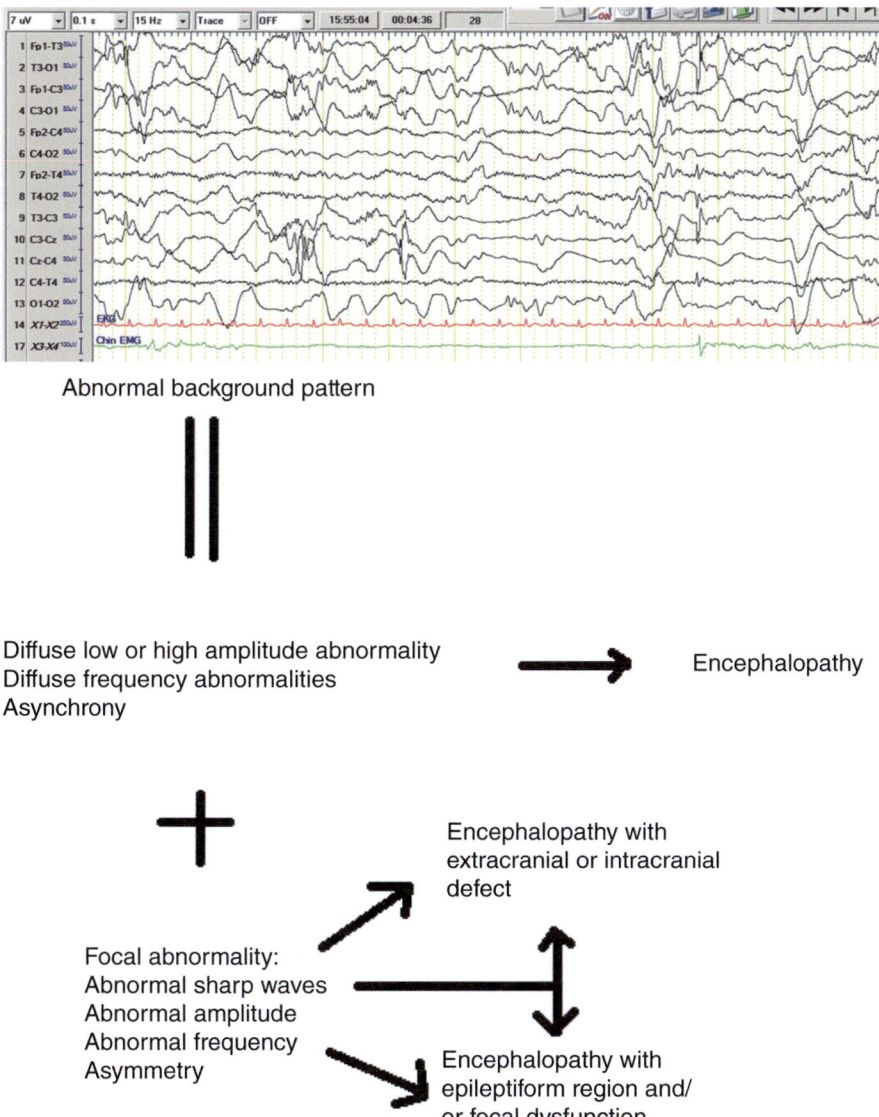

Fig. 3.25 Asymmetrical EEG waveforms in a neonate. The left hemisphere amplitude is higher than the right hemisphere amplitude. In addition, left hemisphere activity is sharply contoured

discontinuity or burst suppression. Voltage or frequency asymmetries may be difficult to discern when the background is overall low voltage due to the nature of the low-voltage activity. Changing sensitivity on the recording to view the waveforms higher on the screen will also show artifact activity, so in some cases, a reader may not be able to accurately or confidently determine amplitude or frequency asymmetries.

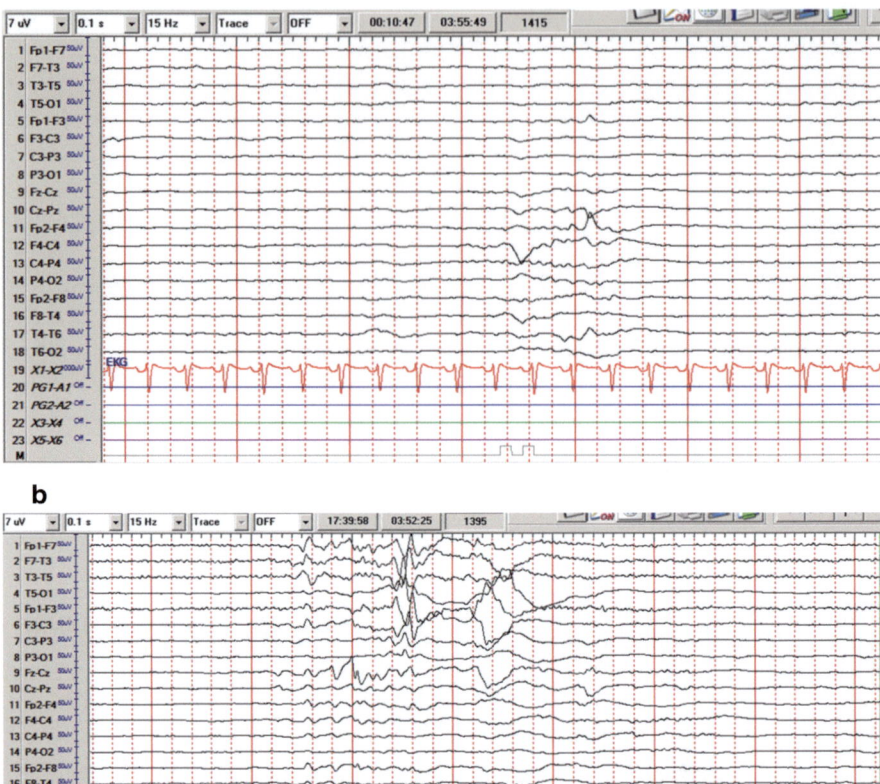

Fig. 3.26 Asymmetrical bursts in neonates with a burst suppression background pattern. (**a**) Higher amplitude activity in the right hemisphere. (**b**) Higher amplitude activity in the left hemisphere, also containing high-amplitude activity in the left frontotemporal region

B. Asynchrony is defined as a greater than 1.5 s interval of burst onset between the left and right hemispheres (Figs. 3.26, 3.27, 3.28, 3.29, and 3.30).
  1. Asynchrony is also a normal developmental finding and is most common during the discontinuous background of neonates around 29–31 WGA. However, even at its peak occurrence, it may only be present about 30% of the time and is most often seen in quiet sleep. Thus, most normal neonatal recordings should be synchronous.
  2. Asynchrony in the setting of normal background patterns suggests a focal hemisphere abnormality. In older children and adults, hemisphere asynchrony can occur with disrupted cortical connections; however, neonates do not typically have such inter-cortical connections developed yet.

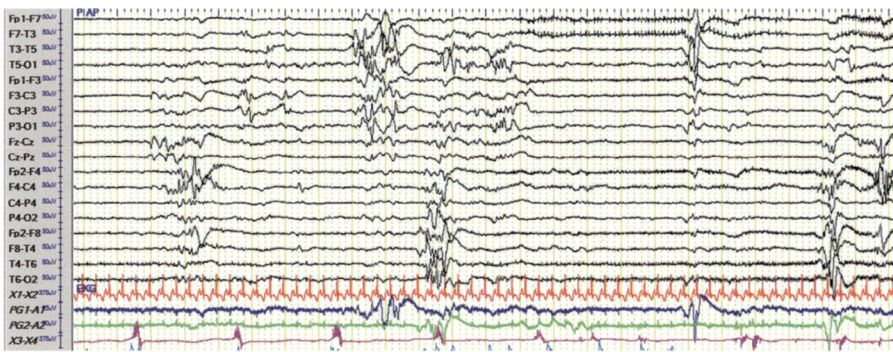

Fig. 3.27 EEG background showing asynchronous bursts in a neonate. Overall, the background activity is symmetric, with an equal amount of activity in each hemisphere. However, the activity does not occur at the same time in a synchronous manner

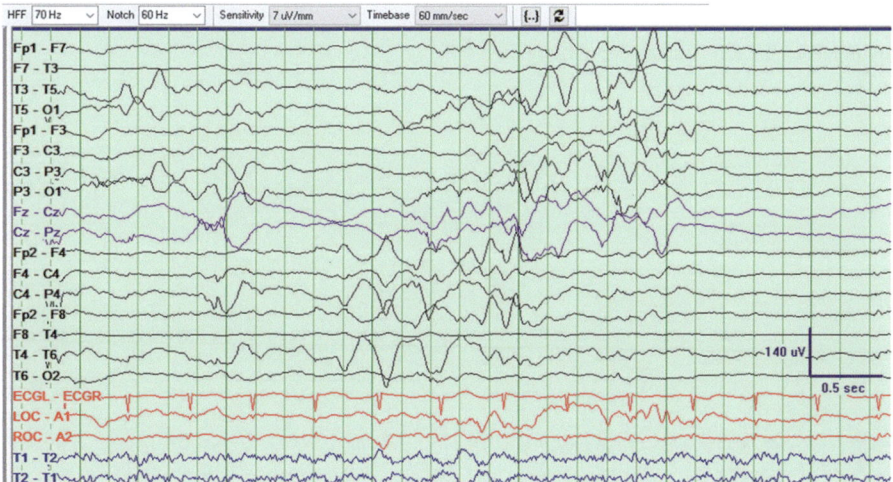

Fig. 3.28 Slight difference between hemisphere activity in a neonate. The burst begins in the right hemisphere and is followed by the left hemisphere activity occurring 1 s later. This difference does not meet definition for asynchrony; however, it is an example of the variety of background patterns. This pattern could be normal for 30 WGA when asynchrony is common in quiet sleep or abnormal for 36 WGA

3. Asynchrony in the setting of encephalopathy (excessive discontinuity or burst suppression) suggests encephalopathy with an additional area of focal dysfunction (either hemisphere).
4. Asynchrony may not be present with all bursts. Some reviewers report it as a percentage, such as the background activity is 50% asymmetric, for example.

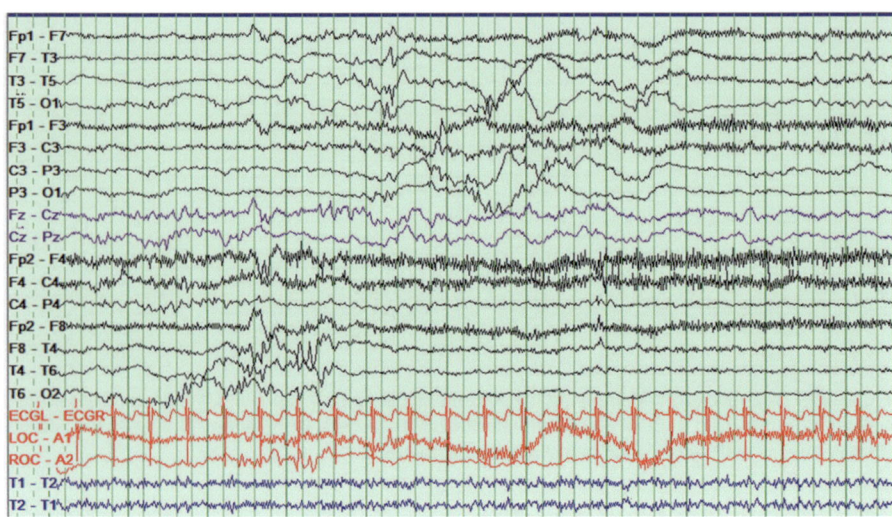

Fig. 3.29 EEG background showing an asynchronous burst in a neonate. Right hemisphere activity precedes the left hemisphere activity by 3 s

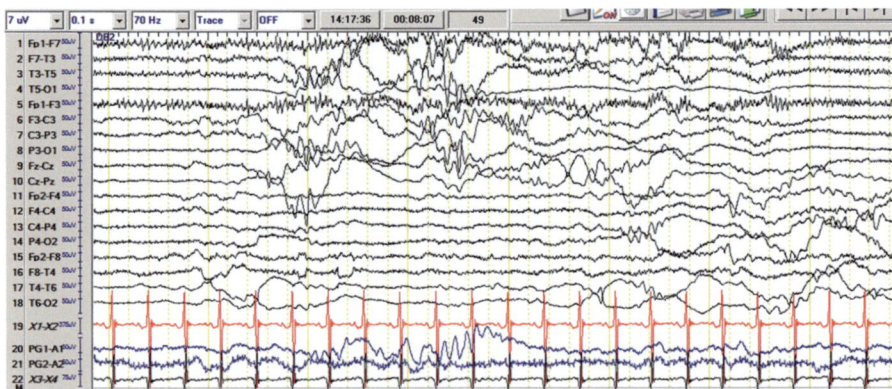

Fig. 3.30 EEG background showing asynchronous bursts in a neonate. The left hemisphere activity precedes the right hemisphere activity by 3 s. This example also shows a case of an overlap in the burst activity

References

1. Almubarak S, Wong P. Long-term clinical outcome of neonatal EEG findings. J Clin Neurophysiol. 2011;28(2):185–9. https://doi.org/10.1097/WNP.0b013e3182121731.
2. Britton J, Frey L, Hopp J, et al. Electroencephalography: an introductory text and atlas of normal and abnormal findings in adults, children and infants. Chicago: American Epilepsy Society; 2016.
3. Chequer R, Tharp B, Dreimane D, et al. Prognostic value of EEG in neonatal meningitis: retrospective study of 29 infants. Pediatr Neurol. 1992;8(6):417–22. https://doi.org/10.1016/0887-8994(92)90001-f.
4. Grigg-Damberger MM, Coker SB, Halsey CL, et al. Neonatal burst suppression: its developmental significance. Pediatr Neurol. 1989;5(2):84–92. https://doi.org/10.1016/0887-8994(89)90032-5.
5. Hahn JS, Monyer H, Tharp BR. Interburst interval measurements in the EEGs of premature infants with normal neurological outcome. Electroencephalogr Clin Neurophysiol. 1989;73:410–8.
6. Holmes GL, Lombroso CT. Prognostic value of background patterns in the neonatal EEG. J Clin Neuophysiol. 1993;10(3):323–52. https://doi.org/10.1097/00004691-199307000-00008.
7. Lobroso CT. Neonatal electroencephalography. In: Niedermeyer E, Lopez da Silva F, editors. Electroencephalography: basic principles, clinical applications and related fields. Baltimore: Urban and Schwarzenberg; 1982. p. 599–637.
8. Mizrahi E, Hrachovy R. Atlas of neonatal electroencephalography. 4th ed. New York: Demos Medical; 2016.
9. Neurophysiology Society, Critical Care Monitoring Committee. J Clin Neurophysiol. 2013;2:161–73. https://doi.org/10.1097/WNP.0b013e3182872b24.
10. Prechtl H. The neurological examination of the full-term newborn infant. Lavenham: J.B. Lippincott Co; 1977.
11. Selton D, Andre M, Hascoet JM. Normal EEG in very premature infants: reference criteria. Clin Neurophysiol. 2000;111(12):2116–24. https://doi.org/10.1016/s1388-2457(00)00440-5.
12. Tsuchida T, Wusthoff C, Shellhaas R, et al. ACNS standardized EEG terminology and categorization for the description of continuous EEG monitoring in neonates. Report of the American Clinical Neurophysiology Society. 2013.
13. Vecchierini MF, d'Allest AM, Verpillat P. EEG patterns in 10 extreme premature neonates with normal neurological outcome: qualitative and quantitative data. Brain Dev. 2002;25:330–7.

Abnormal Background Patterns in Neonatal EEG Recordings: Sharp Waves

Mary Payne

4.1 Introduction

Sharp waves can be a normal or abnormal finding depending on the age and state of the neonatal patient. Sharp waves are also suspected to be abnormal based on their location, frequency, duration, and asymmetry. Inter-reader agreement does not always occur. Abnormal sharp waves may be an indication of an underlying focal region of irritability or epileptogenicity. Following anti-epileptic medication administration, localized sharp waves may be present in that region of seizure origin. This chapter will present guidelines for determining normal and abnormal sharp waves. This chapter is based on Hrachovy et al. [3], Lobroso [4], Mizrahi and Hrachovy [5], Sansavere and Harrar [6].

4.2 EEG Tidbit

In traditional EEG language and in older patients, sharp waves are typically defined as having a duration of 70–200 ms and spikes are defined as having a duration of 20–70 ms. Sharp waves and spike waves both indicate a region of epileptiform potential. However, in neonates, sharp waves can be a normal finding during the process of EEG maturation. Sharp waves can be as long as 2 s, and determining if they are normal or abnormal may be difficult. Spike waves, which are shorter in duration than sharp waves, are more likely to be abnormal in the neonate. Another important uniqueness in neonatal recordings is that abnormal sharp waves and spike waves are not specific to an area of epileptic potential. An area of dysfunction (cellular injury, abnormal cortical signaling) can also create sharp waves and spike waves [5].

M. Payne (✉)
Department of Pediatrics, Division of Pediatric Neurology, Joan C. Edwards School of Medicine, Hoops Family Children's Hospital, Marshall University, Huntington, WV, USA
e-mail: paynem@marshall.edu

© The Author(s), under exclusive license to Springer Nature Switzerland AG 2025
M. Payne, D. Gloss II (eds.), *Neonatal EEG*,
https://doi.org/10.1007/978-3-031-92556-6_4

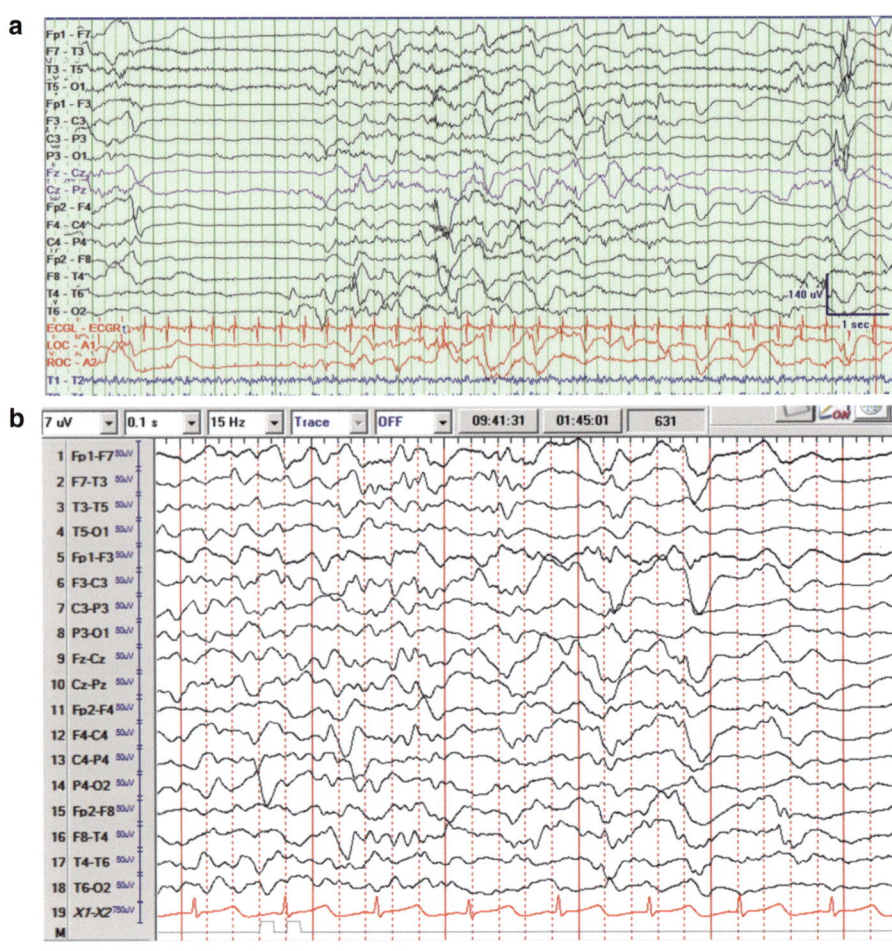

Fig. 4.1 (a) Asymmetric anterior dysrhythmia in a neonate showing dominant waveforms in the left frontal region. This may indicate epileptiform activity or an area of dysfunction in the left frontal region. (b) Normal anterior dysrhythmia showing symmetric frontal activity

A. Frontal region sharp waves (Figs. 4.1, 4.2, 4.3, 4.4, 4.5, 4.6, 4.7, 4.8, and 4.9)
  1. Normal frontal sharp waves are called encoches frontales (EF) and occur in runs that last less than 1.5 s with a waveform that is 0.5 s in duration.
  2. Anterior dysrhythmia (AD) is a similar pattern and qualifies as runs of frontal sharp waves with a frequency of 5–9 Hz that last a few seconds with an amplitude of 50–150 µV. They are seen best between 38–42 WGA during transitional or quiet sleep.
  3. Abnormal frontal sharp waves do not meet the above criteria.
     Below is a chart showing normal features of encoches frontales, anterior dysrhythmia, and traits that suggest abnormal frontal sharp transients. Asymmetric or abnormal feature sharp transients would indicate a region of dysfunction or epileptogenicity of that side where they are located. (Table 4.1)

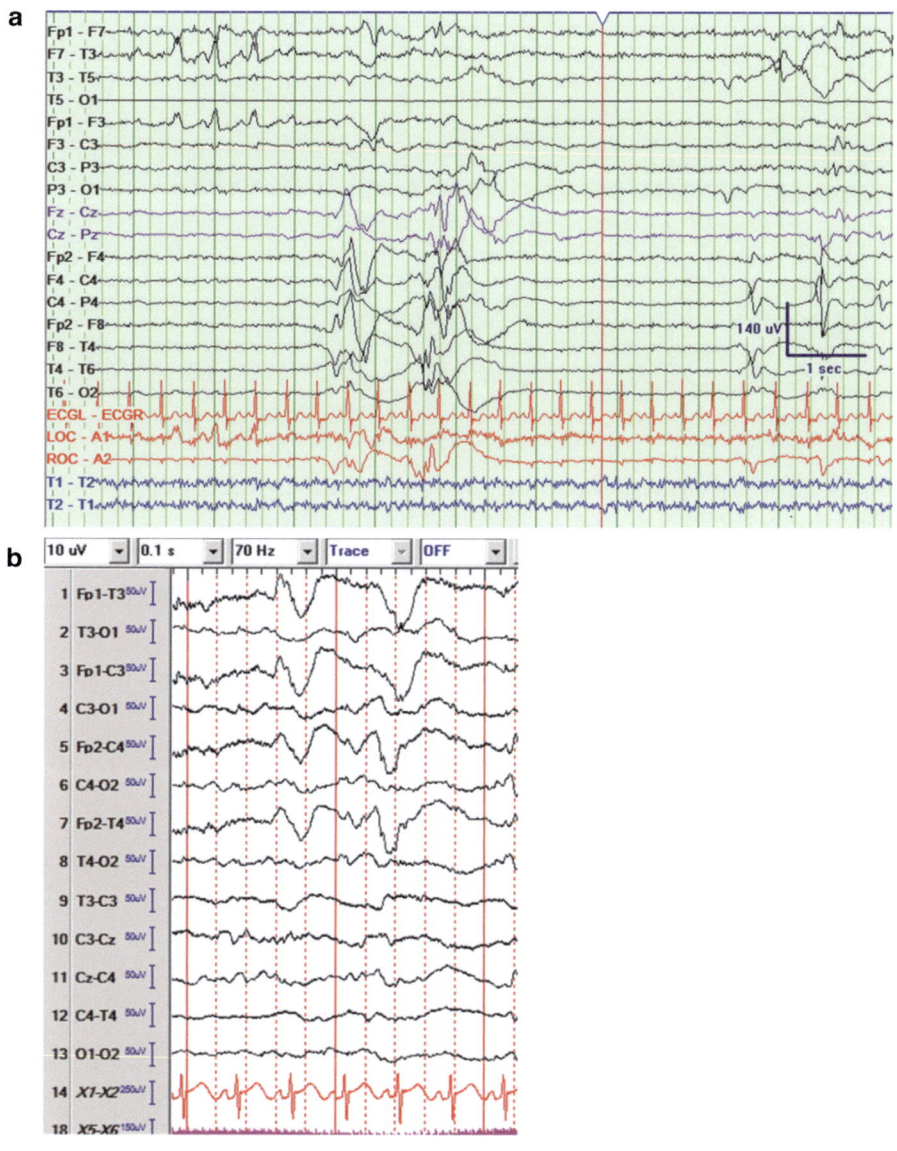

Fig. 4.2 (a) Abnormal left frontal and right frontocentral sharp waves in a neonate. (b) Normal frontal sharp waves seen between 34 and 40 WGA, called encoche frontales

B. Central region sharp waves
   1. Negative central sharp waves (Table 4.2 and Figs. 4.10, 4.11, 4.12, and 4.13)
   2. Positive central sharp waves (positive polarity) have been reported in infants with intraventricular hemorrhage and periventricular leukomalacia [1, 2]. (Figs. 4.14 and 4.15).
   3. Central rhythmic sharp activity (Figs. 4.16, 4.17, and 4.18)

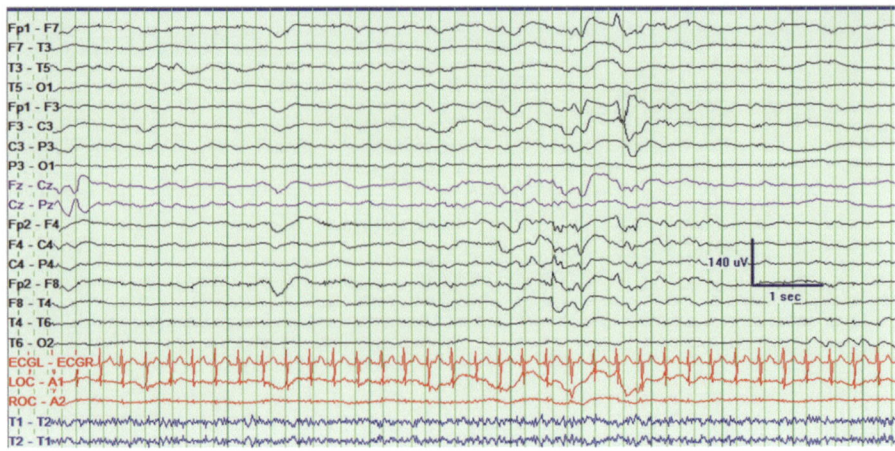

Fig. 4.3 Abnormal left frontotemporal sharp waves in a neonate. Right hemisphere low-amplitude spikes are also occurring

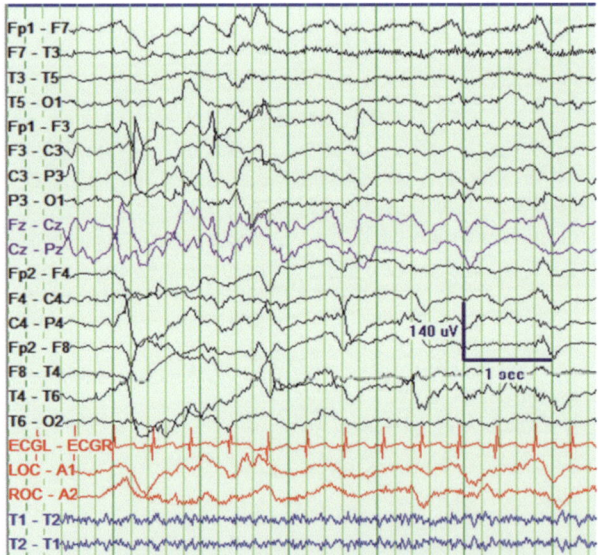

Fig. 4.4 Abnormal frontal transients in the left frontal region in a neonate

Symmetric central rhythmic activity may be seen in normal infants. The central region is the location of sleep architecture as the baby matures, usually around 48 WGA. Early sleep architecture may be asynchronous but should be symmetric. Similar to frontal activity guidelines, if this central activity is asymmetric, it likely represents an abnormal hemisphere function.

4 Abnormal Background Patterns in Neonatal EEG Recordings: Sharp Waves

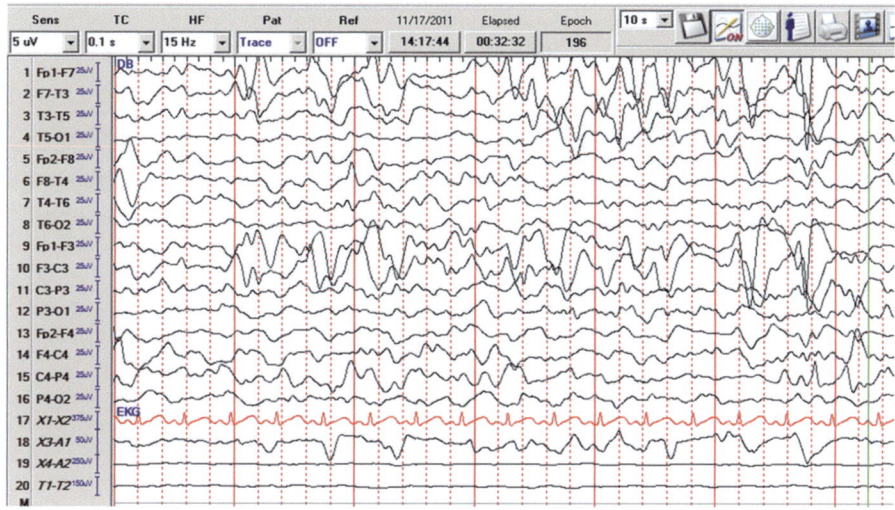

Fig. 4.5 Runs of left frontal sharp waves in a neonate

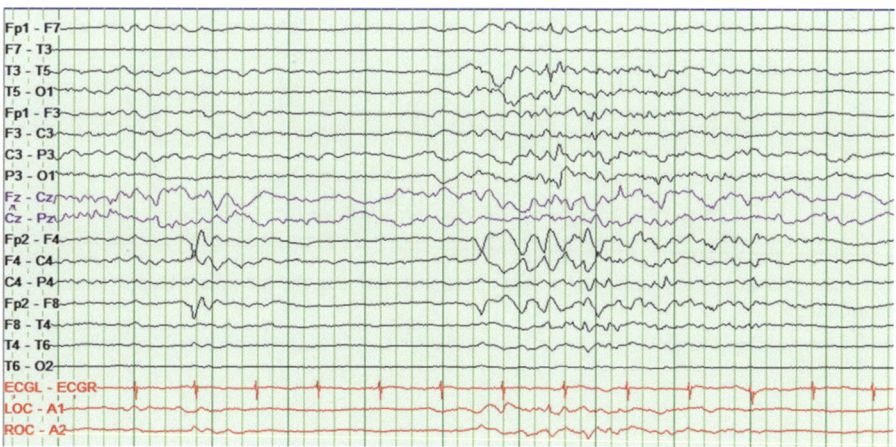

Fig. 4.6 Right frontal sharp waves in a neonate with a discontinuous background pattern

C. Temporal region sharp waves: any abnormal characteristic suggests abnormality (Table 4.3 and Figs. 4.19 and 4.20)
D. Parietal region sharp waves (Fig. 4.21)
   Parietal sharp wave characteristics are not as well described as many neonatal recordings do not contain parietal electrodes. However, abnormal sharp waves are suspected with high-amplitude waveforms, asymmetry of waveforms or occurring beyond 46 WGA.
E. Occipital region sharp waves (Figs. 4.22 and 4.23)

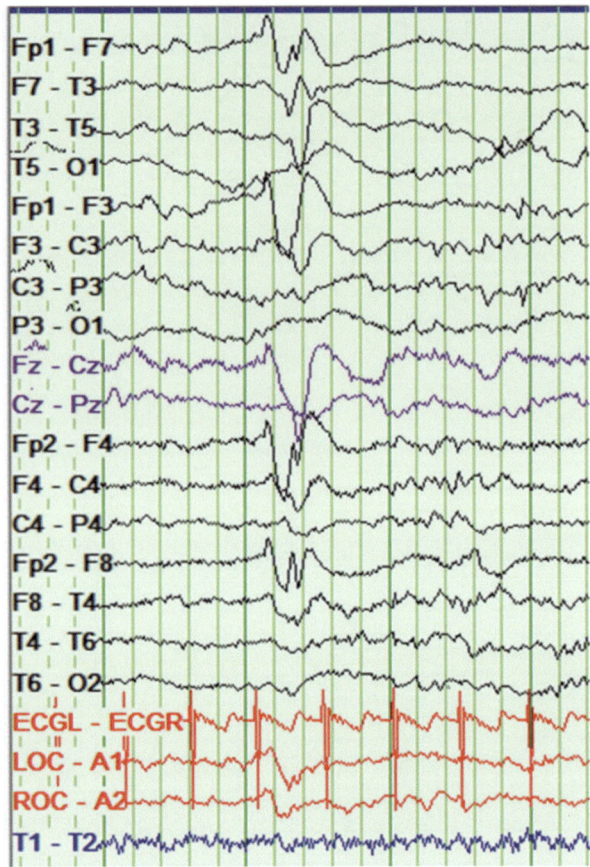

Fig. 4.7 Bilateral frontal sharp waves that are abnormal due to the presence of a polyphasic morphology

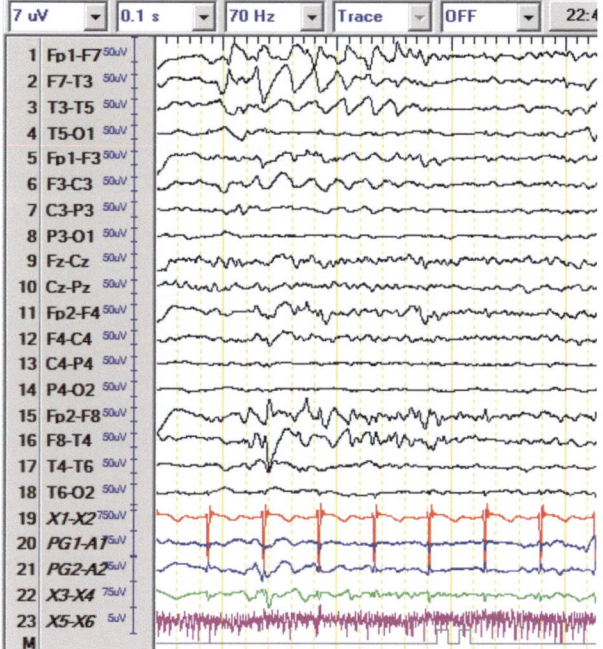

Fig. 4.8 Run of abnormal left frontal sharp waves with spread to the left central and left temporal regions. Notice the right frontal sharply contoured activity. It is unclear in this segment the significance of this activity. However, Fig. 4.9 is of the same patient and provides further information

Abnormal occipital sharp waves are suspected with high amplitude, asymmetric, or occurring beyond 46 WGA.

F. Periodic lateralized sharp wave discharges (PLDs) Can occur in any location but the discharges are consistently in that one location. Seen with focal lesion (infarction, infection such as HSV temporal in the temporal regions) and lateralized and localized to the area of insult. Similar to the finding of frequent epileptiform discharges. In older children and adults, these discharges are often seen in strokes with epileptiform potential. PLDs are not as common in neonates, but when present, also suggest a region of epileptiform potential (Figs. 4.24, 4.25 and 4.26).

G. Putting it all together.

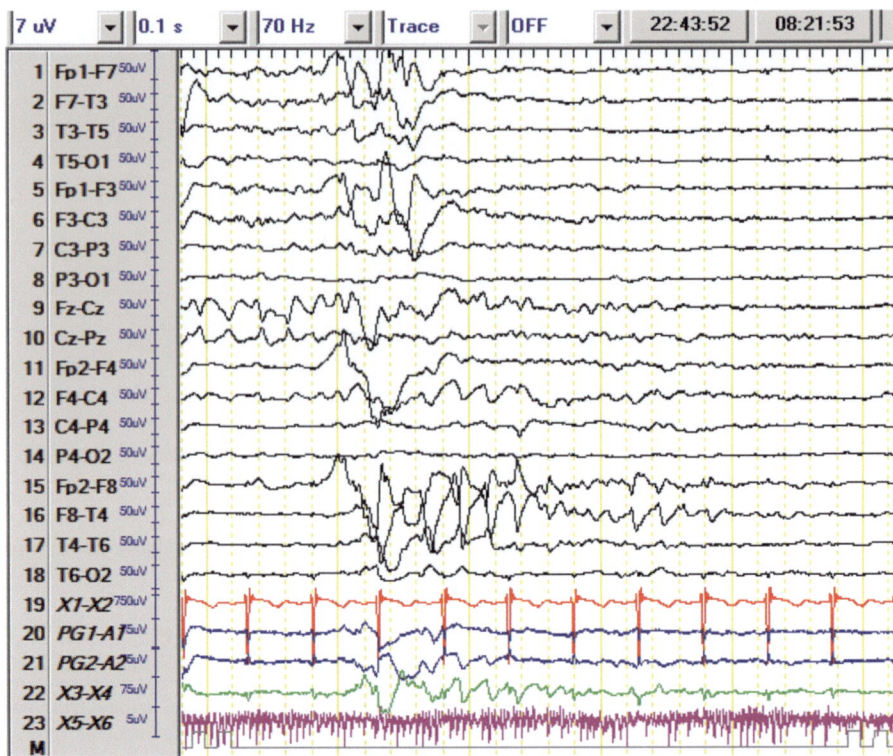

Fig. 4.9 Abnormal frontal waves in a neonate. This is the same patient as in Fig. 4.8. Left frontal sharp waves are present, again. Right frontal waveforms also demonstrate a morphology suggestive of epileptiform potential with this brief run of right frontal spikes. These two figures demonstrate the importance of serial comparisons and monitoring of suspicious waveforms

Table 4.1 Neonatal frontal sharp waves: any abnormal characteristic suggests abnormality

	Normal—EF	Normal—AD	Abnormal
Symmetry	Symmetric	Symmetric	Asymmetric
Frequency of waveform	2–4 Hz	1.5–2 Hz	4 Hz
Duration of waveform	<2 s	2–5 s	5 s
Amplitude	<200 µV	50–150 µV	200 µV
State	Transitional/quiet sleep	Transitional/quiet sleep	Any
Age	<42/44 WGA	38–44 WGA	42/44 WGA

Mizrahi and Hrachovy [5] and Lobroso [4]
AD anterior dysrhythmia, *EF* encoches frontales, *Hz* Hertz, *WGA* weeks gestational age

Table 4.2 Central sharp waves: any abnormal characteristic suggests abnormality

	Normal	Abnormal
Amplitude	< 75 µV	50–250 µV
Initial polarity	Negative	Positive
Symmetry	Unilateral or bilateral	Unilateral or asymmetric
Morphology	Mono- or diphasic	After going surface wave is negative and low voltage
Age	35–44 WGA	< 36 WGA

Mizrahi and Hrachovy [5]
Hz Hertz, *WGA* weeks gestational age

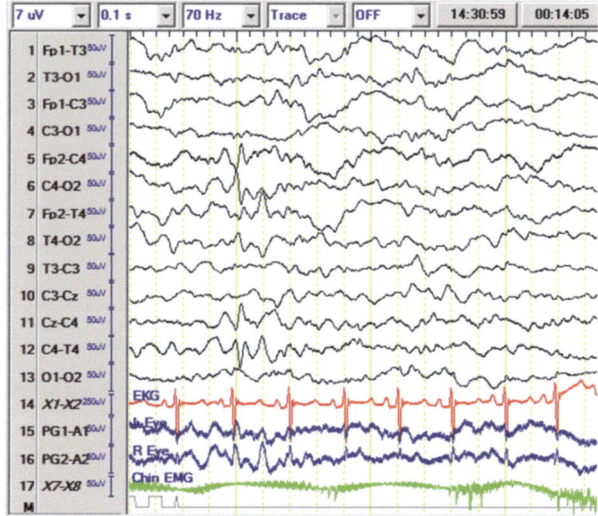

Fig. 4.10 Right central sharp waves in a neonate with a middle cerebral artery infarction. These waves are short in duration, higher amplitude compared to the background activity, and asymmetric

Combination of abnormal background patterns and abnormal sharp waves usually seen with encephalopathy with focal regions of dysfunction and/or epileptogenicity (Figs. 4.27 and 4.28).

The following examples demonstrate a few more examples of abnormal focal findings with encephalopathy.

A neonate with encephalopathy from hypoxia and an additional focal region of ischemia causing seizures shows electrographic low-amplitude background activity and focal right occipital sharp waves (Fig. 4.29).

A neonate of 28 WGA with meningitis and later found to have an infarction in the right occipital lobe. EEG shows extreme discontinuity and high-amplitude

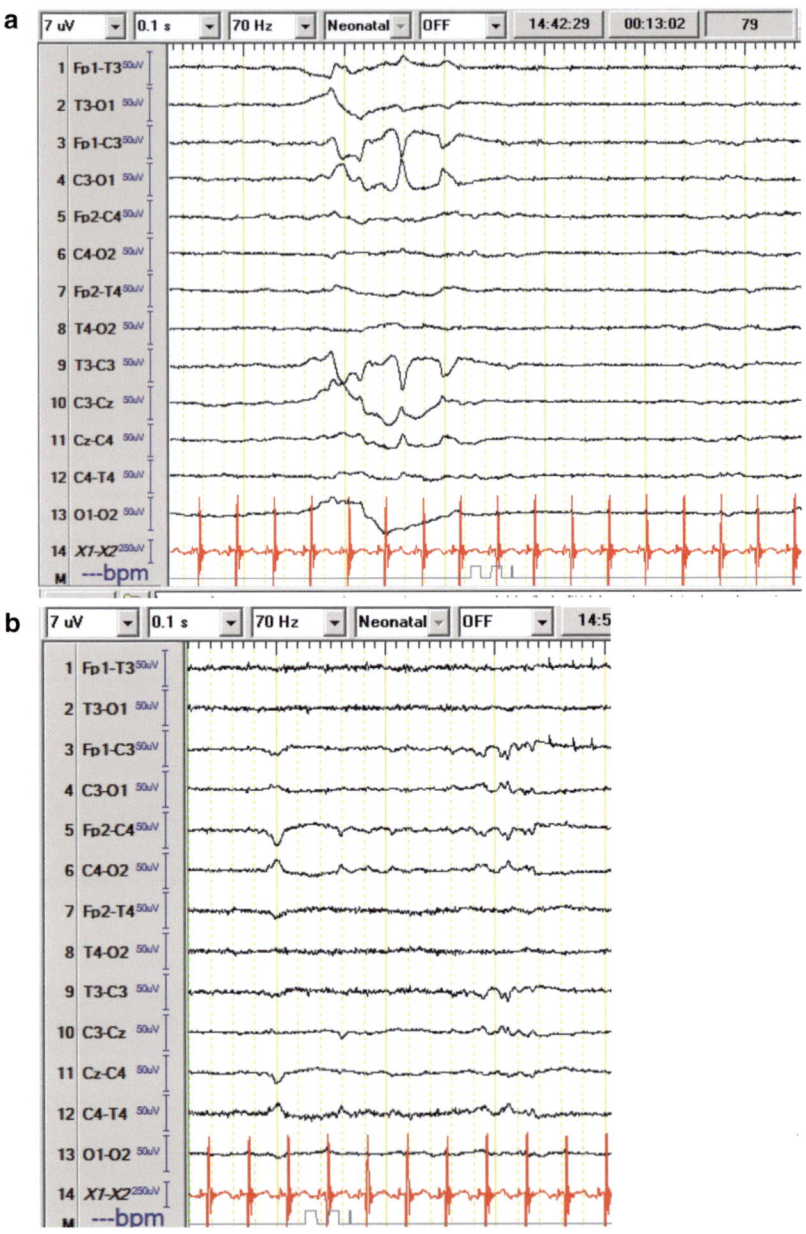

Fig. 4.11 (a) Bilateral abnormal central sharp waves in a neonate in a 35 WGA infant with hypoxic-ischemic encephalopathy. (b) Normal Rolandic dips in a neonate between 28 and 29 WGA. Compared to the picture (a), these Rolandic dips are lower amplitude. Also, the spikes in picture (a) show a field, an area where the sharp activity spreads. The maximal negativity is in the C3 electrode, but involvement of the Cz electrode also occurs. This suggests abnormality. The overall background environment changes with the presence of the spike; sharper activity is noted in the leads and disruption of T3 and O1 electrodes is noted

4 Abnormal Background Patterns in Neonatal EEG Recordings: Sharp Waves

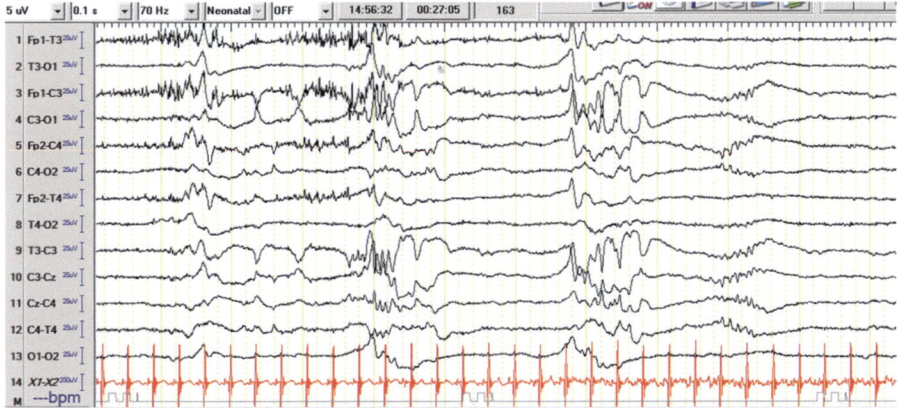

Fig. 4.12 Bilateral central spikes, occurring in runs of 1.5–4 s in a 35 WGA neonate with hypoxic-ischemic encephalopathy. This is the same patient as shown in Fig. 4.11. However, this segment shows repetitive sharp waves, considered a run. Notice the delta waves with superimposed alpha waveforms on the right side of the image. This pattern is normal in a neonate younger than 30 WGA but for this neonate would be considered to be abnormal

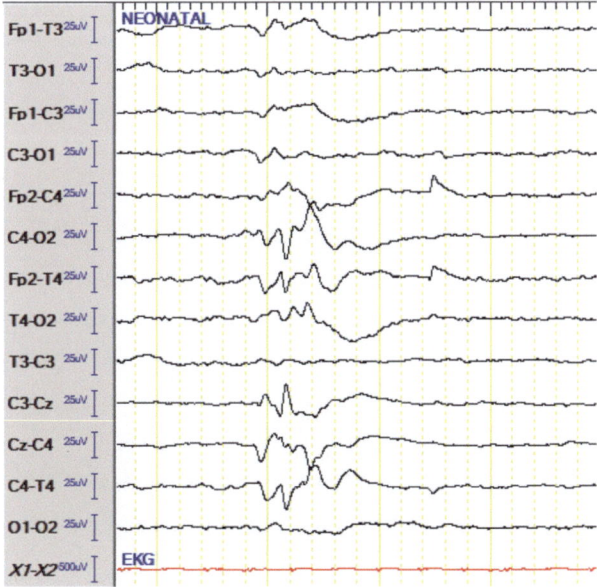

Fig. 4.13 Abnormal right centrotemporal sharp waves in a 27 WGA neonate with right centrotemporal seizures

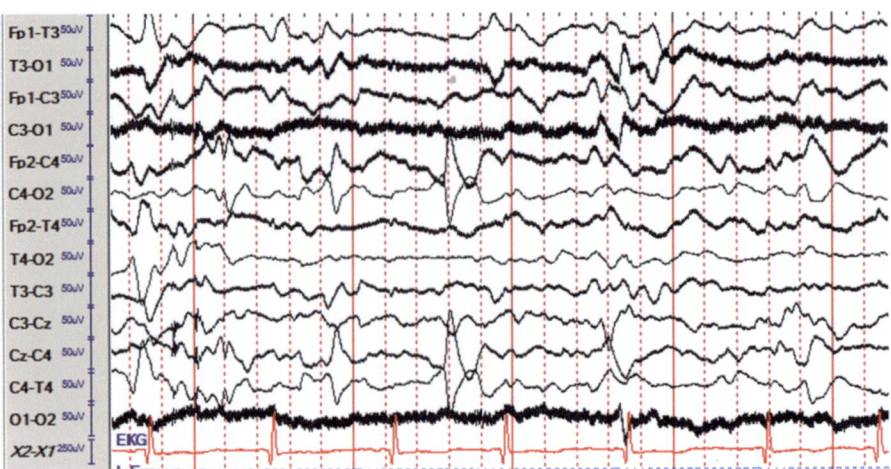

Fig. 4.14 Neonate with right side grade II intraventricular hemorrhage at 30 WGA showing right central positive sharp waves on the EEG recording

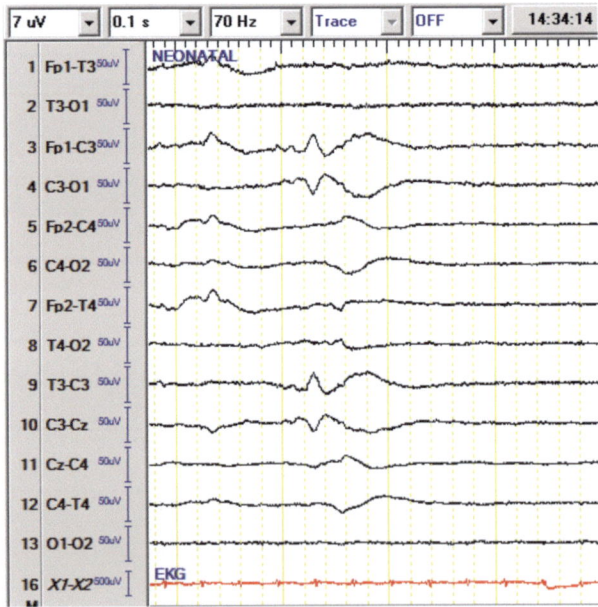

Fig. 4.15 Neonate with left-side intraventricular hemorrhage and EEG recording showing left central positive sharp waves

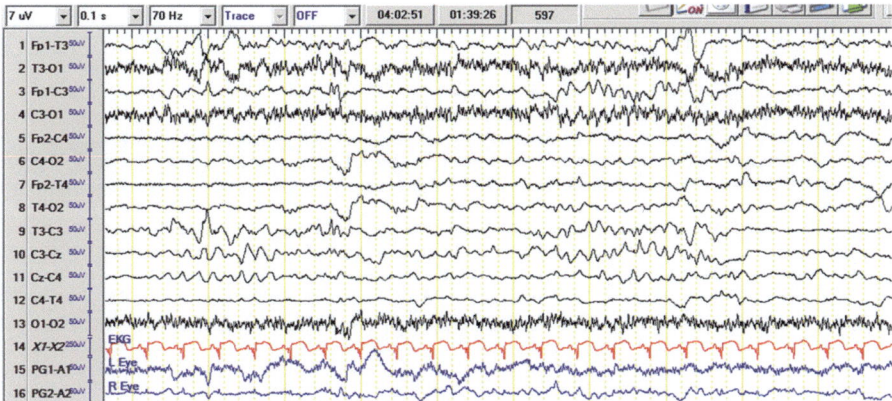

Fig. 4.16 Normal central rhythmic activity in a neonatal EEG. Rhythmic activity is monomorphic, meaning the waveform does not show a sharper component in one area. In addition, this central rhythmic activity occurs in the left central region with extension to the vertex (Cz electrode) region and right central region. As the neonate matures, central activity becomes the location of sleep activity and normal central activity is seen in both central regions, sometimes maximal in the vertex region (Cz electrode), which represents the region along the falx and detects electrical activity in central regions along the hemispheres

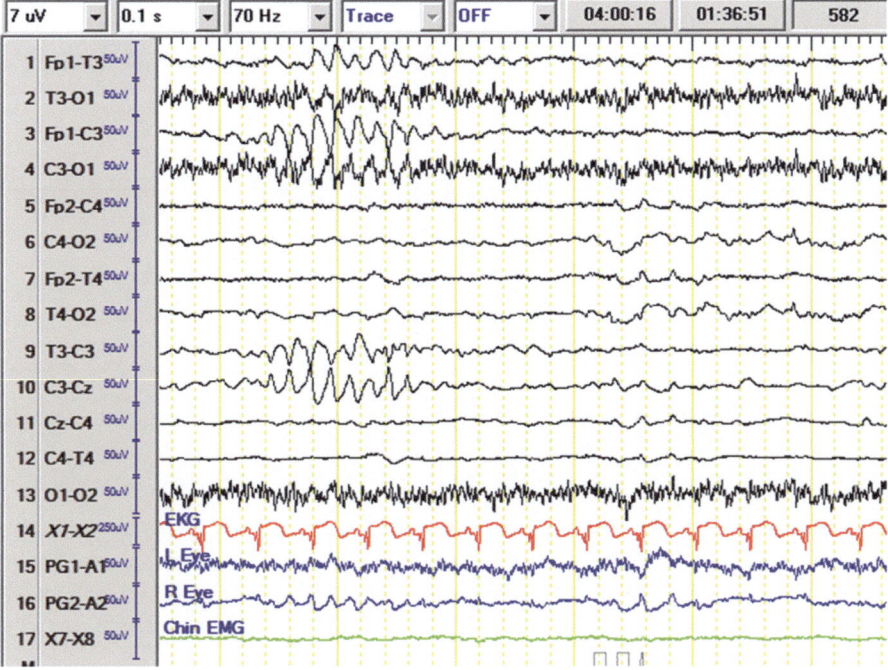

Fig. 4.17 Abnormal central rhythmic activity in a neonate. These central rhythms are focal and persistently localized to the one area of the C3 electrode. Extension to the left temporal region occurs, which also suggests abnormal activity

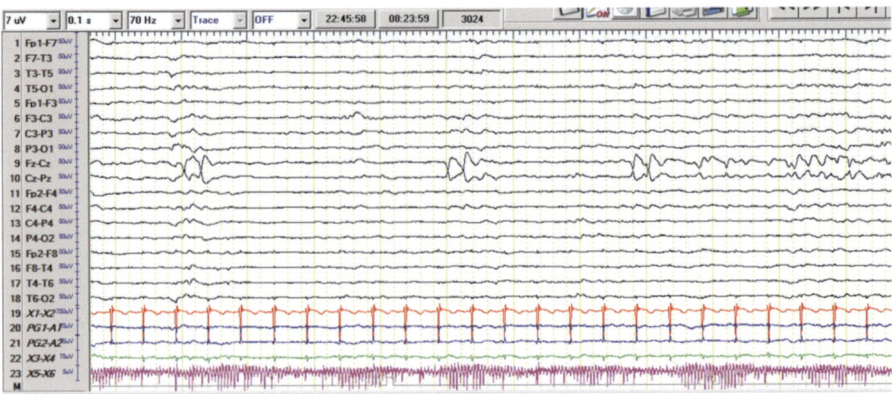

Fig. 4.18 Abnormal central sharp waves in a neonate. Central sharp waves, occurring as a brief couplet or as a longer pattern of semi-rhythmic 4–6 Hz frequency

Table 4.3 Temporal sharp waves

	Normal	Abnormal
State	Sleep	Awake
Amplitude	<75 µV	150 µV
Symmetry	Bilateral, +/− synchronous	Asymmetric
Initial polarity	Negative	Positive
Morphology	Mono or diphasic	Polyphasic or followed by slow waves
Gestational age	Less than 46 WGA	Beyond 46 WGA

Mizrahi and Hrachovy [5]
WGA weeks gestational age

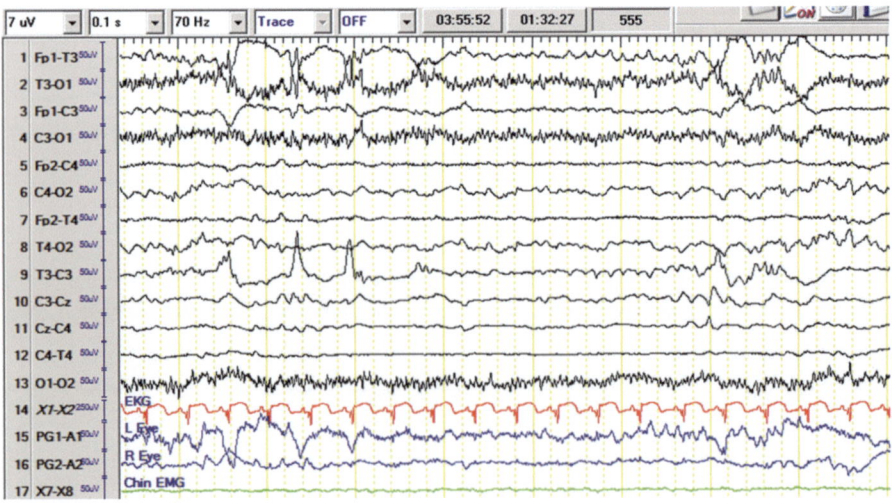

Fig. 4.19 Abnormal left temporal sharp waves in a neonate with left temporal seizures. Notice the "end of chain" phenomenon of the T3-C3 electrode chain. Sharp waves are in the left temporal region, and the waveform is reflected in the positive direction since there is not a partner electrode in that montage

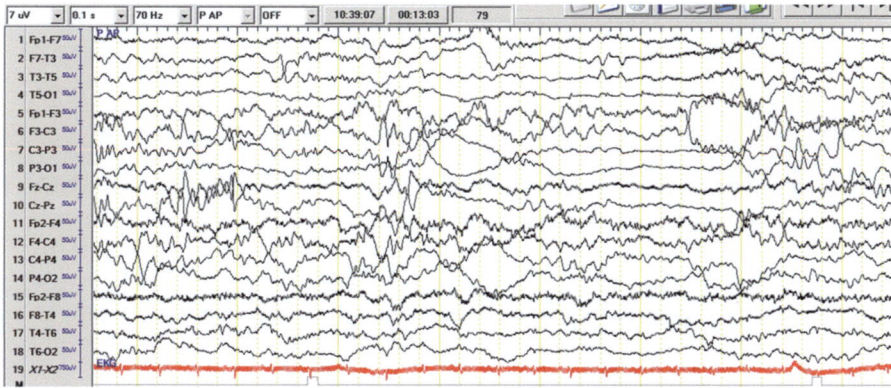

Fig. 4.20 Abnormal left temporal sharp waves in a neonate. These are low amplitude and persistent

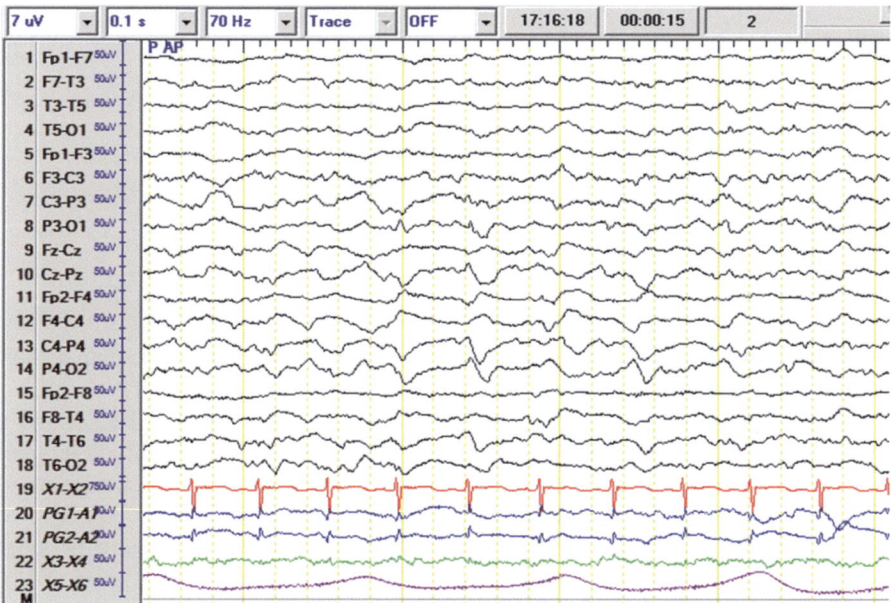

Fig. 4.21 Asymmetric parietal sharp waves in a neonate with encephalitis. Neonatal EEGs do not always contain parietal electrodes as the parietal region is not as common to be associated with seizures. This patient likely has bilateral areas of dysfunction, thus causing bilateral parietal sharp waves. Presence of asymmetry of higher amplitude and better defined parietal sharp waves on the right region indicates a slightly more dysfunction right parietal region compared to the left parietal region

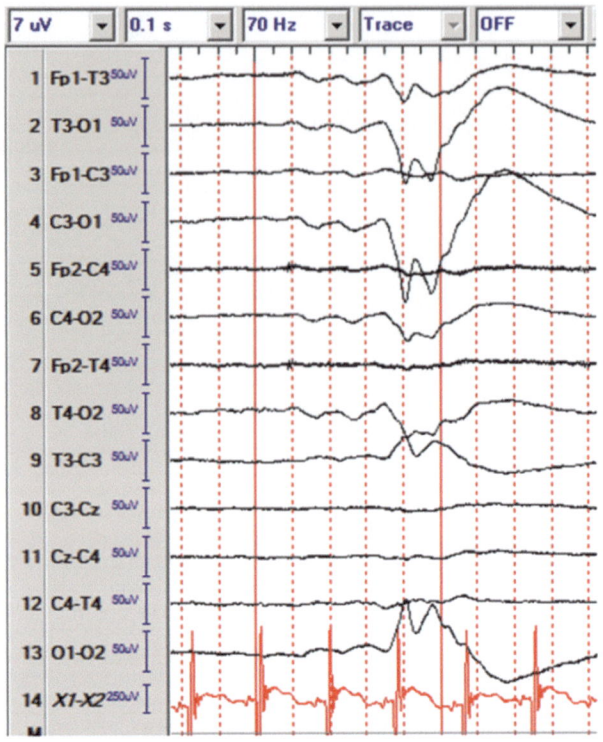

Fig. 4.22 Abnormal left occipital sharp waves, showing high amplitude and diphasic morphology in a neonate

occipital sharp waves. Right occipital sharp waves are higher amplitude than the left occipital sharp waves, indicating right occipital dysfunction (Fig. 4.30).

A full-term neonate with radiographic findings of lissencephaly. EEG shows a discontinuous and asynchronous background activity with high-amplitude left and right temporal sharp waves. The abnormal cortex and cortical connections caused asynchrony and bilateral regions that were epileptiform (Fig. 4.31).

Full-term neonate with bilateral closed-lip schizencephaly showing bilateral regions of epileptiform activity and bilateral regions of attenuation (Fig. 4.32). Seizures were not detected but the EEG shows the potential in both hemispheres.

Neonate at 30 WGA with respiratory distress and seizure-like activity. Background activity is symmetric but asynchronous, which could be normal for age. However, left and right sharp waves were extremely high amplitude and persistent, suggestive of regions of focal dysfunction or epileptic potential (Fig. 4.33).

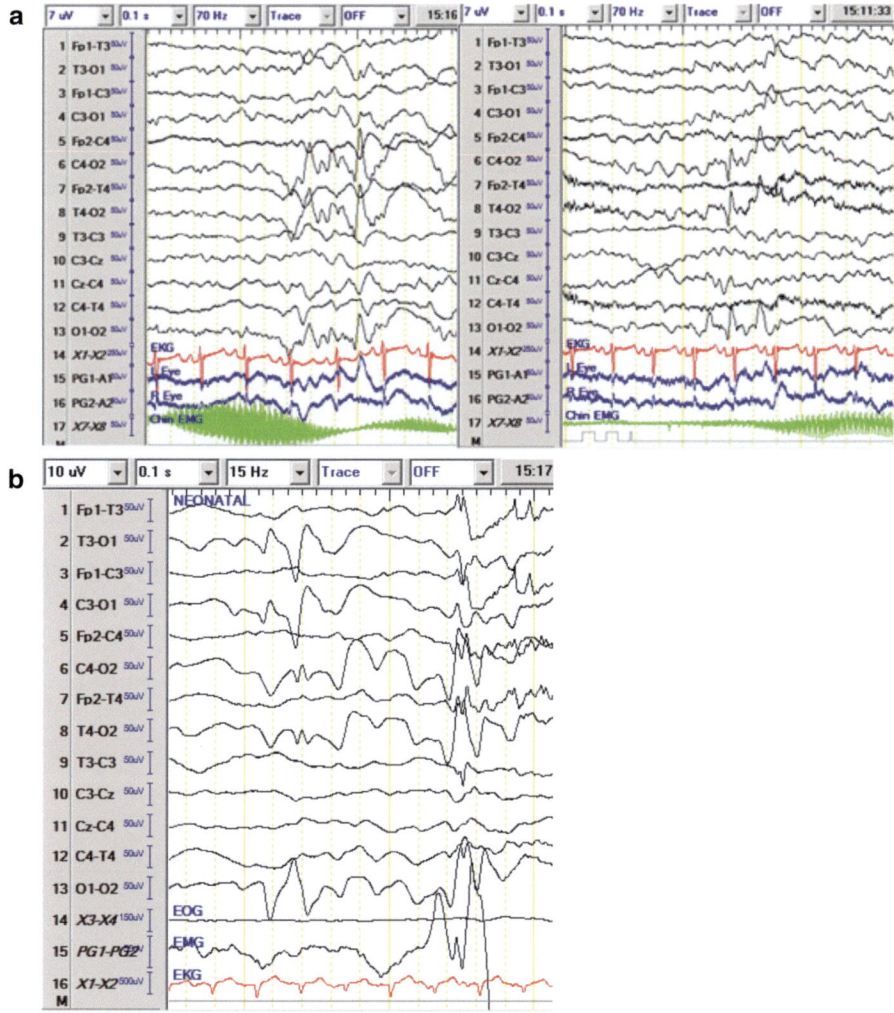

Fig. 4.23 (a) Abnormal right occipital sharp waves in a neonatal patient with a right hemisphere infarction. (b) Normal occipital sharp transients

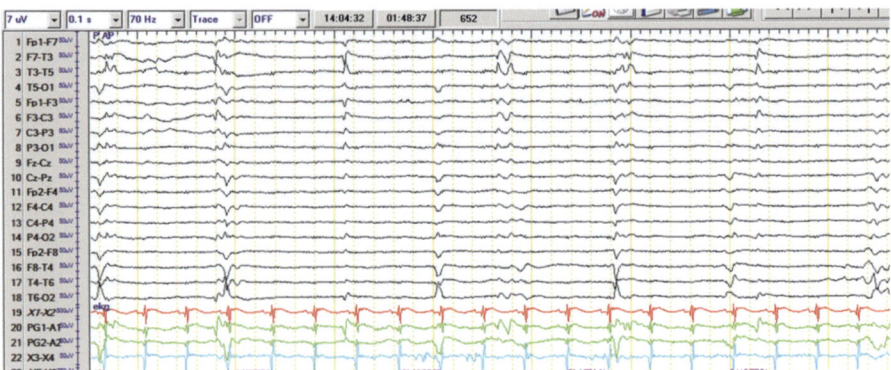

Fig. 4.24 Periodic lateralized epileptiform discharges in the left and right temporal regions in a neonate with hypoxic-ischemic encephalopathy. These discharges are frequent spikes or sharp waves that are *periodic* in that they occur in a repeated pattern but are not organized in a way to be considered sustained rhythmic. *Lateralized* implies that they occur in one region. For this particular patient, PLDs are present in bilateral hemispheres, indicating independent bilateral regions of dysfunction and epileptogenicity. There is spread to the contralateral region but the left and right temporal PLDs do not occur in synchrony; therefore, the PLDs represent two distinct regions of abnormality

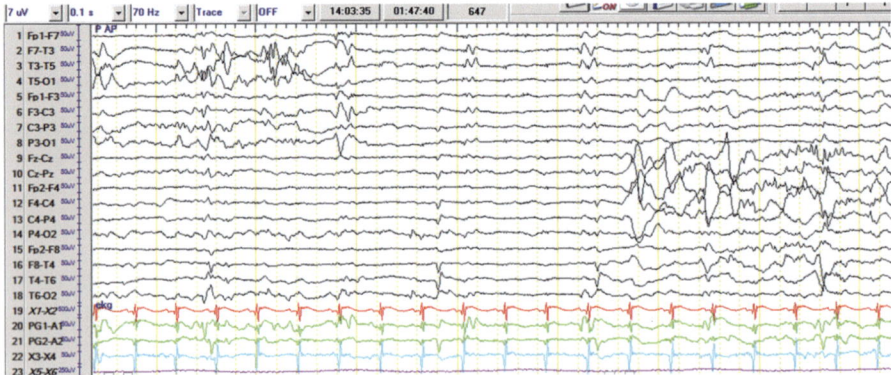

Fig. 4.25 Another example of left and right temporal PLDs in a neonate. In this segment, a discontinuous background is also present

4 Abnormal Background Patterns in Neonatal EEG Recordings: Sharp Waves

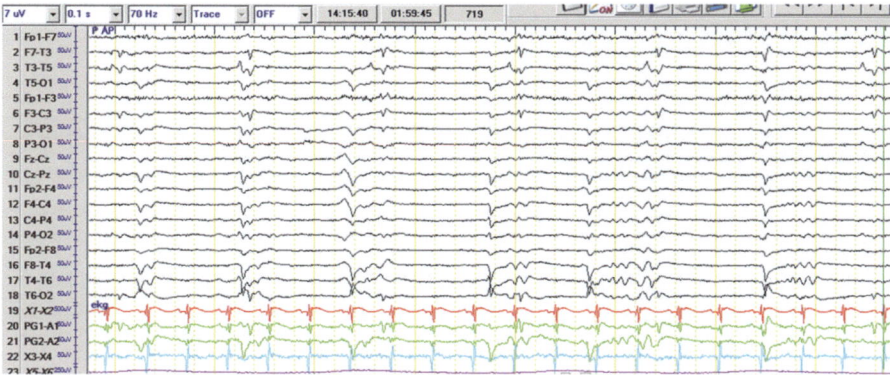

Fig. 4.26 Progression of PLDs to brief rhythmic discharges (BRDs) in the right temporal region in a patient with hypoxic-ischemic encephalopathy

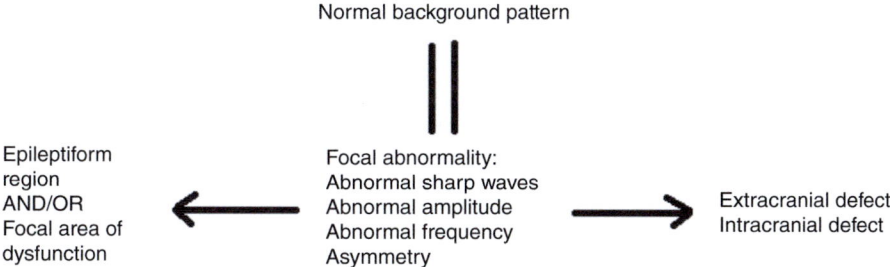

Fig. 4.27 Schematic outlining the variety of abnormal findings in a neonate with abnormal EEG findings in the setting of an otherwise normal background pattern

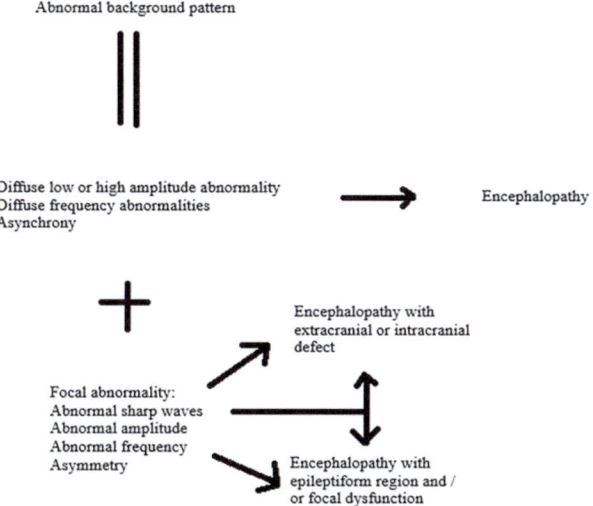

Fig. 4.28 Schematic outlining the variety of abnormal findings in a neonate with abnormal EEG background activity

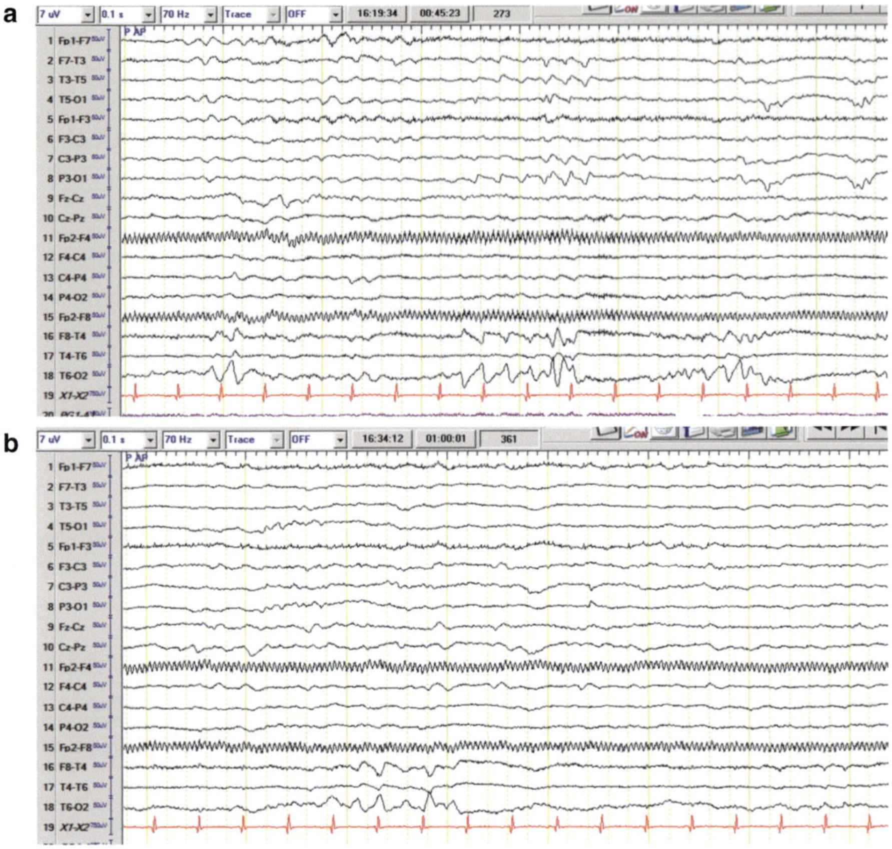

Fig. 4.29 (**a**, **b**) 38 WGA neonate with an encephalopathic background activity and focal sharp waves. Background activity shows waveforms less than 20 µV and right occipital sharp waves with voltages of 40 µV

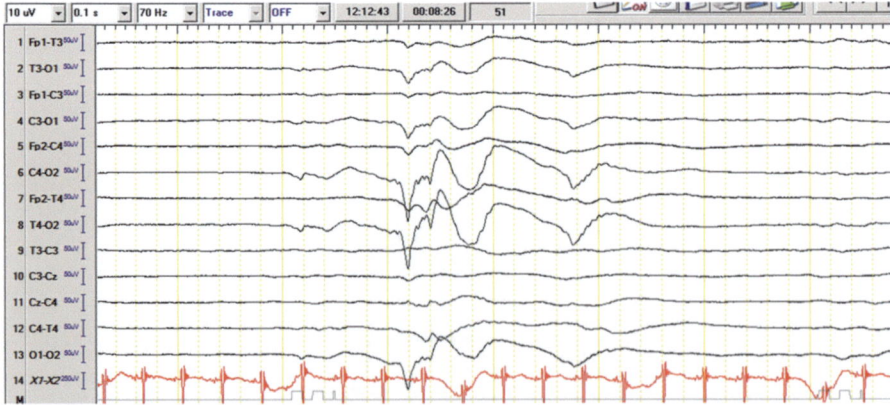

Fig. 4.30 28 WGA neonate with extremely discontinuous background activity and asymmetrical right occipital sharp waves. *WGA* weeks gestational age

4 Abnormal Background Patterns in Neonatal EEG Recordings: Sharp Waves 125

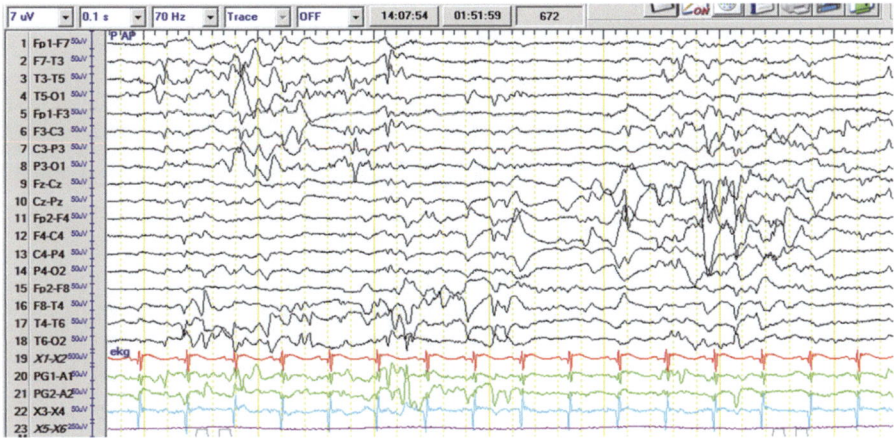

Fig. 4.31 Neonate with background of discontinuous asynchrony and abnormal left and right temporal sharp waves

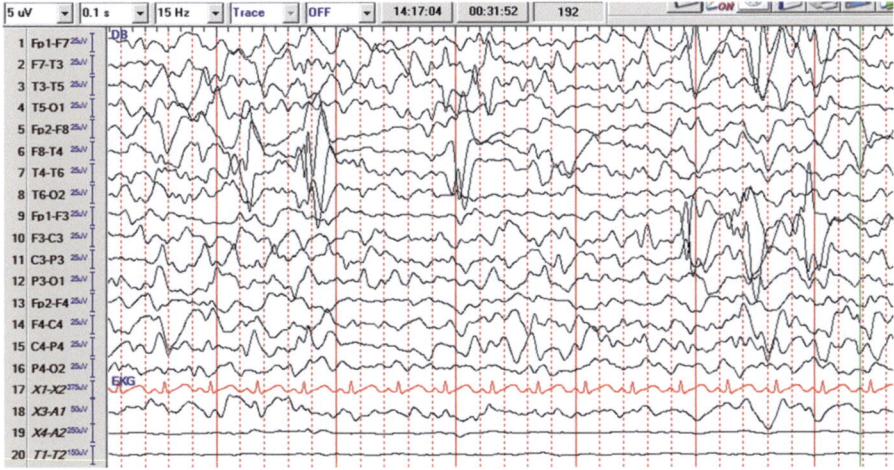

Fig. 4.32 Neonate with multiple regions of high-amplitude sharp waves and suppression. This patient has bilateral schizencephaly

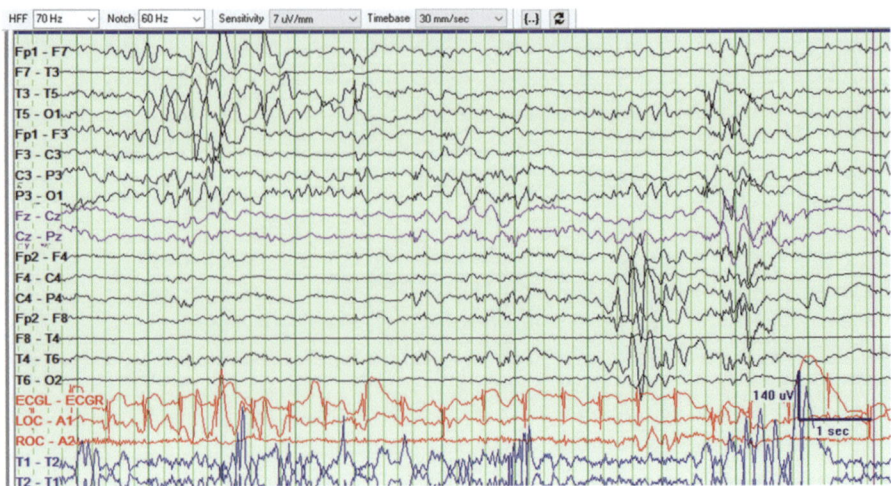

Fig. 4.33 Neonate with discontinuous background activity. Shown are symmetric bursts, asynchronous bursts, and left and right hemisphere high amplitude abnormal sharp waves

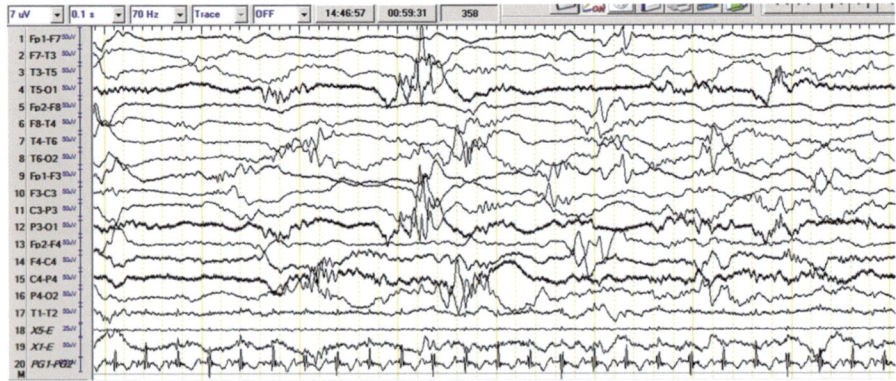

Fig. 4.34 Neonate at 40 WGA with multiple venous infarctions and EEG showing diffusely slow background activity with multiple regions of high-amplitude abnormal sharp waves

Neonate at 40 WGA with multiple venous infarctions and seizures. The EEG showed diffusely slow background activity with multiple regions of high-amplitude abnormal sharp waves. Seizures were later captured in the left occipital region (Fig. 4.34).

44 WGA neonate with viral encephalitis. The below EEG segments show continuous activity with periods of asymmetric attenuation and slowing. Left and right frontal sharp waves occurred with spread to adjacent regions. Central sharp waves were also present. Seizures were captured from these focal regions (Fig. 4.35).

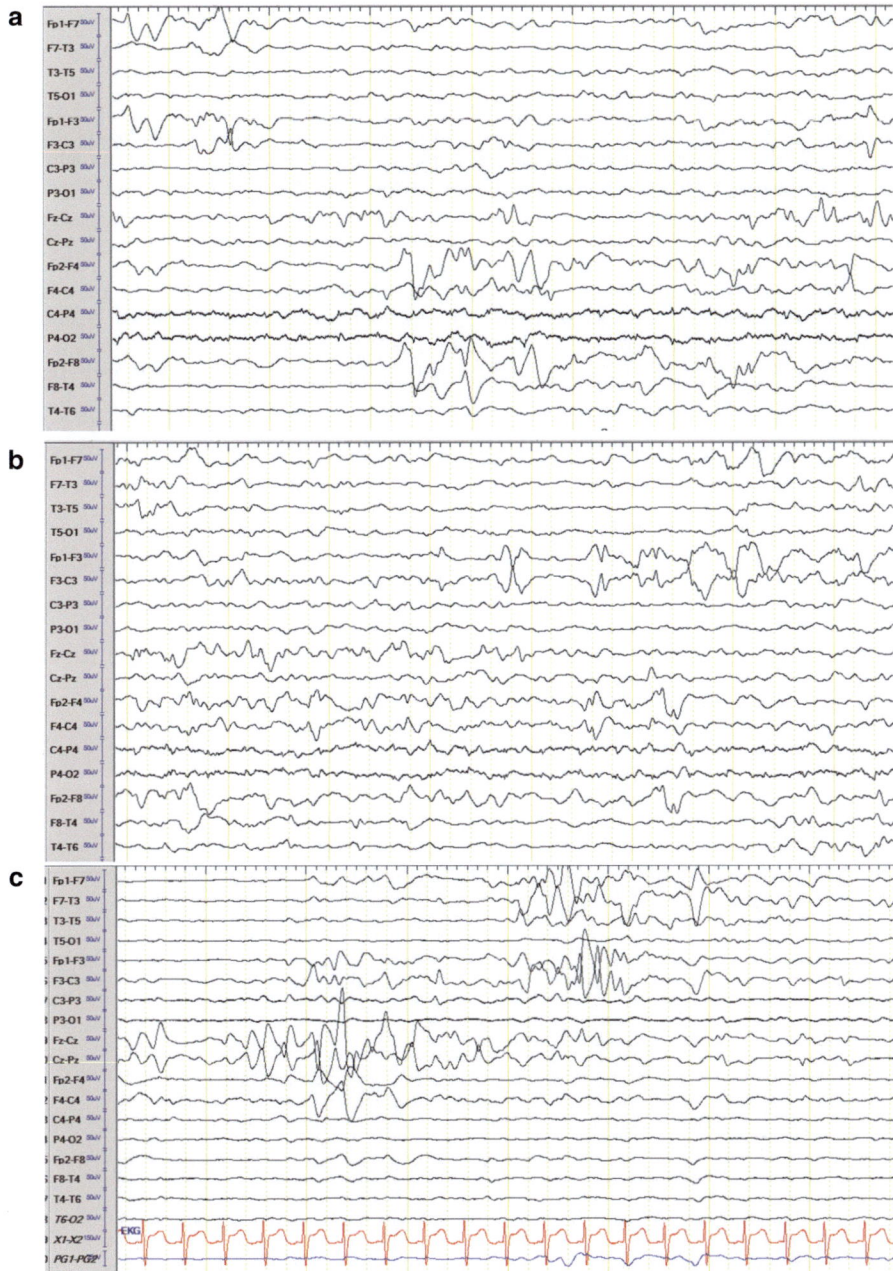

Fig. 4.35 (**a**–**c**) Neonate with encephalitis and EEG shows continuous activity with periods of asymmetric attenuation and slowing with left and right frontal sharp waves. (**b**) Left frontal sharp waves occur in a run of semi-rhythmic activity. (**c**) High-amplitude (vertex) central sharp waves are present with spread to the right central region. Separately, high-amplitude left frontal sharp waves are present

References

1. Blume WT, Dreyfus-Brisac C. Positive Rolandic sharp waves in neonatal EEG. Types and significance. Electroencephalgr Clin Neurophysiol. 1982;53:277–82.
2. Clancy RR, Tharp BR. Positive Rolandic sharp waves in the electroencephalogram of premature neonates with intraventricular hemorrhage. Electroencephalogr Clin Neurophysiol. 1984;57:395–404. https://doi.org/10.1016/0013-4694(84)90068-3.
3. Hrachovy RA, Mizrahi EM, Kellway P. Electroencephalography of the newborn. In: Daly D, Pedley TA, editors. Current practice of clinical electroencephalography. 2nd ed. New York: Raven Press; 1990. p. 201–41.
4. Lobroso CT. Neonatal electroencephalography. In: Niedermeyer E, Lopez da Silva F, editors. Electroencephalography: basic principles, clinical applications and related fields. Baltimore: Urban and Schwarzenberg; 1982. p. 599–637.
5. Mizrahi E, Hrachovy R. Atlas of neonatal electroencephalography. 4th ed. New York: Demos Medical; 2016.
6. Sansavere AJ, Harrar DB. Atlas of pediatric and neonatal ICU EEG. New York: Demos Medical; 2021.

Electrographic Findings of Neonatal Seizures

5

Mary Payne

5.1 Introduction

5.1.1 What Is a Seizure?

An abnormal clinical event that occurs with a set of signs and symptoms different from baseline activity originating from the cortex of the brain is a seizure. During this event, the EEG shows a corresponding electrographic change. The seizure semiology (seizure depiction) represents the cortical region of epileptic activity. The homunculus is a type of map used to correlate the cortical location of seizure activity to patient movements. EEG electrodes placed on the scalp represent certain areas of the underlying cortex. In this way, the electrodes show us where the abnormal cortical signals likely originate. Using this schema, we can reasonably deduce where the seizure activity originates and propagates. However, detecting seizures and distinguishing seizure events can be challenging. This chapter will discuss how seizures are defined, the interictal-ictal continuum, and status epilepticus.

5.2 Part 1: Epileptic Discharges and Seizures on a Cellular Level

We know that an abnormal spike tends to be epileptiform. But how does a seizure actually occur on a cellular level? How are these negative cortical potentials depicted on the EEG recording?

Principles of neurophysiology:

M. Payne (✉)
Department of Pediatrics, Division of Pediatric Neurology, Joan C. Edwards School of Medicine, Hoops Family Children's Hospital, Marshall University, Huntington, WV, USA
e-mail: paynem@marshall.edu

© The Author(s), under exclusive license to Springer Nature Switzerland AG 2025
M. Payne, D. Gloss II (eds.), *Neonatal EEG*,
https://doi.org/10.1007/978-3-031-92556-6_5

Sodium entering a cell depolarizes the cell.
Potassium leaving a cell repolarizes the cell.

Glutamate is an excitatory neurotransmitter, so it causes depolarization in its cellular environment. It can potentiate spread of depolarization.

GABA is an inhibitory neurotransmitter, so it causes repolarization of neurons. Repolarizing will restore a neuron to its resting potential and thus inhibit further seizure-inducing changes. However, in neonates, GABA receptors have been shown to have an excitatory effect at times. In addition, the neonate also has less GABA stores than an older child or adult would have.

In the setting of ischemia or metabolic derangements, neuronal injury occurs. The ATP-dependent sodium-potassium pump functioning may be interrupted and causes depolarization of the cell (Fig. 5.1). In addition, glutamate may be released into the intracellular web, further propagating the negative potentials (Fig. 5.2). The areas of damage or derangement then spread on a cellular level and create an excitatory environment that leads to the electrographic and clinical seizures that we can detect by EEG and clinical change.

The EEG waveforms seen on the screen represent the direction of the dipole. Current flows from positive to negative areas (Fig. 5.3).

- When the electrode closer to the surface is more negative than the deeper electrode, a negative signal is produced, which is plotted as an upward deflection. (Convention of EEG)
- When the electrode closer to the surface is more positive than the deeper electrode, a positive signal is produced, which is plotted as a downward deflection. (Convention of EEG)

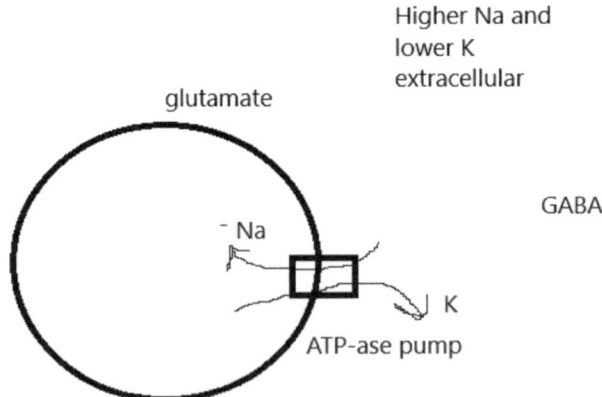

Fig. 5.1 Schematic detailing the ATP-ase pump and directions of sodium and potassium flow in a neuron. *Na* sodium, *K* potassium, *GABA* gamma-aminobutyric acid, *ATP-ase* adenosine triphosphate enzyme

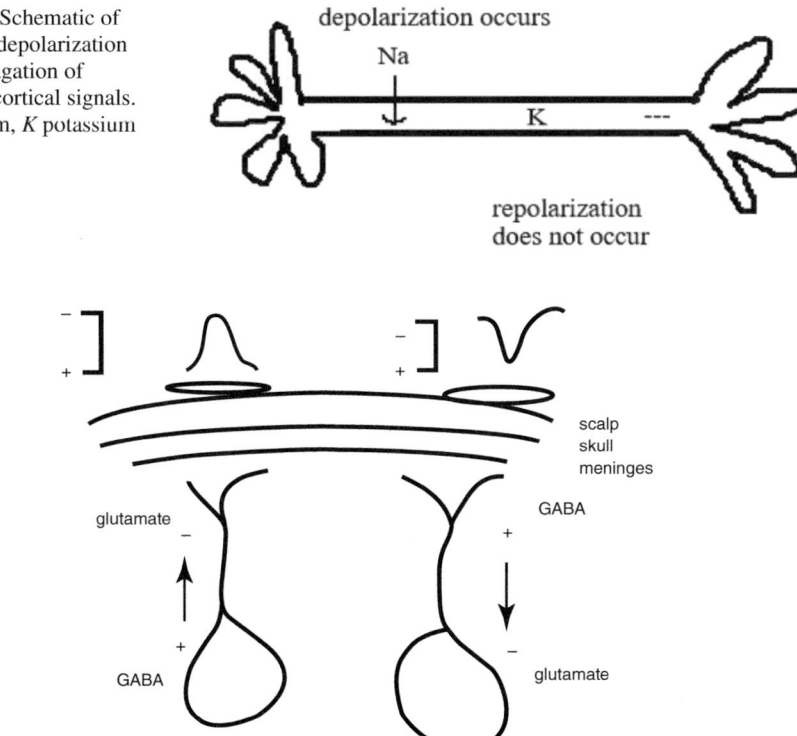

Fig. 5.2 Schematic of neuronal depolarization and propagation of negative cortical signals. *Na* sodium, *K* potassium

Fig. 5.3 Schematic showing electrical potentials and relation of the neurons to the scalp EEG electrodes and signal they produce. Scalp electrodes represent potentials from cortical pyramidal neurons oriented perpendicularly to the scalp. *GABA* gamma-aminobutyric acid

In each chain (F8 to T4 to T6 in this example), an electrode's voltage is compared to that of the electrode above it, so each tracing line represents a pair of electrodes in which the voltage of the second electrode is subtracted from the voltage of the first. Because of this, in bipolar montage, if the first electrode in the tracing line is more positive or higher than the second, then there is a positive, downward deflection. If the second electrode is more positive or higher, then there is a negative, upward deflection. A phase reversal is created, where the downward and upward deflections meet. Using these calculations for a bipolar montage, the electrode in common (in this case T4) has the maximum negativity compared to surrounding electrodes (Fig. 5.4).

Depolarization of neurons causes changes that create epileptic activity with an imbalance between excitatory and inhibitory synapses. In this case, excitatory postsynaptic potentials (EPSPs) outnumber inhibitory postsynaptic potentials (IPSPs) causing an excess in excitation, which is detected by the scalp electrodes as continued negative activity [2].

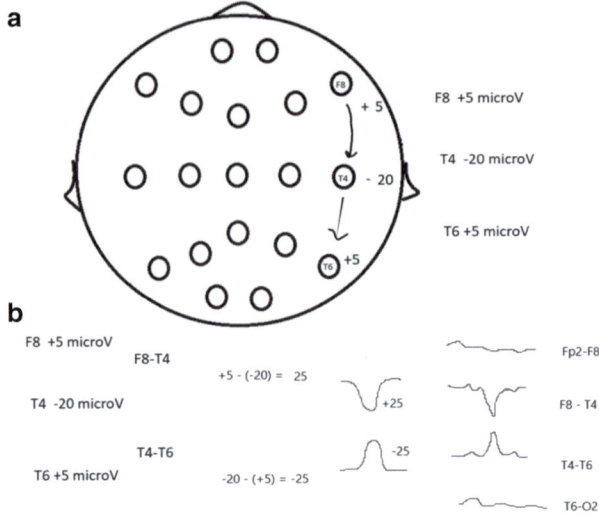

Fig. 5.4 (**a, b**) Examples of how the montage and electrode differences show the phase reversals as maximal negativity on the display

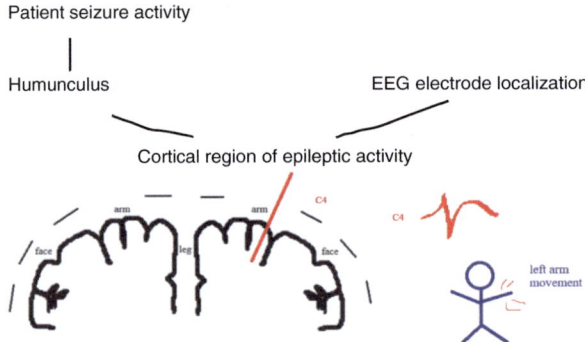

Fig. 5.5 Schematic of seizure activity correlating with EEG electrodes and cortical origin

5.3 Part 2: Epileptic Discharges and Seizures on a Clinical and Electrographic Level

The clinical seizure activity correlates with the region of cortical epileptic activity. The homunculus, a map of motor function, can provide imagery for clinical seizure correlation (Fig. 5.5).

In older infants, children, and adults, a typical electrographic epileptic pattern (seizure) shows a change and progression in the frequency of epileptiform discharges, voltage (amplitude), morphology, and/or location during the seizure (Fig. 5.6). These changes, or *evolution*, correlate with cellular changes with propagation of the negative cortical potentials and are depicted with predictability and reliability on the digital screen. However, neonatal epileptic seizures may not show these changes clearly, so reliance on the repetitive or rhythmic nature of epileptiform discharges is important.

Nevertheless, these EEG changes are termed *evolution* and are mentioned here for presentation:

– *Morphology:* The shape of the wave changes. For example, the wave may start as a smooth wave, then becomes sharper with a spike and wave character as the seizure continues.
– *Frequency:* The frequency or a rhythmic event, or seizure, may increase or decrease, for example, 2–3 Hz activity changes to 7–8 Hz activity during the seizure.
– *Amplitude:* Beyond the neonatal period, the amplitude may increase or decrease; however, a neonatal seizure may not demonstrate this change.

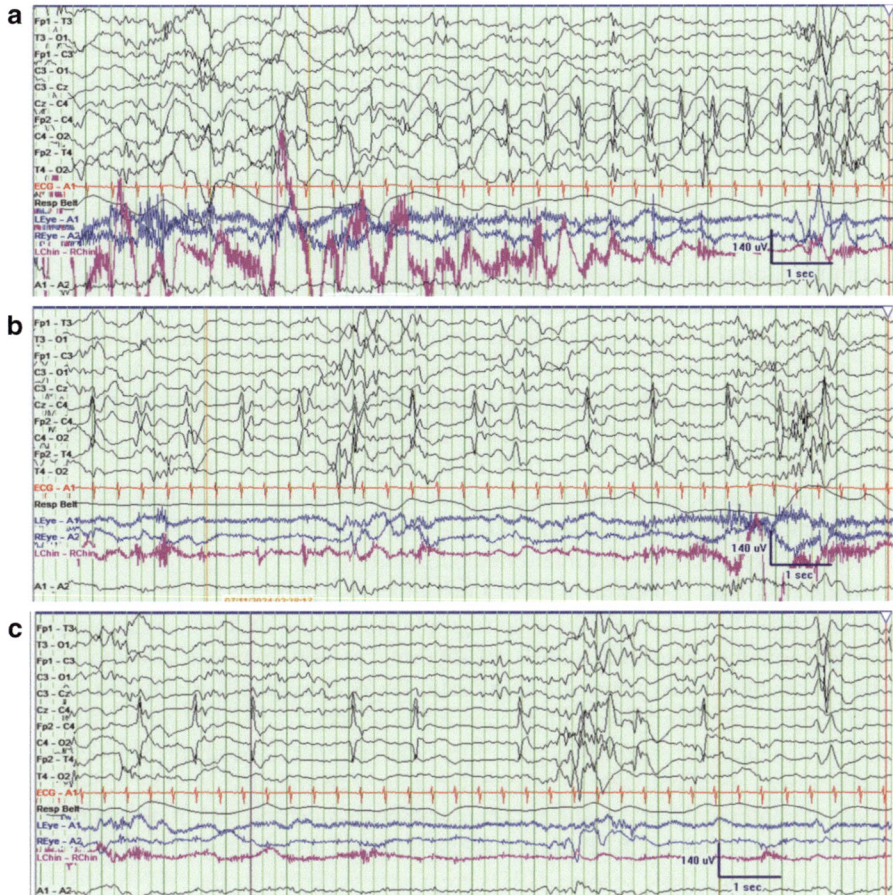

Fig. 5.6 (**a–c**) Electrographic seizure originating in the right central region. Change in amplitude, sharp wave morphology, and frequency (2 Hz then 3 Hz) occurs. This overall pattern change as the electrical epileptic activity propagates is termed *evolution*

- *Location:* Electrographic activity beginning in one region, then spreading to another cortical adjacent region. Also, location may spread to the opposite hemisphere. However, as mentioned above, neonates may not display spread of rhythmic activity and often neonatal rhythmic seizure activity may be contained to one lead only.
- *Duration:* At least 10 s (unless myoclonic) per ACNS. ILAE seizure criteria do not state a minimum duration to be considered an epileptic (seizure) event. Older patients' seizures have a consensus that 10 s duration is minimum to be considered an epileptic event (see below).

In 2013, the American Clinical Neurophysiology Society defined a neonatal seizure as "a sudden abnormal EEG event, defined by a repetitive and evolving pattern with a minimum of 2 μV in amplitude as measured by the peak-to-peak voltage and having a duration of at least 10 seconds" [4].

In 2021, the International League Against Epilepsy further changed the criteria to not require a minimum duration. Their definition states a neonatal seizure is "an electrographic event with a pattern characterized by sudden, repetitive, evolving stereotyped waveforms with a beginning and end. The duration is not defined but has to be sufficient to demonstrate evolution in the frequency and morphology of the discharges and needs to be long enough to allow recognition of onset, evolution, and resolution of an abnormal discharge" [3].

Currently, an ILAE Task Force is working with the World Health Organization (WHO) to update the WHO 2011 guidelines on neonatal seizures. Many developing countries do not have access to EEGs, so clinical characteristics are often the only defining feature.

Note also how neither the ACNS or ILAE require or mention the presence of a clinical change in the patient to occur during a seizure. This is another outcome of the widespread use of prolonged EEG recording in neonates. As many as 80% of seizures in hypoxic-ischemic encephalopathy are subclinical, so observation of seizures alone may not be sufficient for patient care. ILAE definition also leaves open the presence of brief rhythmic activity to count as epileptic seizure. Per ACNS, these brief runs are considered to be BRDs. Thus, brief runs less than 10 s are felt by some to be defined as a seizure. How does this affect treatment?

This brings us to the ictal interictal continuum …

Brief rhythmic discharges (BRDs) or brief interictal/ictal rhythmic discharges are less than 10 s and may be electrographically identical to an epileptic event. Since neonatal seizures may consist of rhythmic activity in one lead without a significant change in frequency or amplitude, the occurrence of BRDs can be very confusing as to identifying and delineating a seizure (epileptic event). BRDs are seen in patients with seizures as part of the ictal–interictal spectrum. This term best characterizes a patient who is encephalopathic with frequent seizure activity and frequency interictal abnormalities. The exact beginning and end of a seizure event may be difficult to identify. Frequent BRDs may in a way coalesce to appear identical to an electrographic seizure. BRDs are a term accepted by the ACNS. However, the ILAE does not distinguish between BRDs and seizures, so briefer events (less than 10 s) may be considered to be epileptic.

In clearly defined settings, there are interictal epileptiform discharges that indicate a region of epileptogenicity and separately, there occurs an electrographic seizure (ictus). However, in patients with encephalopathy and/or a high seizure burden, the separation is not straightforward.

- Frequent spikes can coalesce to become rhythmic runs, occurring repetitively for a period of time (BRDs) (Fig. 5.9).
- Periodic lateralized discharges (PLDs) are frequent interictal epileptiform spikes that occur repeatedly, but are not rhythmic. These seem more often in older children and adults; however, they also represent part of the ictal–interictal continuum. Treatment of PLDs varies as well, based on clinical scenario (Fig. 5.10).
- This rhythmic activity may become longer in duration and show features of a seizure, such as change in morphology, frequency, and spread to adjacent regions. (seizure)
- Use of anti-epileptic medications may shorten seizures to give them the appearance of these in-between epochs, improving to presence of only BRDs, spikes or PLDs (Fig. 5.7).

Now that we have discussed the spectrum of spike and seizure, how does knowledge of this effect treatment? Why make a delineation that a seizure exists for a certain amount of time?

Do we treat seizures? Yes.

Do we treat spikes? Yes and no.

Do we treat rhythmic activity? Yes and no.

WHY THE 10 SECOND DELINEATION: Controversies …

With the advent of continuous EEG monitoring, we are detecting subclinical seizures and with longer monitoring, more subclinical seizures can be noted. Implications of treatment thus ensue, and as medical providers, we are inclined to treat seizures, subclinical and clinical. For example, the seizures associated with HIE tend to occur at 24–48 hours of age and are often subclinical. However, it is easy to fall into the trap of treating interictal abnormalities and perhaps doing more harm than good with administering high doses of sedatives and anti-epileptic medications. Often in sick patients there is an ictal–interictal continuum, when the EEG shows frequent spikes, some rhythmic at times, perhaps even showing brief evolution. Thus, it can be difficult to discern exactly seizure onset and ending.

This manifests to the art of medicine and balancing the interictal–ictal continuum with the overall medical plan of the patient in mind. Some who promote the 10 s minimum feel that every epileptic rhythmic discharge occurrence does not need to be treated and thus the brief rhythmic runs (less than 10 s) do not reach a threshold for seizure treatment. However, the mark of 10 s is useful for treating providers and reading epileptologists to aid in an appropriate, clinically significant number of epileptic events to be counted as seizure without being overly sensitive and possibly causing morbidity with higher AED dosing administration.

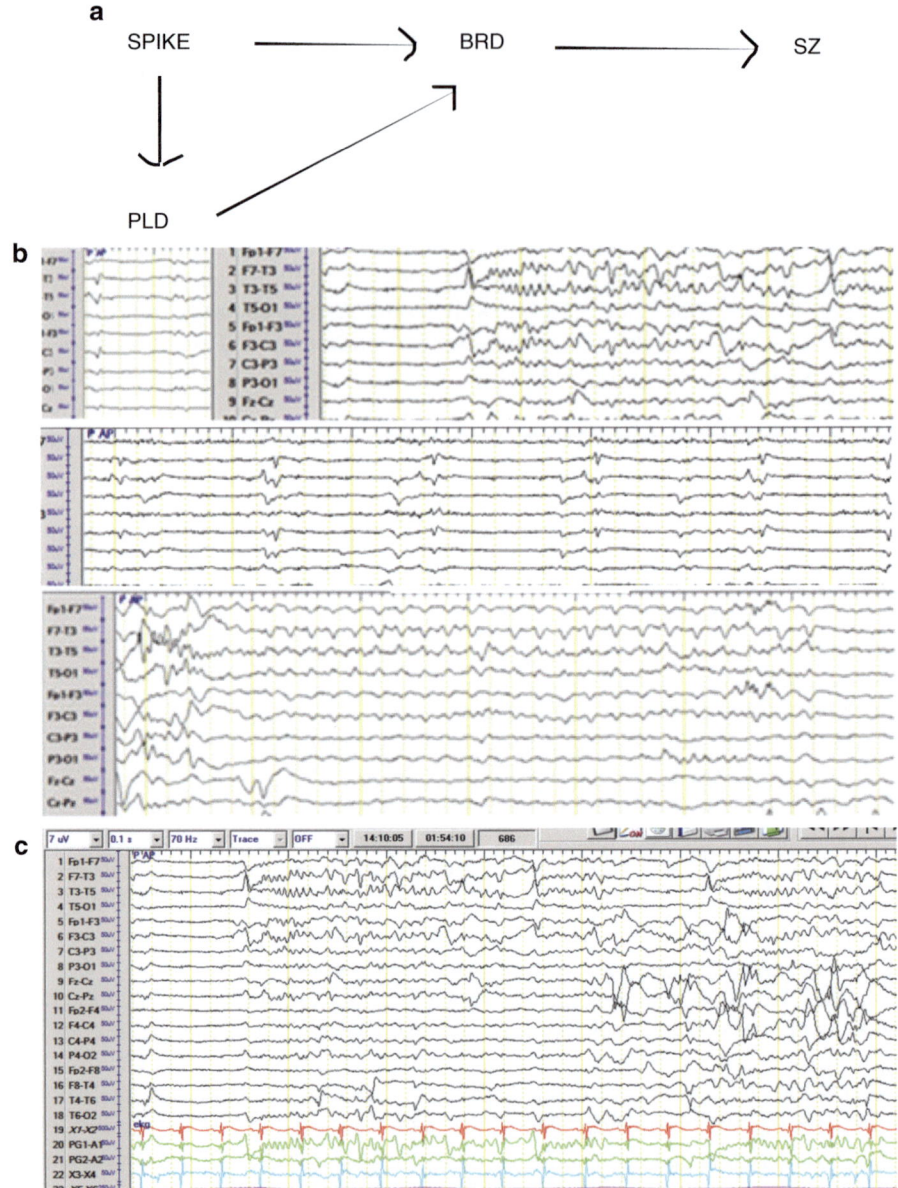

Fig. 5.7 (a) Electrographic progression from spike to brief rhythmic discharge or PLD to seizure. (b) Pictures showing spike (top left), BRD (top right), PLDs (center), and seizure (bottom). *BRD* brief rhythmic discharge, *PLD* periodic lateralized discharge. (c) Example of brief rhythmic discharges (BRDs) in the left temporal region in a neonate with left temporal lobe seizures. This is an expanded view of the BRD discharges shown in (b). (d) Example of right temporal brief epileptiform discharges (BRDs) in a neonate with right temporal lobe seizures. Left hemisphere periodic lateralized discharges (PLDs) are also present. Expanded view of the PLDs in section (b)

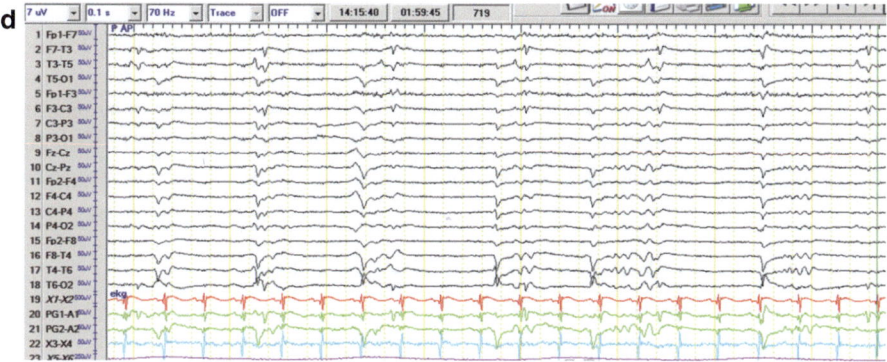

Fig. 5.7 (continued)

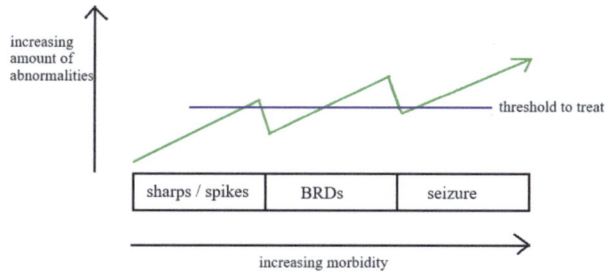

Fig. 5.8 Schematic of treatment options and patterns in patients along the ictal–interictal continuum. Presence of interictal spikes only may warrant monitoring only, but as spike frequency increases, neurologists may opt to treat with anti-epileptic medications. Occurrence of BRDs is slightly more concerning and threshold to treat may be lower than for interictal spikes alone. However, seizure occurrence will likely lead to prompt and continued treatment

Those who do not separate 10 s epileptic events view the overall activity as a measure of seizure burden.

However, a way to measure epileptic activity is to look at the recording in terms of seizure burden. This may be calculated as a percentage of seizures or rhythmic discharges in a given period of time. One might make the decision on how to treat based on the percentage of interictal and ictal spike occurrence.

Seizure burden—ictal electrographic activity in a given period of EEG recording, stated as electrographic seizure seconds or minutes. This is a term used to quantify and guide treatment per hospital /physician preferences. For example, a prior to anti-epileptic medications, a patient may have a seizure burden of 70% and following medications may have improved to a seizure burden of 30%.

Either way, the decision to treat and how to treat is based on each unique clinical scenario (Fig. 5.8). Presence of interictal epileptiform spikes does not warrant the same plan of treatment as the presence of electrographic seizures.

Status epilepticus, or the occurrence of a prolonged seizure or seizures with altered mental status, is difficult to discern in neonates. Neonates with frequent seizures often have a background showing encephalopathy and frequent brief rhythmic discharges, along the interictal continuum. Recent ACNS criteria suggest the occurrence of status epilepticus in a neonate can be documented if more than 50% of an hour segment contains epileptic activity.

5.3.1 Interictal Sharp Transients: Interictal Abnormality Considerations

Interictal epileptiform abnormalities, also referred to as spikes or sharp waves, in older children and adults indicate an epileptiform region. Neonates demonstrate sharp waves as part of the expected developmental process and are referred to as sharp transients or graphoelements. Morphology of these sharp transients is nearly identical to that of interictal epileptiform spikes seen in older patients. This dichotomy can easily cause confusion for a reader who is not accustomed to interpreting neonatal EEGs as normal for neonatal age sharp waves may appear to be erroneously abnormal and epileptiform. Learning about EEG developmental maturation can explain the natural progression of these sharp transients and criteria that can be used as a guide to help identify normal or abnormal sharp waves.

An additional confusing aspect of neonatal sharp wave transients is that their presence may indicate a region of dysfunction and a region of potential epileptogenicity. In older patients, the presence of sharp waves is considered to be epileptiform and thus suggests a region that is potentially epileptogenic. However, in neonates, abnormal sharp waves may simply indicate a region of focal dysfunction, such as that seen with ischemia. Not all regions with focal dysfunction are epileptogenic, and the sharp waves may abate as neuronal healing occurs [1].

5.4 Part 3: Seizure Examples

As it is with anything in medicine, determining the presence of seizure activity is not always straightforward.

- We know that not all abnormal involuntary movements are seizures and there are many seizure mimics.
- Clinical semiology does not always correlate with the location of scalp EEG abnormalities.
- Patients can have subclinical seizures, so no apparent clinical sign of an epileptic event.

Other electrographic seizure features (Figs. 5.9, 5.10, 5.11, 5.12, 5.13, 5.14, 5.15, 5.16, 5.17, 5.18, and 5.19):

5 Electrographic Findings of Neonatal Seizures

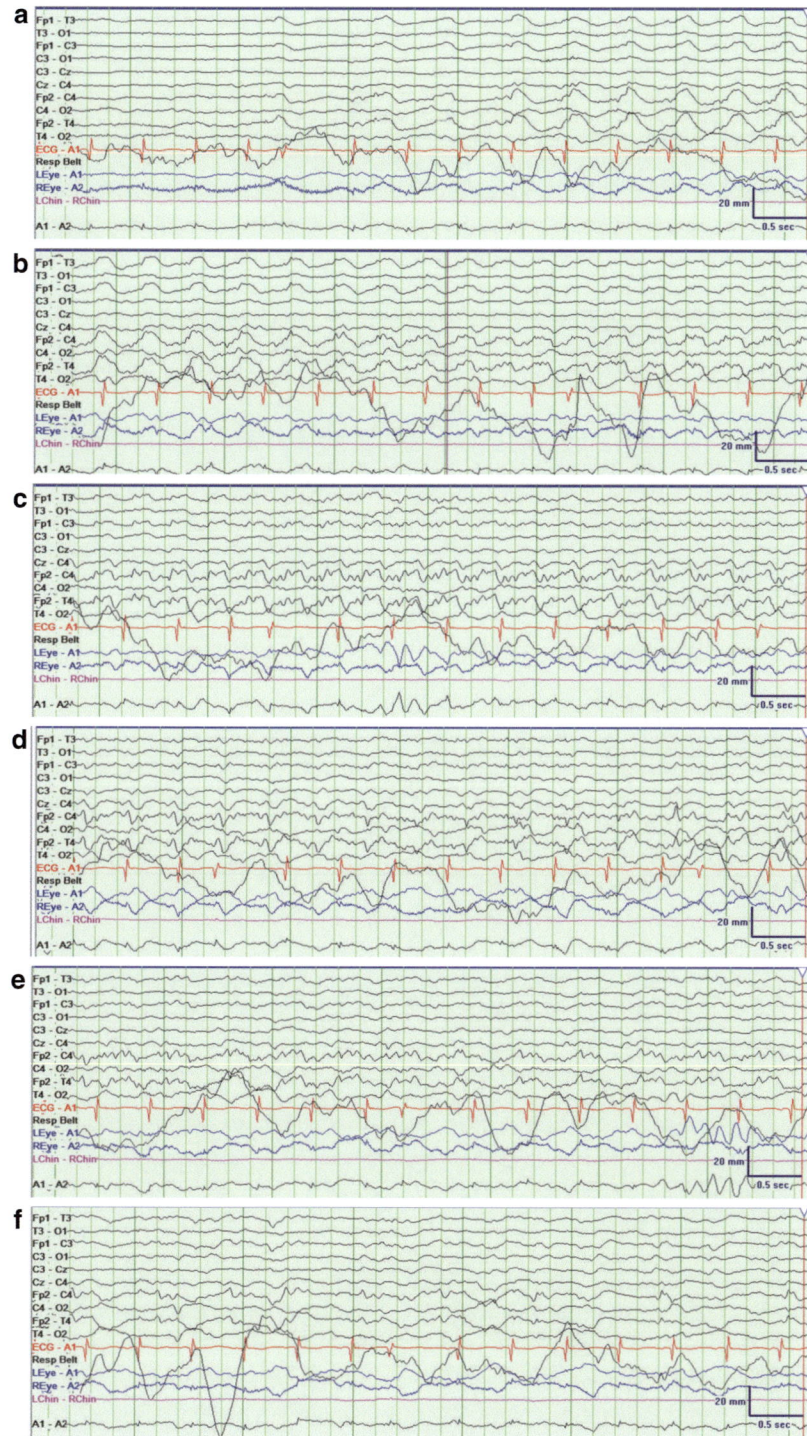

Fig. 5.9 (**a–f**) Example of a seizure in the right centrotemporal region with evolution. Spread to the left frontal region is also occurring

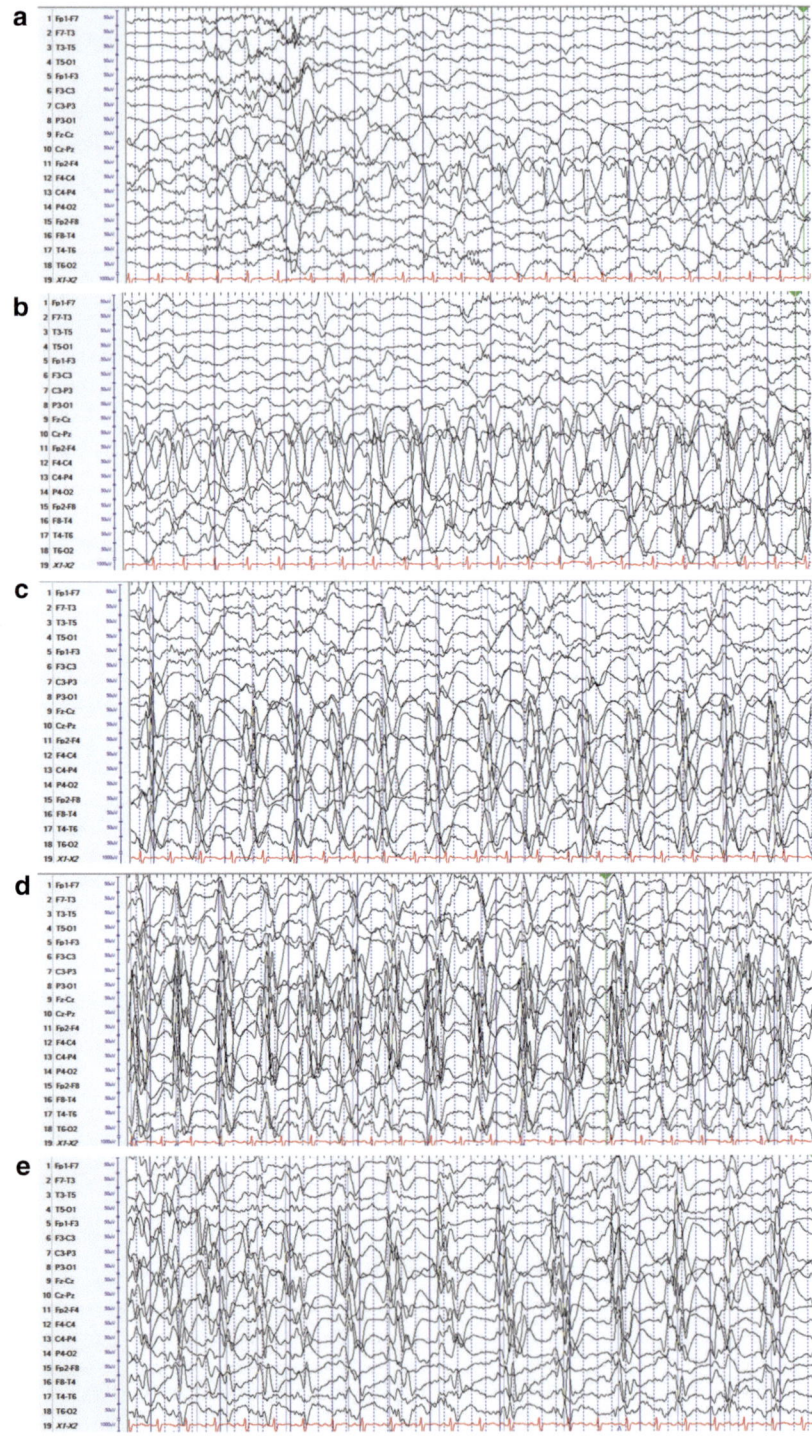

Fig. 5.10 (a–e) Right frontal focal seizure with spread to adjacent cortical regions seizure. In this case, spread to the left hemisphere also occurs

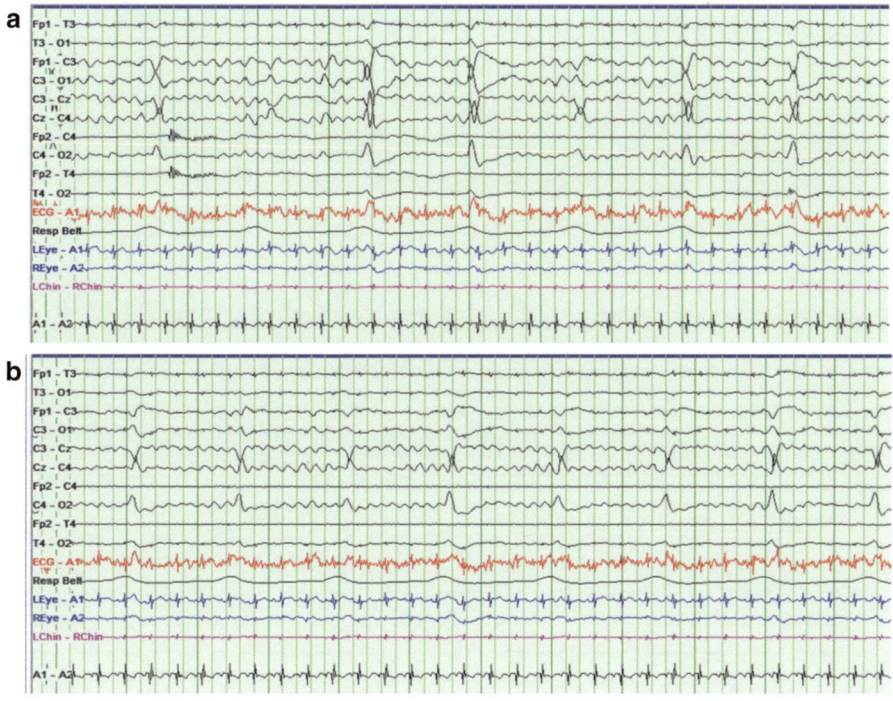

Fig. 5.11 (a, b) Left central seizure in a neonate with spread to the right central region and right occipital region

- Lower-voltage activity tends to be higher frequencies.
- Higher-voltage activity tends to be lower frequencies.
- Often seizures consist of a combination of spikes, sharp waves, and slow waves as the evolution occurs. More mature brains (after the neonatal period) show this evolution very well.

5.4.1 EEG Tidbit

- Seizure in a severe CNS insult tends to be low voltage, long duration, localized, with minimal spread or evolution and is subclinical.
- Alpha seizure that consists of rhythmic 8–12 Hz activity and 20–70 µV in amplitude in central or temporal regions suggests a poor prognosis and is usually subclinical.
- Paralyzed infant will not show clinical seizure activity, so EEG is often run continuously to identify seizures for optimal treatment.
- If a clinical event is present, the type of event correlates anatomically with the region of cortical electrographic focus.

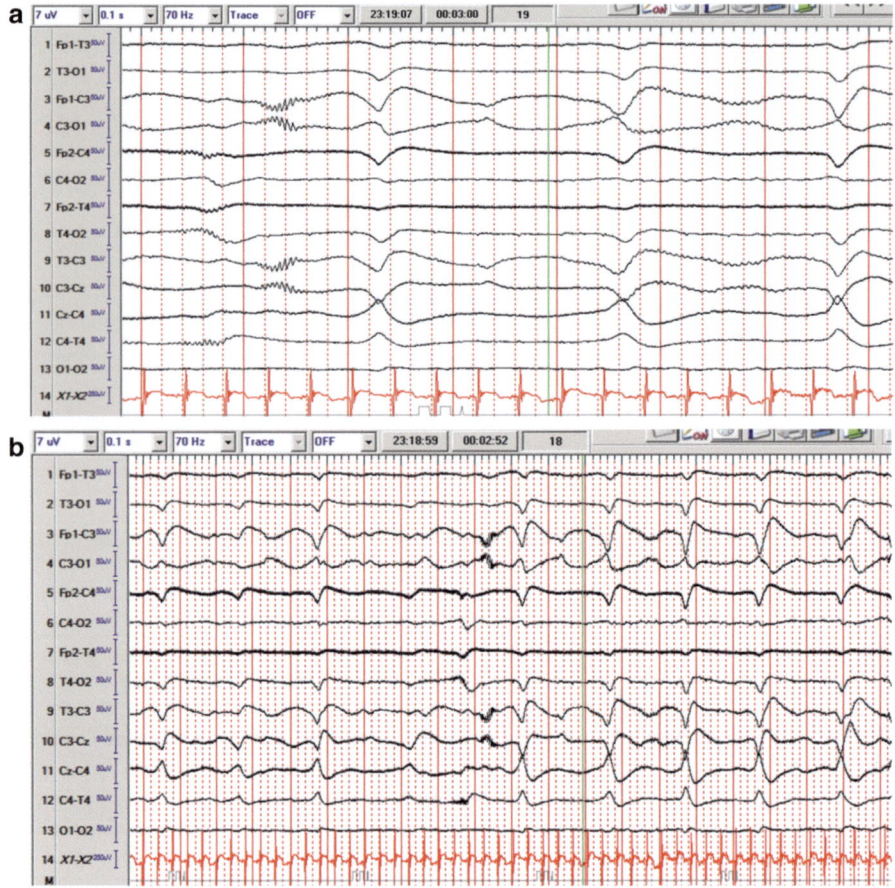

Fig. 5.12 (**a**, **b**) Neonate at 24 WGA with a focal seizure in the central region. (**a**) Paper speed showing 7 s in the clip and (**b**) paper speed showing 20 s in the clip

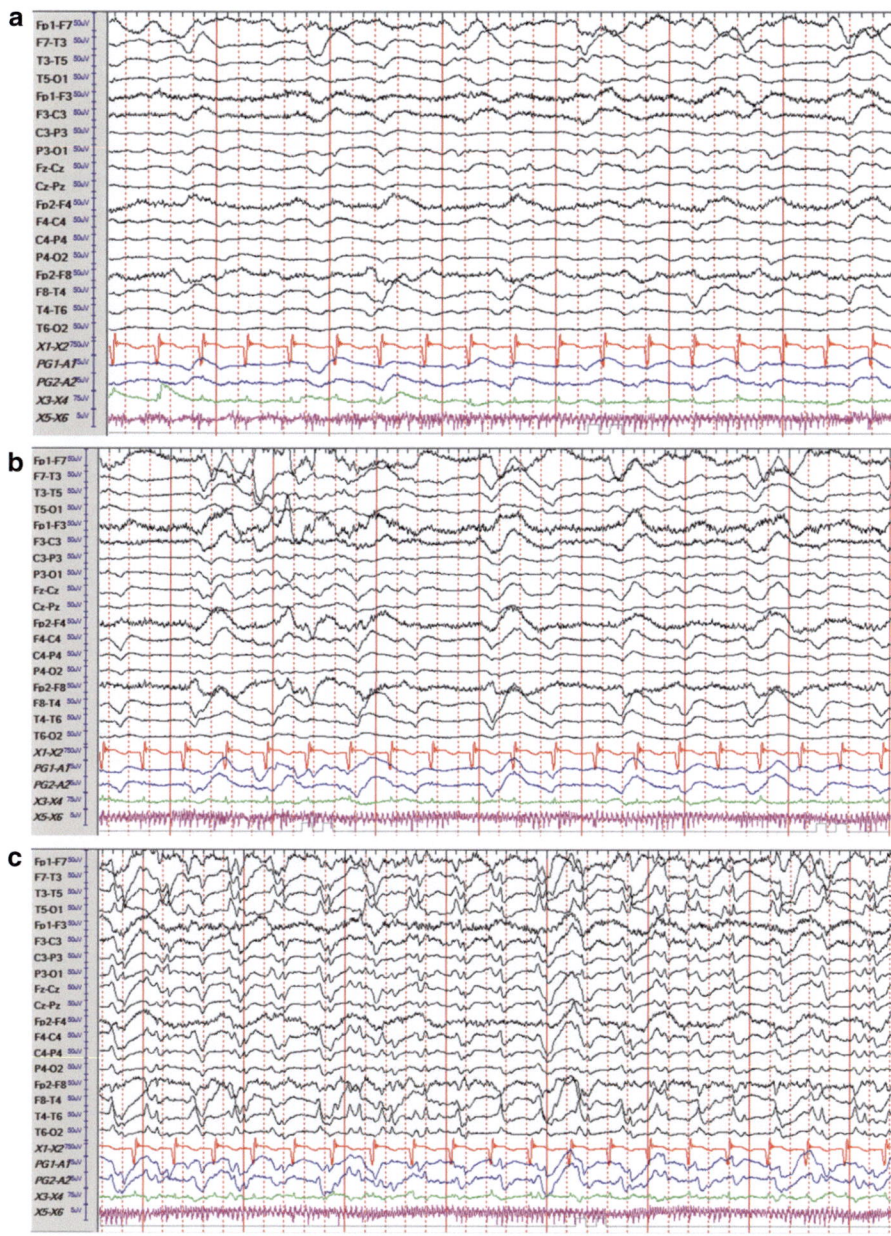

Fig. 5.13 (**a–f**) Evolution of left frontal seizure in a neonate with rapid spread to the right frontal region and quickly seen in both hemispheres

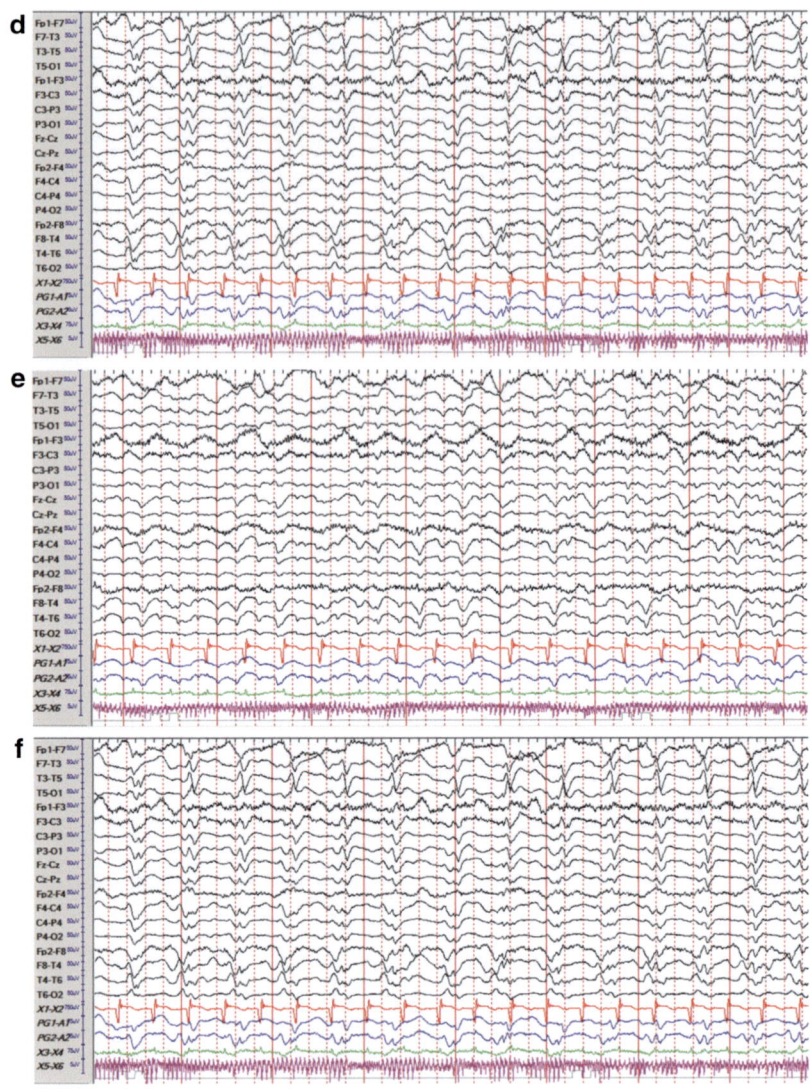

Fig. 5.13 (continued)

5 Electrographic Findings of Neonatal Seizures

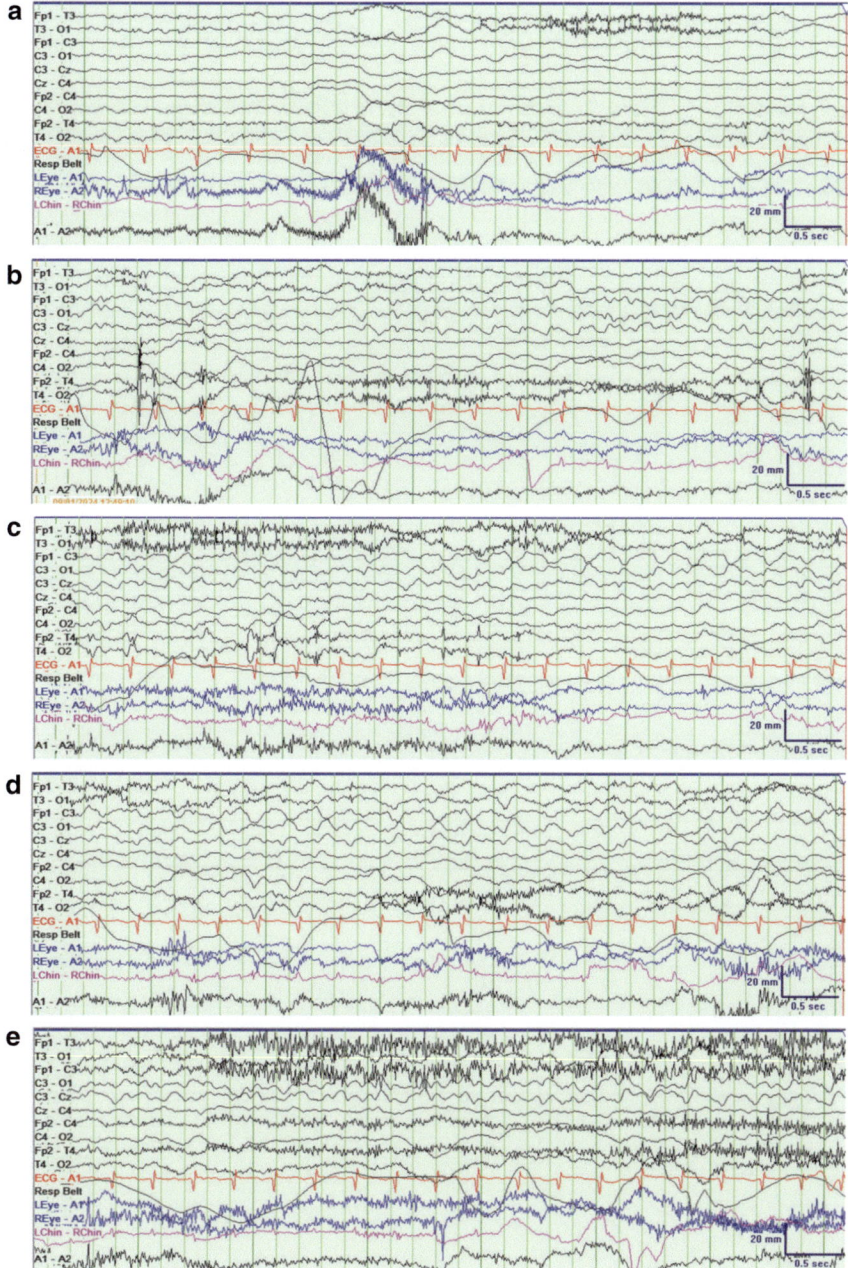

Fig. 5.14 Example of left central seizure in a neonate with anti-epileptic treatment. (**a–n**) before treatment and (**o**) After treatment with anti-epileptic medications (**o–s**) after treatment. Epileptic activity is lower voltage and less sharp, although remains rhythmic

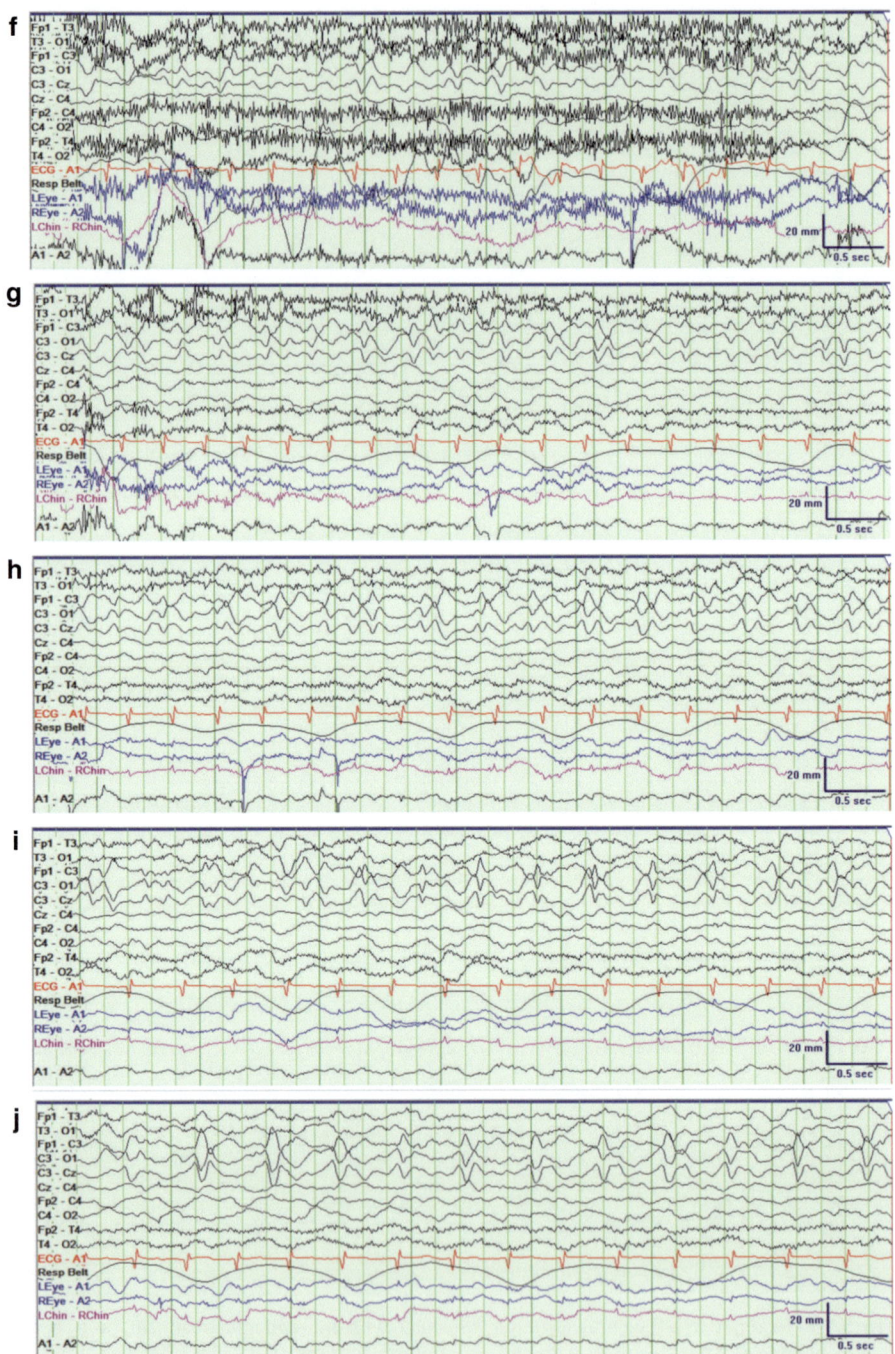

Fig. 5.14 (continued)

5 Electrographic Findings of Neonatal Seizures

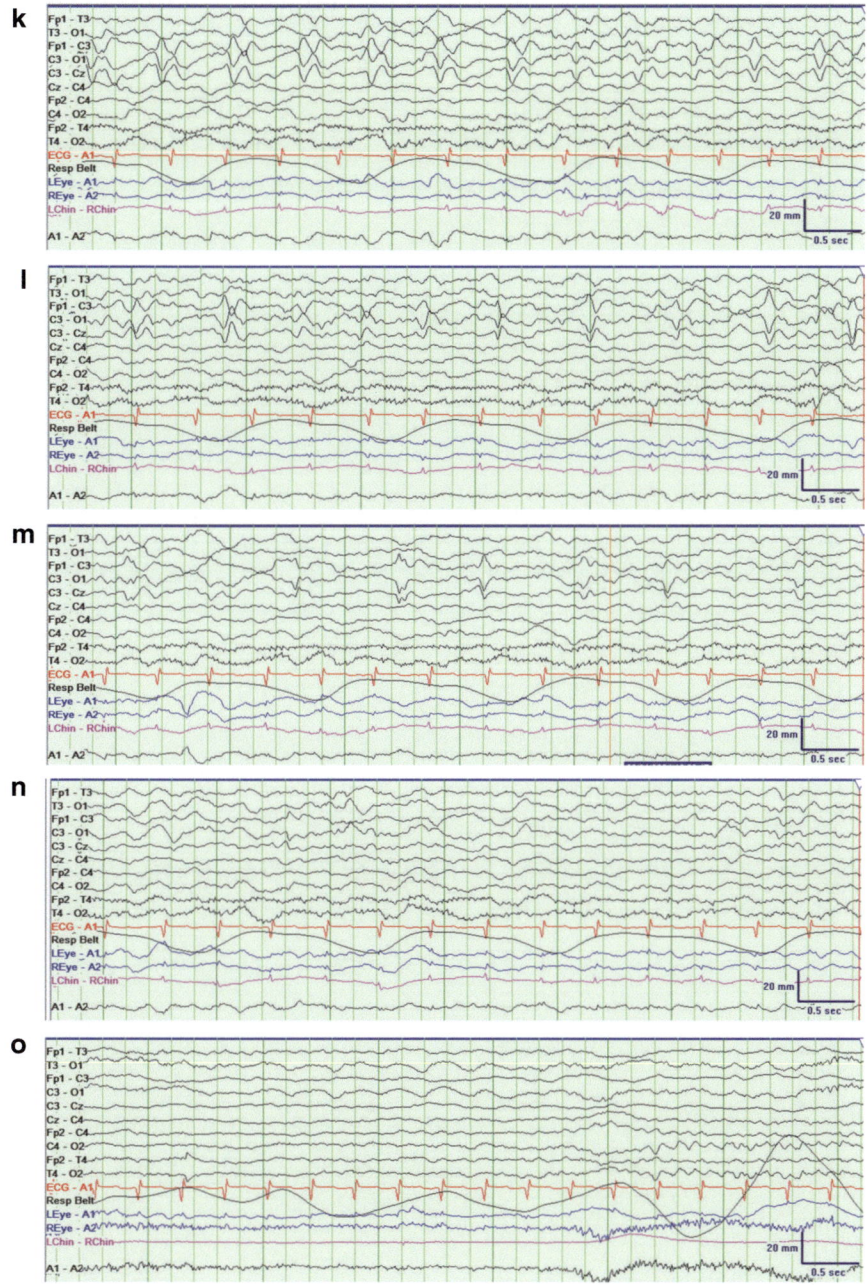

Fig. 5.14 (continued)

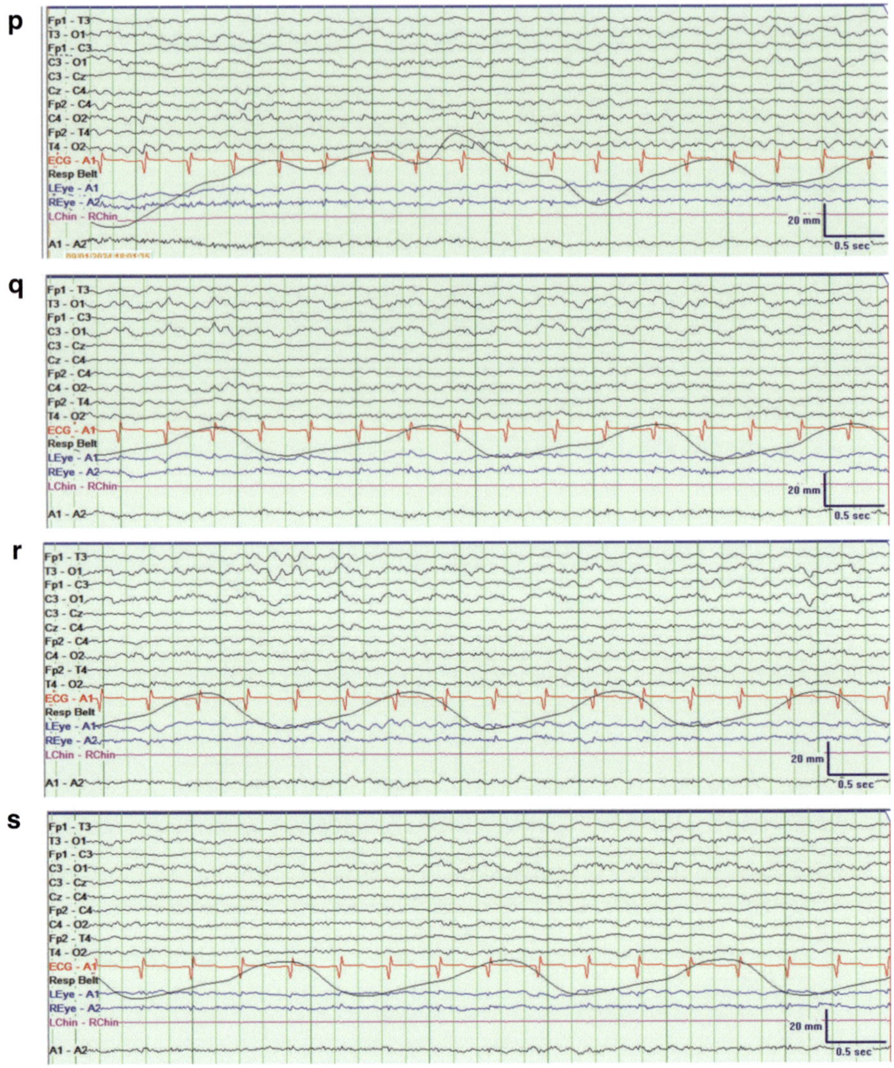

Fig. 5.14 (continued)

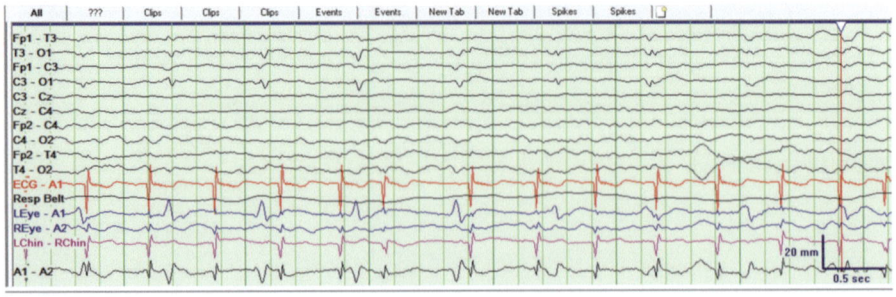

Fig. 5.15 Left occipital focal seizure showing artifact in the left eye lead

5 Electrographic Findings of Neonatal Seizures

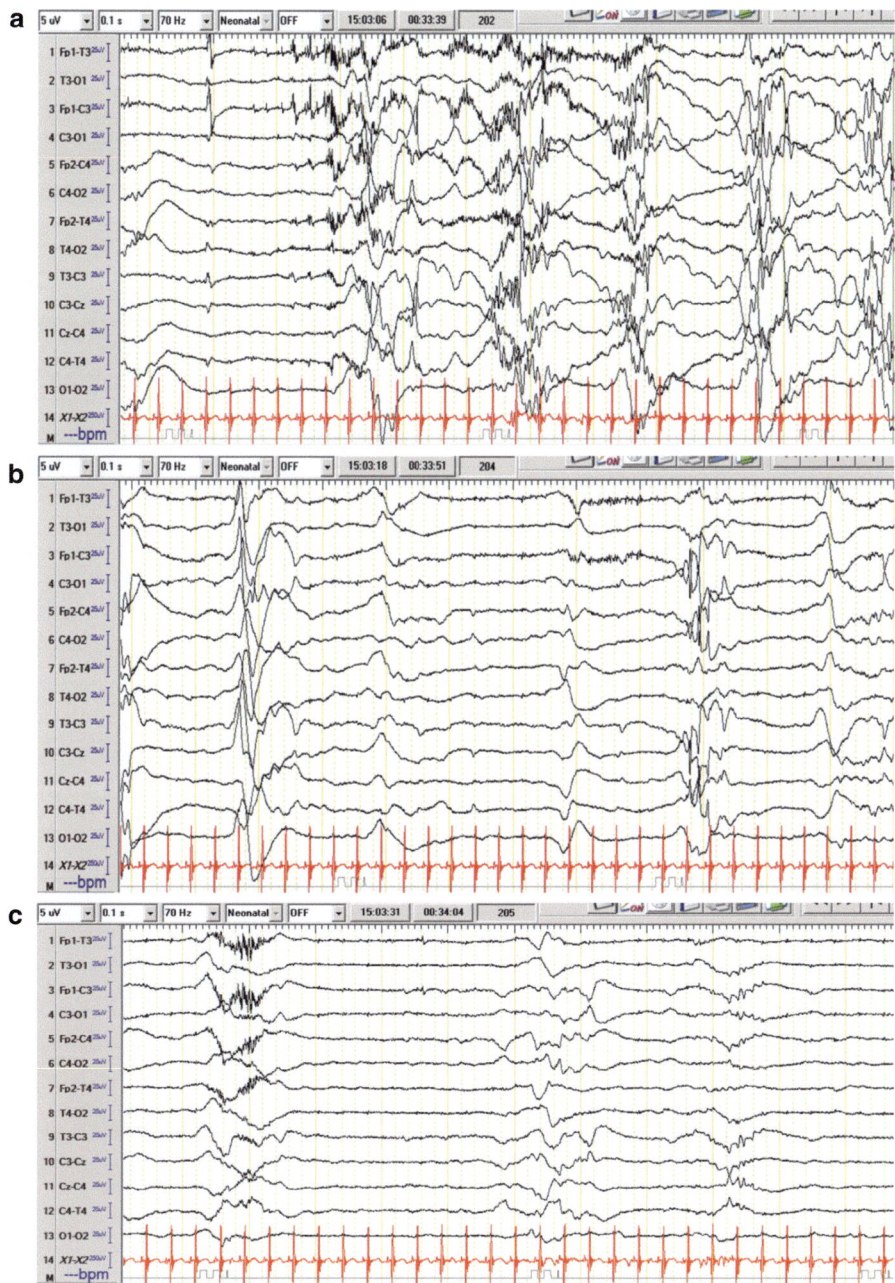

Fig. 5.16 Generalized discharges in a neonate with myoclonic seizures (**a**–**c**)

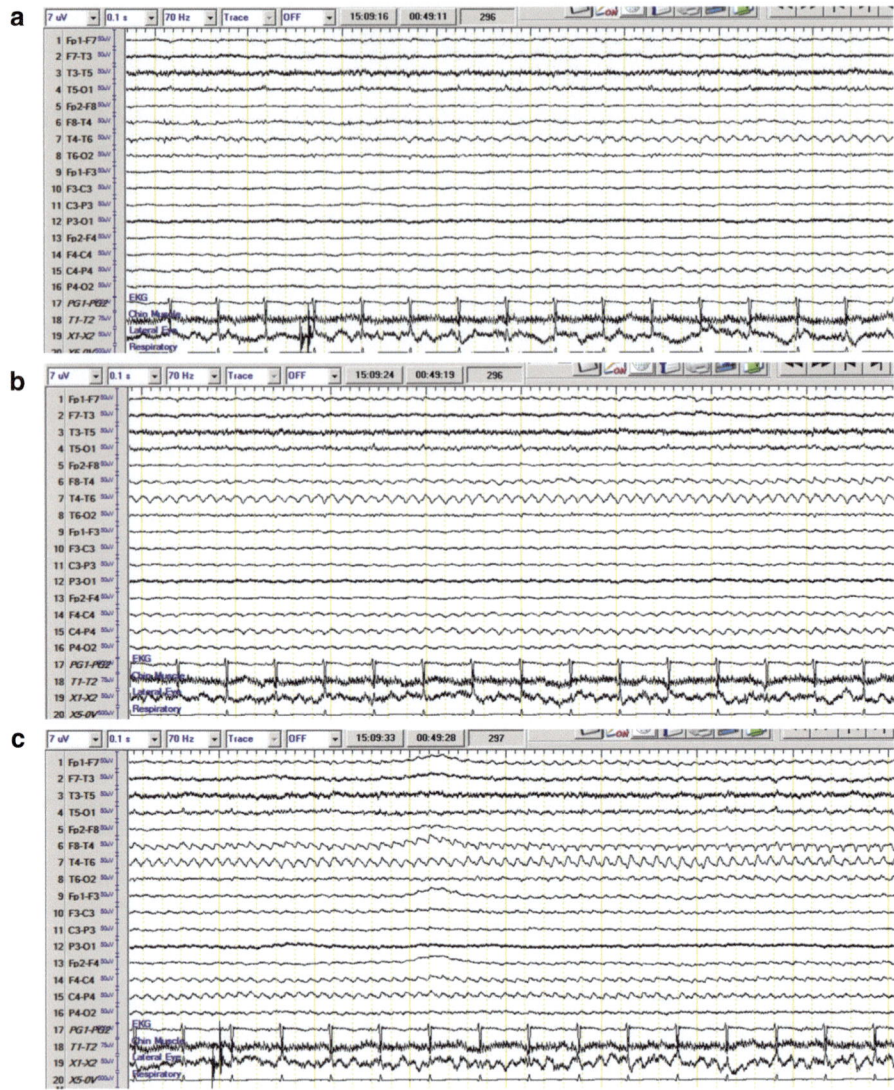

Fig. 5.17 Right temporal seizures as low-voltage rhythmic activity evolving with frequency, amplitude, and location (**a–f**)

5 Electrographic Findings of Neonatal Seizures 151

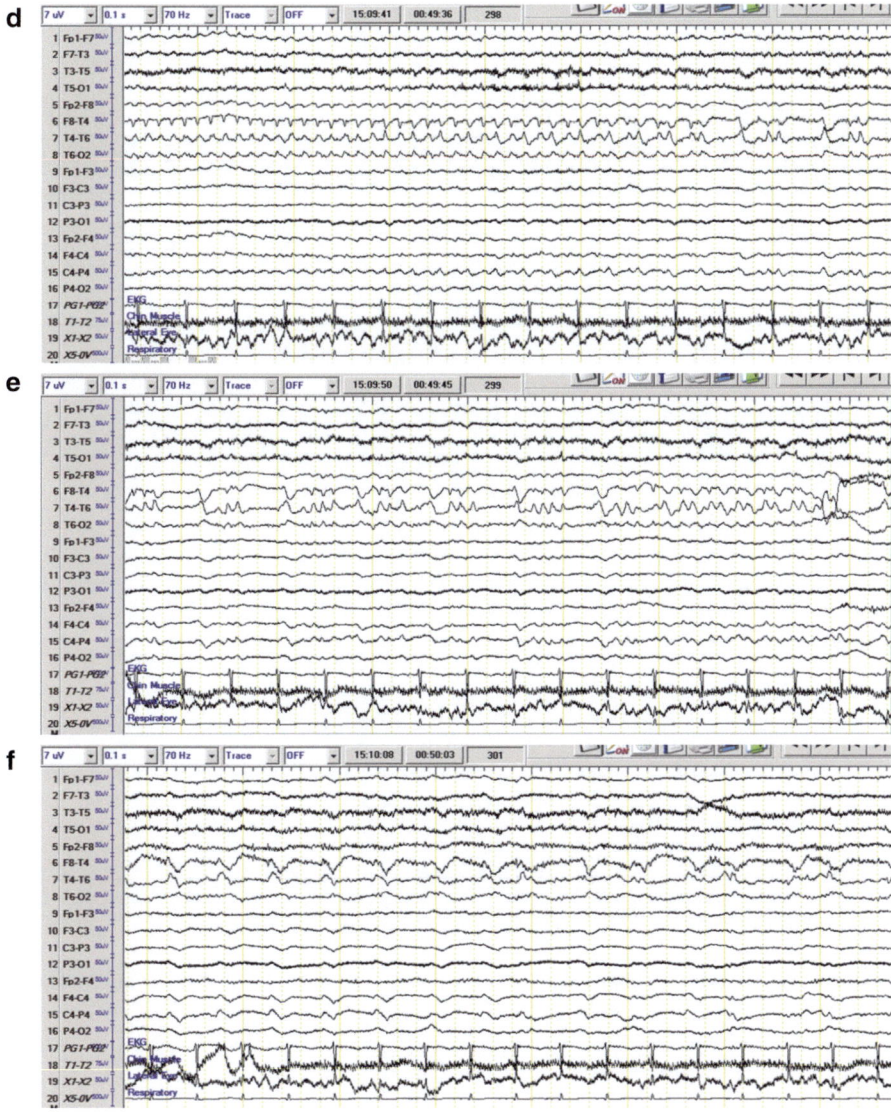

Fig. 5.17 (continued)

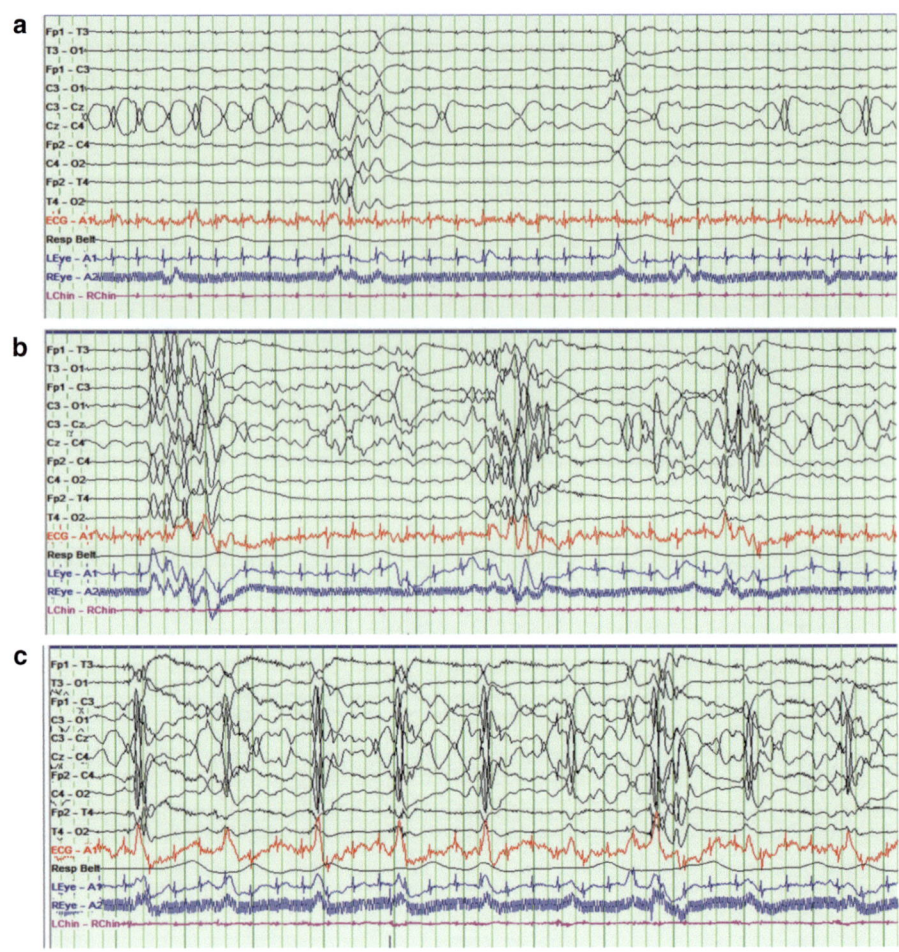

Fig. 5.18 (**a–c**) Central rhythmic activity organizing into an electrographic and clinical seizure

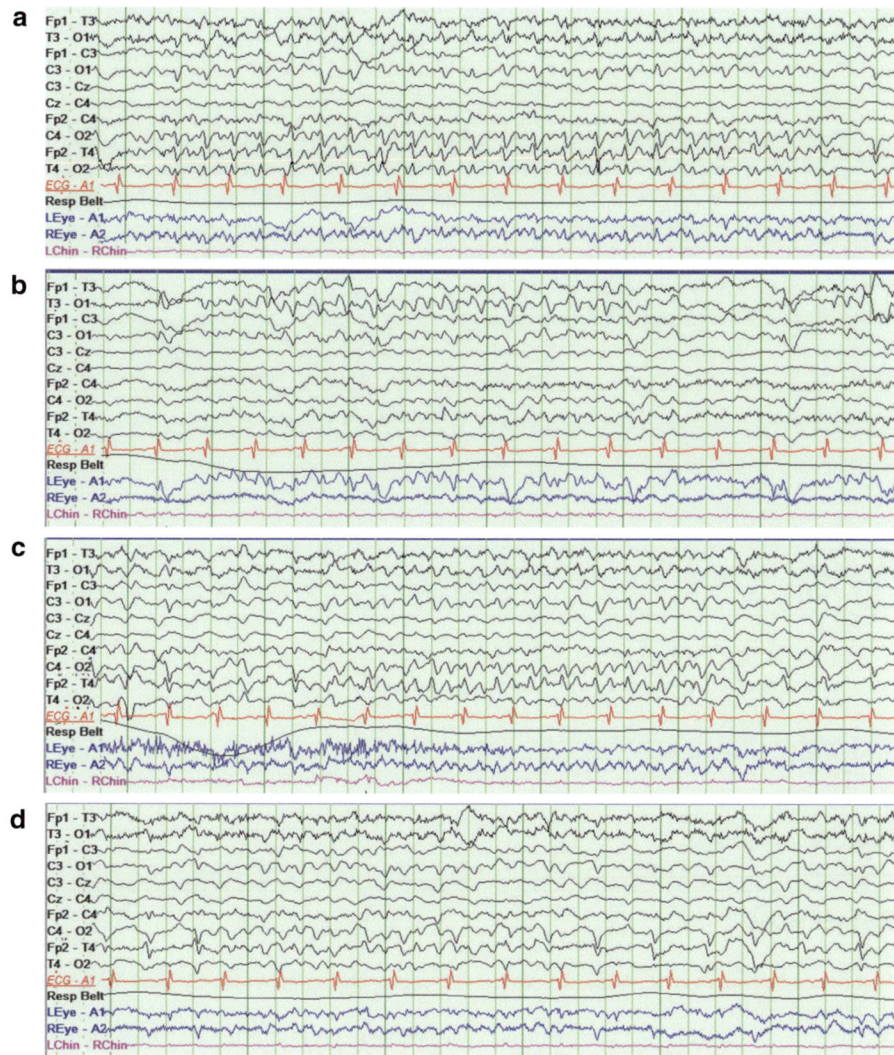

Fig. 5.19 Alpha frequency seizures in a neonate. This usually signifies a poor prognosis. Apnea is also present, as seen with the flattening of the respiratory lead (**a–g**)

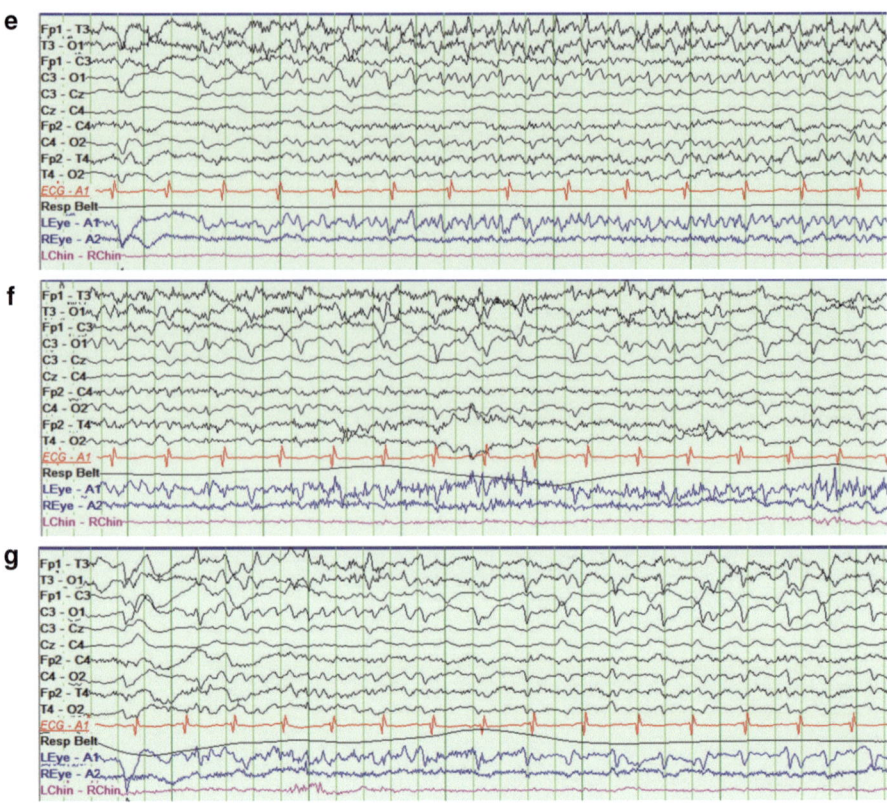

Fig. 5.19 (continued)

References

1. Mizrahi E, Hrachovy R. Atlas of neonatal electroencephalography. 4th ed. New York: Demos Medical; 2016.
2. Niedermeyer E, De Silva FL. Electroencephalopagraphy, basic principles, clinical applications and related fields. Philadelphia: Williams and Wilkins; 1993.
3. Pressler RM, Cilio MR, Mizrahi EM, et al. The ILAE classification of seizures and the epilepsies: modification for seizures in the neonate, position paper by the ILAE Task Force on Neonatal Seizures. Epilepsia. 2021;62(3):615–28.
4. Tsuchida TN, Wusthoff CT, Shellhaas RA, et al. American clinical neurophysiology society standardized EEG terminology and categorization for the description of continuous EEG monitoring in neonates: report of the American clinical neurophysiology society critical care monitoring committee. J Clin Neurophysiol. 2013;30:161–73.

Seizures in Neonates: Clinical Manifestations and Etiology Timeline

6

Jonathan Hanson and Mary Payne

6.1 Introduction

Eighty percent of neonatal seizures occur within the first week of life, regardless of gestational age at birth. Seizures are higher in preterm infants due to the increased risk of hypoxia, infection, and intracranial hemorrhage. This chapter will discuss clinical manifestations of seizures, etiologies, and time frame of occurrence.

6.2 Part 1: Seizure Characteristics—Clinical Manifestations

A. Neonatal seizures are often labeled by their appearance as a description of the type of seizure activity. Certain seizure types are associated with particular pathologies. Meanwhile, there are similar appearing movements that are not epileptic (Table 6.1).

6.2.1 EEG Tidbit

6.2.1.1 Notes About Generalized Seizures

A generalized seizure in an older child or adult can occur from spread through myelinated networks of epileptic activity from a single epileptic focus. Neonates have immature myelination and thus an inability for an epileptic signal to spread from a focal region to bilateral cortical hemispheres. However, neonates can present

---

J. Hanson
University Hospital Center, Bridgeport, WV, USA

M. Payne (✉)
Department of Pediatrics, Division of Pediatric Neurology, Joan C. Edwards School of Medicine, Hoops Family Children's Hospital, Marshall University, Huntington, WV, USA
e-mail: paynem@marshall.edu

Table 6.1 Clinical characteristics of neonatal seizures, EEG findings of neonatal seizures, and considerations for other (nonepileptic) etiologies

Type	Clinical characteristics	EEG findings	Nonseizure etiologies (similar clinical presentation)
Tonic	Stiffening: may be entire body or one limb	Fast-frequency spikes Focal discharges correlating to clinical event and correlate with anatomy	Can also be posturing (response to abnormal brainstem or cortical functioning) or back arching seen with irritability, gastric reflux
Clonic	Rhythmic, repetitive contractions One limb, multiple limbs	Focal epileptiform discharges at the same time as the clonic movements of the seizure and correlate with anatomy	Clonus, stimulated or spontaneous
Myoclonic	Rapid muscle contraction, may be one limb or generalized	Focal or generalized epileptic discharges Typically high amplitude and slow frequency	Exaggerated startle reflex, spinal myoclonus, benign sleep myoclonus
Subtle/automatisms[a]	Chewing, sucking, bicycling of legs	Focal epileptiform discharges	Nonepileptic behaviors
Autonomic[a]	Change in heart rate, pupil reaction, temperature, blood pressure, or presence of apnea	Focal epileptiform discharges	Other systemic issues
Behavioral arrest[a]	Pause of movement	Focal epileptiform discharges	Nonepileptic behavior, encephalopathy
Sequential seizure	Any of the above seizure types either moving to one body part to another or a mixture of seizure types occurring concurrently or consecutively	Focal epileptiform discharges, changing cortical location within the same seizure event, correlating with the clinical change	Not applicable
Electrographic only seizure	No clinical change noted, only EEG shows seizure activity, also in paralyzed neonates	Focal discharges, fast-frequency spikes, generalized spikes	Not applicable

[a]Subtle, autonomic, and behavioral arrest seizures are typically associated with other seizure types (tonic, clonic, myoclonic). Similar appearing movements may occur without an electrographic epileptic correlate and thus not considered to be an epileptic event. In this case, an EEG can help distinguish epileptic and nonepileptic events and help guide treatment. In addition, if behaviors such as automatisms, autonomic changes or behavioral arrest occur with stimulation or can be suppressed by stimulation, they are likely not epileptic

with a sequential seizure [International League Against Epilepsy (ILAE)] in which there is spread of seizure activity from one cortical region to another, as seen electrographically and clinically. Seizures can spread in this way rather quickly, sometimes to two different regions showing two distinct epileptic activities at the same time. At the bedside, the infant may appear to have a generalized convulsive seizure as what would be recognized as generalized in an older child/adult. This distinction may be confusing to the medical staff and family.

An exception to the above generalization is myoclonic seizures, which can be focal or truly generalized. The generalized myoclonic movements correlate with generalized epileptiform discharges (involving both hemispheres simultaneously at onset). However, this phenomenon is thought to be due to the rapid spread of deeper neural networks and not from secondary spread through myelin networks.

B. Correlating cortical, electrographic, and clinical seizure semiology.

Scalp electrode location correlates with the underlying brain region that produces electrical signals and seizure activity (Figs. 6.1 and 6.2). The use of continuous video EEG monitoring can help identify the exact time frame of electrographic waveforms and clinical changes in the patient. For example, electrographically, a seizure may start in the left temporal region, then spread to the

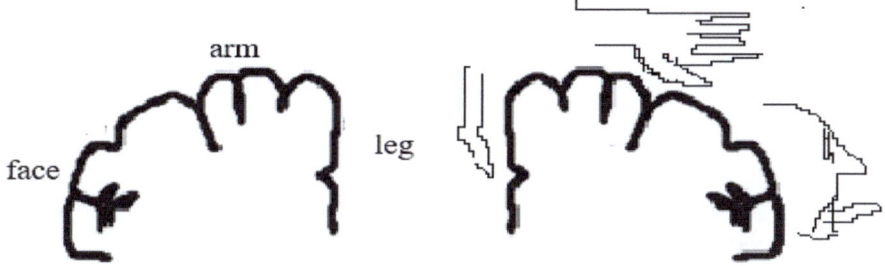

Fig. 6.1 The homunculus is an anatomical representation of the motor movements correlating with cortical regions. The feet are midline and deeper along the frontal lobe, so the EEG leads may not show initial epileptiform activity in these deeper frontal regions

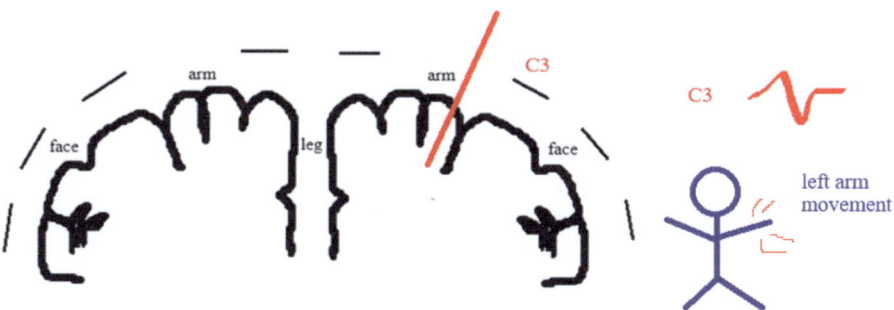

Fig. 6.2 Humunculus with EEG scalp electrodes and seizure focality

left frontal region. Clinical change in the patient may not be apparent until the seizure has spread to the left frontal region, the left motor cortex, producing right-side clonic activity.

6.3   Part 2: Etiologies and Time Course of Neonatal Seizures

A. List of Seizure Etiologies in Neonates [2, 5]
- Hypoxic-ischemic encephalopathy—Most common cause of neonatal seizures, approximately as frequent as occurring in 50% of neonates with seizures. These seizures occur within the first 12–24 h of life. However, seizures may also occur during therapeutic hypothermia or while rewarming from therapeutic hypothermia. In addition, up to 80% of these seizures are subclinical (only detected by EEG recording). Seizures tend to be multifocal, so they originate in many regions due to the underlying pathology of diffuse ischemic injury.
- Ischemic stroke—Second most common cause of neonatal seizures, about 10–20% of seizure patients and etiology can be arterial or venous infarctions. These seizures tend to occur after the first 12 h of life. These babies may or may not be encephalopathic and seizure location correlates with area of lesion, manifesting as focal clonic.
- Intracranial hemorrhage—Third most common cause of neonatal seizures, accounting for 10–15% of full-term neonatal seizures and 30% of preterm neonatal seizures. Seizures correlate with the region of hemorrhage and are typically focal clonic. Time of seizure onset varies [3].
- Types of hemorrhages:
  - Intracerebral
  - Subarachnoid
  - Germinal matrix/intraventricular
  - Subdural—associated with trauma often, so timing correlates with time of trauma
  - Subpial—bleeding within the space between the cortex and the pia
- Intracranial infection—Congenital infections or acute, new-onset infections. These seizures typically present at infection onset or peak. Seizure origin can be focal or multifocal, depending on the extent of infectious injury and other related factors.
- Bilirubin encephalopathy—Seizures with kernicterus start 2–7 days after birth, likely due to the time required for unconjugated bilirubin to accumulate in the brain after crossing the blood–brain barrier. Deposits of bilirubin cause localized epileptic regions.
- Glut 1 deficiency—Glucose transporter deficiency, in which there is poor transport of glucose into the CSF by the glucose transporter. CSF shows extremely low glucose levels. These seizures usually occur within a few days of birth. In addition to traditional anti-epileptic medications, the ketogenic diet is used as a treatment and may help seizure control.
- Seizures associated with ECMO extracorporeal membrane oxygenation—Use of ECMO in neonates with congenital heart disease or other causes of

cardiopulmonary disease. Frequent seizures (up to 10%) postoperatively on ECMO and most seizures are subclinical. Challenges for diagnosis and treatment may be compounded by the use of sedatives and paralytics. Seizures are likely related to the combination of many factors, including hypoxia, infection, inflammation, and stroke.
- Drug withdrawal—Typically from in utero exposure to opiates, benzodiazepines, and barbiturates.
- Cortical dysplasia, neurocutaneous syndrome—Tend to begin after immediate postnatal time period.
- Metabolic abnormalities/inborn errors of metabolism [1, 9]
  – Hypocalcemia—Seizures tend to begin on the day of life 2 or 3 and occur in low-birthweight babies and babies of diabetic mothers. Later onset, weeks to months later, hypocalcemia seizures are from the infant drinking milk with low calcium.
  – Hypoglycemia—Seizures tend to occur on day of life 2 and occur in small newborns or infants of diabetic mothers.
  – Hypomagnesemia—Seizure onset 2–6 weeks of age, occurs from a defect of magnesium absorption.
  – Hyponatremia—May co-occur with other cerebral pathology leading to inappropriate antidiuretic hormone secretion or in an older infant with intake of excessive free water.
  – Vitamin K deficiency-related seizures: Due to insufficient vitamin K at birth (breastfed infants who did not get prophylaxis at birth). Seizures will start 24–72 h after birth. Seizures are usually due to intracranial hemorrhage or infarction from vitamin K deficiency coagulopathies.
  – Vitamin D deficiency: Causes include maternal vitamin D deficiency, inadequate sun exposure, or poor intake of vitamin D. Seizures usually start weeks to months after birth and may be associated with tetany, irritability, and hypocalcemia.
  – Pyridoxine (B6)-dependent epilepsy. Seizures usually start within hours to days after birth. Seizures are often refractory and do not respond well to anti-epileptic medications. Trial of intravenous or oral pyridoxine can be performed.
  – Thiamine (B1) deficiency: Results from maternal malnutrition, hyperemesis gravidarum, and exclusive breastfeeding in a B1-deficient mother. Seizures usually start days to weeks after birth. Seizures can occur in the setting of encephalopathy and metabolic acidosis.
  – Folinic acid (B9) deficiency: Cerebral folate deficiency syndromes, very rare. These respond to folinic acid 0.5–1.0 mg daily. Cause includes disorder of autoimmune folate antibodies: Seizures around 4 months of age, with irritability and sleep disturbances. Later, patients develop movement disorders. Serum contains antibodies to folate CSF shows low MTHF levels.
  – Biotinidase (B7) deficiency: Autosomal-recessive inheritance of a mutation of biotinidase gene on chromosome 3 and is considered a neurocutaneous metabolic disorder. Patients present with seizures, hypotonia, auditory and visual abnormalities, eczema, and alopecia. Neurocutaneous

features (atopic/seborrheic dermatitis, alopecia, hypopigmentation of the hair or skin, fungal skin infections) develop around 2–5 months but presentation could be as late as adulthood.
- B12 deficiency—Patients of vegan mothers who exclusively breastfeed infants and seizures present around 4–8 months of age. Other symptoms include neurodevelopmental delay, failure to thrive, irritability, hypotonia, tremor, choreoathetosis, and microcephaly.
- Other inborn errors of metabolism.
- Amino acidopathies, organic acidemias urea cycle disorders, peroxisomal disorders, and lysosomal storage disorders usually present with lethargy and poor feeding prior to seizure onset. Symptoms tend to occur within the first 72 hours of birth; however, if feeding initiation has been postponed due to other medical reasons, presentation of lethargy and seizures may be delayed.
- General timeline of specific disorders
  - Within 24 h: urea cycle disorders, maple syrup urine disease, pyruvate dehydrogenase deficiency, and nonketotic hyperglycinemia.
  - 24–72 h: urea cycle disorders (after feeding), organic acidemias, galactosemia, and nonketotic hyperglycinemia.
  - Beyond 72 h: phenylketonuria, mitochondrial disorders, peroxisomal disorders, lysosomal storage disorders, late-onset urea cycle disorders, and organic acidemias.
- Diagnostic clues based on the time of seizure onset
  - Immediate or soon after birth: severe metabolic acidosis, hypo/hyperglycemia, and hyperammonemia.
  - Post-feeding seizures: galactosemia, maple syrup urine disease, and organic acidemias.
  - Progressive seizures: mitochondrial and lysosomal storage disorders.
- Nonketotic hyperglycinemia—One of the amino acid disorders. Important to acknowledge separately due to the occurrence of seizures in utero, which may be interpreted to be hiccoughs. NKH tends to produce a burst suppression background pattern with myoclonic seizures. Treatment includes traditional anti-epileptic medications and the ketogenic diet.
- Specific epileptic syndromes, to be discussed in Part 3.

B. Time of Seizure Onset Based on Etiology

Time of seizure occurrence varies based on etiology and the underlying metabolic, neuronal, and synaptic dysregulations. For example, some genetic disorders with epilepsy are due to abnormal receptors or signaling pathways, creating abnormal responses to inhibitory neurotransmitters and poor ability for neuronal repolarization. Time of onset of seizure presentation can vary based on the impact of these underlying abnormalities. This chart (Table 6.2) is for general purposes only, and there may be times when a certain seizure etiology has a different time of seizure onset than what is listed below. Thus, clinical scenarios may warrant evaluation of other etiologies that may not correspond with the time frames below.

Table 6.2 Time of neonatal seizure onset based on etiology

Etiology	<24 h	24–72 h	>72 h
HIE	✓	✓	✓
Ischemic stroke	✓	✓	✓
SAH		✓	✓
SDH	✓	✓	✓
IVH (term)	✓		
IVH (preterm)	✓	✓	
Intracranial hemorrhage (all types in general)	✓	✓	
Intracerebral infection	✓	✓	✓
Hypocalcemia		✓	✓
Hypoglycemia	✓	✓	✓
Hypomagnesemia			✓
Hyponatremia	✓	✓	✓
Vitamin K deficiency	✓	✓	✓
Vitamin D deficiency			✓
Vitamin B6 related	✓	✓	✓
Vitamin B1 deficiency			✓
Vitamin B12 deficiency			✓
Vitamin B9 deficiency			✓
Vitamin B7 deficiency			✓
Bilirubin encephalopathy			✓
Glut 1 transporter	✓	✓	✓
Aminoacidopathies	✓	✓	✓
Organic acidopathies	✓	✓	✓
Intrauterine infection, sepsis	✓	✓	✓
Cortical dysplasia			✓
Neurocutaneous syndrome			✓
Drug withdrawal			✓
SELFNE/SELFNIE/SELNE			✓
EIDEE, EIMFS	✓	✓	✓

EIDEE early infantile developmental epileptic encephalopathy, *EIMFS* epilepsy in infancy with migrating focal seizures, *HIE* hypoxic-ischemic encephalopathy, *IVH* intraventricular hemorrhage, *SAH* subarachnoid hemorrhage, *SELFNE* self-limited familial neonatal epilepsy, *SELFNIE* self-limited familial neonatal infantile epilepsy, *SELNE* self-limited nonfamilial neonatal epilepsy, *SDH* subdural hematoma

C. Seizures in the Setting of Encephalopathy

Encephalopathy is a term describing an altered mental state and is depicted by abnormal background activity in the EEG recording. In a neonate, altered mental status of lethargy, abnormal feeding, irritability, and poor consoling are associated with a slow or immature background pattern. Sedative medications can alter mental state, which would also correlate with an encephalopathic background. Medication effects should always be considered when assessing for underlying encephalopathy. Sometimes it is not possible to determine baseline mental status until the sedative medications are withdrawn.

The presence of an encephalopathic background activity in a patient with seizures indicates a more severe case of underlying brain dysfunction and can be seen in patients with high seizure burden. Encephalopathy is also present in patients with epileptic encephalopathies and epileptic developmental disorders discussed later in this chapter.

6.4 Part 3: Neonatal Epileptic Syndromes

In any case of neonatal seizures, imaging and infectious and metabolic evaluation is performed to determine the cause of seizures and genetic testing is not usually performed initially. Genetic factors may be considered based on clinical presentation, especially in the case of no other known cause. However, HIE, infections, or other provoking factors can also occur in patients with genetic neonatal epilepsy, and some studies report a higher rate of chromosome abnormalities in neonates with HIE [11]. Neonatal seizures from genetic causes can fall into two main categories based on prognosis. In the self-limited epilepsies, seizures resolve in infancy and development is normal. In the severe types, seizures are usually lifelong and neurodevelopmental outcomes are poor. Self-limited genetic epilepsies tend to present with seizures after the first day of life, seizures are usually focal, and baseline EEG background activity is normal. Conversely, seizures in patients with severe genetic epilepsy can begin on the first day of life, be of mixed type, and occur amidst an abnormal baseline EEG background activity [4].

Diagnosis of a syndrome is based on

- Patient demographics—in this case neonate
- EEG findings
- Clinical seizure characteristics

Benefit of identifying a syndrome

- Helps guide treatment
- Helps guide prognosis
- Improves accuracy of counseling for families and medical team

A. Neonatal Epilepsies with Normal EEG Background Patterns and a Good Prognosis

These cases of genetic neonatal seizures are fortunately benign, in the way that these neonates may not need treatment with anti-epileptic medications or, if they do, treatment duration is brief (Tables 6.3 and 6.6). The infants have normal development, and the seizures resolve within a few months of life. Important, however, to realize is that the interictal EEG tracing is normal. That is, the EEG will show state changes between wakefulness, active sleep, and quiet sleep. Likewise, the infant will clinically show these state changes as well. If the background activity appears to be immature or encephalopathic, then reconsideration of the diagnosis is warranted.

1. Self-limited familial neonatal epilepsy (SELFNE), previously known as benign familial neonatal seizures (Figs. 6.3 and 6.4)
2. Self-limited nonfamilial neonatal epilepsy (SELNE)
   Difference between SELFNE and SELNE is the presence of family history. SELFNE has a family history and SELNE does not. Both can be from genetic etiologies, however.
3. Self-limited familial neonatal-infantile epilepsy (SELFNIE)

Table 6.3 Characteristics of self-limited neonatal epilepsies

	SELFNE/SELNE	SELFNIE
Onset of seizures	First week of life but may be later	Day 1 to 7 months of age
Seizure clinical typical	Focal tonic	Focal tonic
Other seizure type	Focal clonic, apneic	Focal clonic
Seizure frequency	Multiple times per day	Multiple times per day
Seizure duration	1–2 min	1–2 min
Ictal EEG	Flattening with apnea and motor movements, then bilateral discharges correlating with clonic activity	Flattening with apnea or focal discharges
Interictal EEG background	Normal	Normal
Interictal EEG epileptiform findings	Focal epileptiform discharges	Focal epileptiform discharges
Prognosis	Good, seizures resolve by 6 months of age. May not need AED, may have febrile seizures later	Good, seizures resolve by 2 years of age. May not need AED
Etiology (genes)	KCNQ2, KCNQ3, SCNA2A	SCN2A
Family history	Yes/no	Yes

AED anti-epileptic drugs, *SELFNE* self-limited familial neonatal epilepsy, *SELFNIE* self-limited familial neonatal infantile epilepsy, *SELNE* self-limited nonfamilial neonatal epilepsy

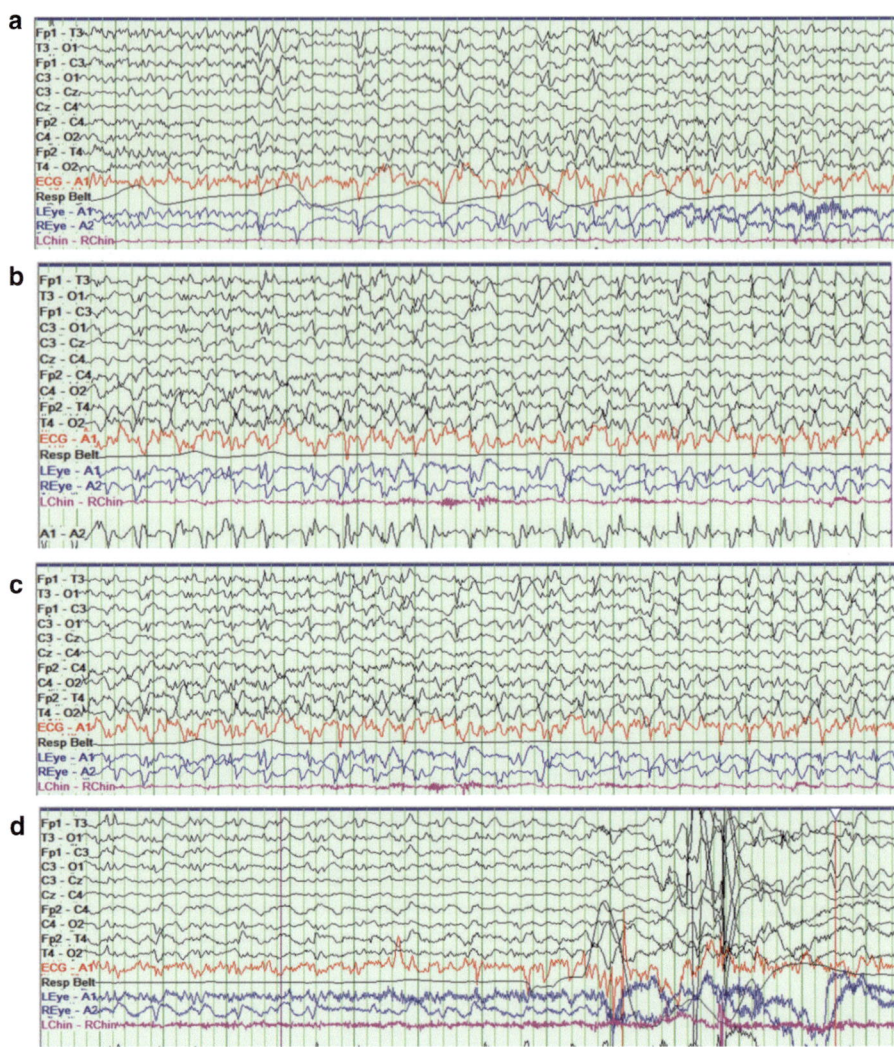

Fig. 6.3 (**a–d**) Self-limited familial neonatal epilepsy (SELFNE) example of electrographic seizure. During this seizure, there is significant apnea as seen by no movement in the respiratory lead. Bilateral discharges are seen within the seizure and patient's seizure is reported to be right, then left, clonic activity with apnea

6.4.1 Note About Benign Nonfamilial Neonatal Convulsions (Fifth-Day Fits) or Benign Idiopathic Neonatal Seizures

This syndrome is no longer considered an epilepsy syndrome by the ILAE; however, it is still recognized as a constellation of findings that are included in those of the self-limited epilepsies defined by the ILAE. Seizures begin in the first week of life, typically the fifth day. Seizures are clonic or tonic, with apnea and neonates often present

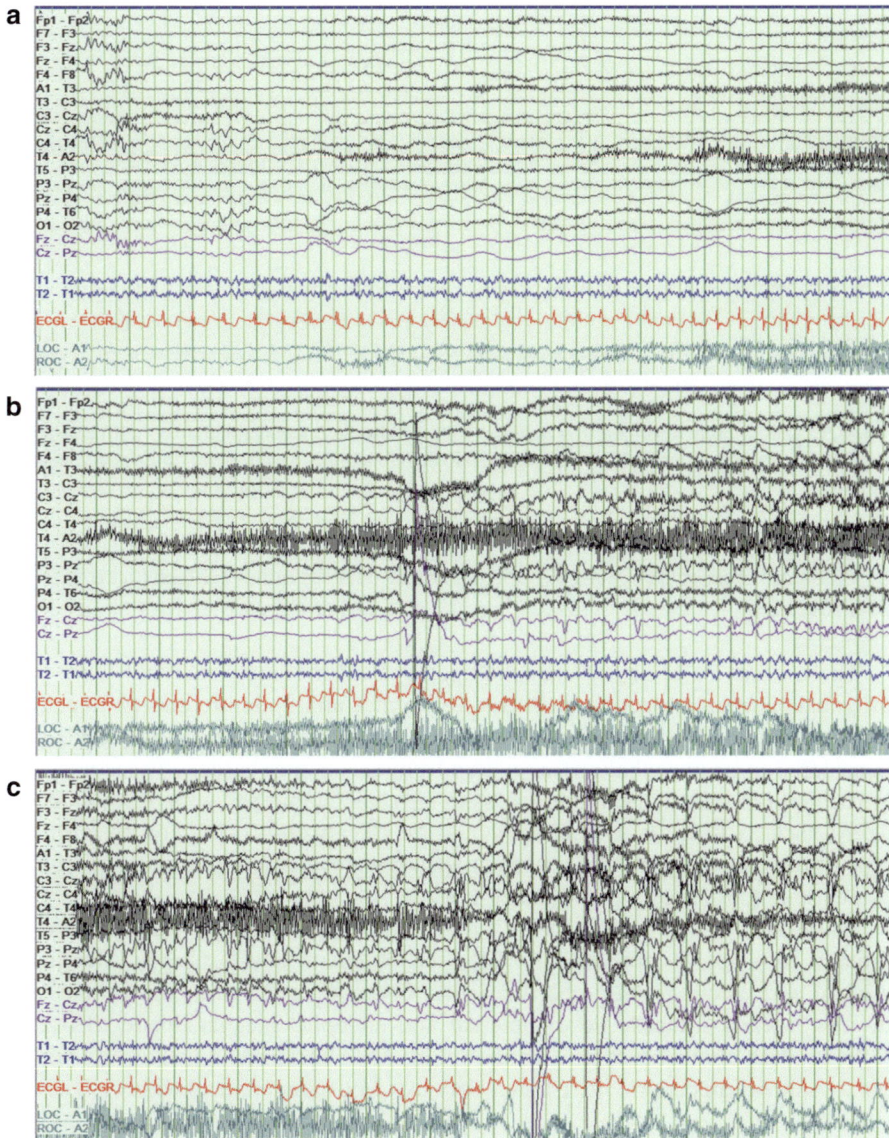

Fig. 6.4 (a–c) Self-limited familial neonatal epilepsy (SELFNE) example of electrographic seizure with attenuation. During this seizure, generalized attenuation precedes the electrographic epileptic event. Patient's seizures were described as clonic

with status epilepticus. This ictal EEG can show attenuation (Fig. 6.4) while a distinctive interictal background finding has been termed theta pointu alternant, in which bursts of sharply contoured theta activity are interrupted by low-amplitude periods of attenuation (Fig. 6.5). Early studies identifying this syndrome may have misidentified neonates with viral encephalitis or a nonfamilial type of epilepsy [4].

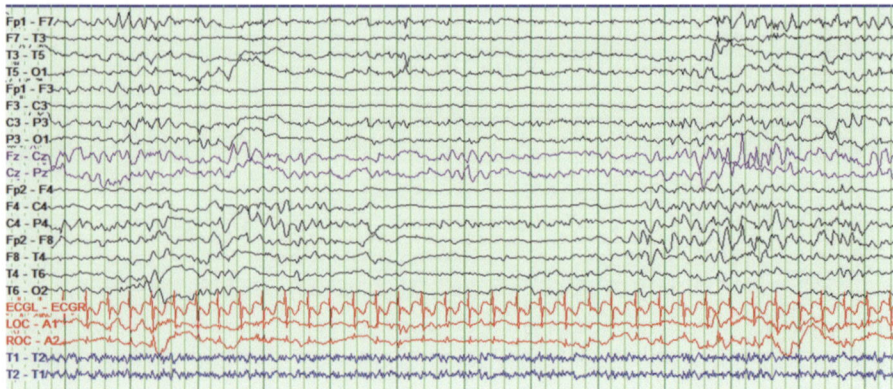

Fig. 6.5 Theta pointu alternant in a neonate with self-limited neonatal epilepsy. Diffuse sharply contoured theta activity is interrupted by generalized attenuation, an interictal finding seen in these patients

B. Neonatal Epilepsies with Abnormal EEG Background Patterns and a Poor Prognosis

These cases of epileptic encephalopathy are fortunately rare but have poor prognosis and are categorized as developmental and epileptic encephalopathies (DEE) by the updated ILAE criteria in 2022 (Table 6.6). The background is thus considered to be encephalopathic with a frequent seizure burden. These neonates are difficult to treat and often progress to intractable epilepsy with developmental delay, such as in Lennox–Gastaut syndrome. Evaluation of a neonate with this type of presentation includes extensive metabolic evaluations, cerebrospinal fluid evaluation, neuroimaging, and genetic testing.

The ILAE in 2022 combined early myoclonic encephalopathy (EME) and early infantile epileptic encephalopathy (EIEE or Ohtahara) due to frequent overlap in clinical and electrographic characteristics. The new term comprising both syndromes is early infantile developmental and epileptic encephalopathy (EIDEE). Both of these clinical scenarios consist of an EEG background activity showing a burst suppression pattern, interrupted only by electrographic ictal activity. There is

Table 6.4 Comparison of Ohtahara and EME epileptic syndromes, now combined to be termed early infantile developmental and epileptic encephalopathy (EIDEE)

	Ohtahara (EIEE)	EME
Time of onset of seizures	First week of life	First week of life
Gender	Male more common	No gender difference
Interictal pattern	Burst suppression	Burst suppression
Length of bursts	5–10 s	1–5 s
Length of suppression	3–5 s	3–10 s
Seizures—clinical typical	Tonic mostly, 1–20 s	Myoclonic mostly
Seizures—electrographic	Low-amplitude fast activity Multifocal discharges	High-amplitude spikes Multifocal discharges
Seizures—clinical also seen	Focal clonic Fragmented tonic	Focal clonic Fragmented myoclonic
Etiology	Genetic and/or IEM	Genetic and/or IEM
Prognosis	Poor, developmental delay, epilepsy, encephalopathy	Poor, developmental delay, epilepsy, encephalopathy

Panayiotopoulos [6] and Volpe et al. [10]
EIEE early infantile epileptic encephalopathy, *EME* early myoclonic encephalopathy

no state change, so the neonate does not clinically demonstrate waking and sleep and the EEG does not show state changes either.

Listed in the chart below are the typical EME and EIEE features, which historically have been distinguished as two separate syndromes (Table 6.4).

1. Ohtahara syndrome (early infantile epileptic encephalopathy).
2. Early myoclonic encephalopathy (Figs. 6.6 and 6.7).
3. Epilepsy in infancy with migrating focal seizures (EIMFS), previously malignant migrating partial seizures of infancy (Tables 6.5 and 6.6 and Figs. 6.8 and 6.9).

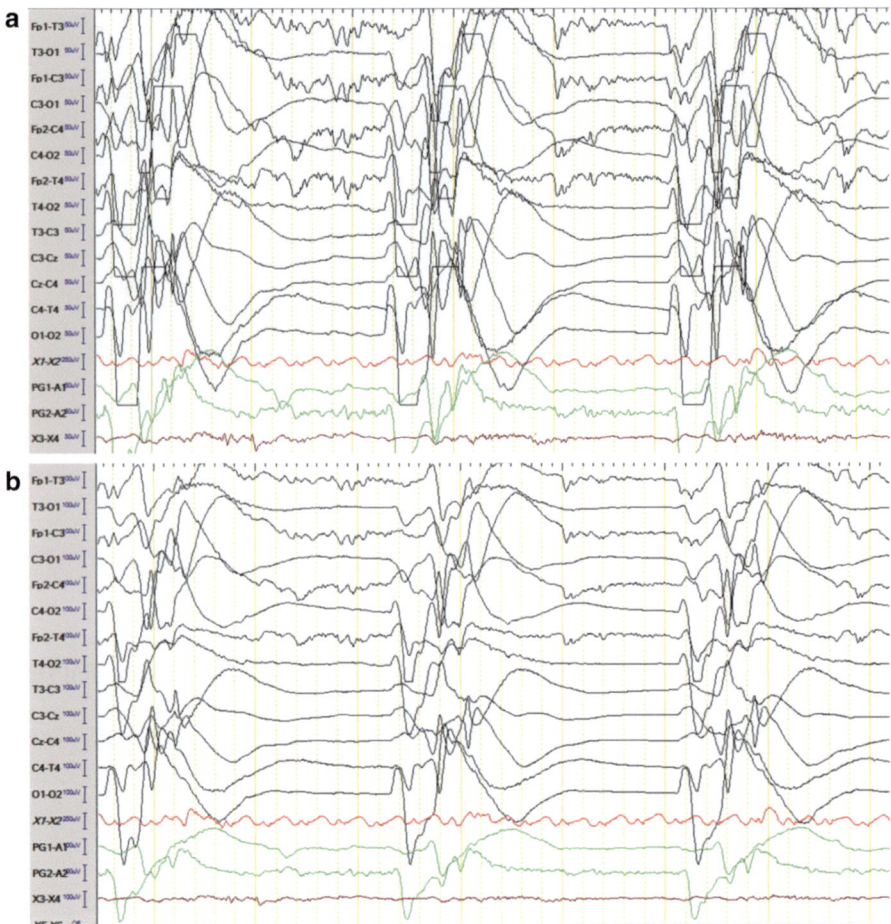

Fig. 6.6 (**a**, **b**) Early myoclonic encephalopathy. Background activity is burst suppression and bursts are high-amplitude epileptiform spikes associated with myoclonic movements. (**a**) (sensitivity = 7 μV). (**b**) Early myoclonic encephalopathy. Background activity is burst suppression and bursts are high-amplitude epileptiform spikes associated with myoclonic movements. (**b**) (sensitivity = 20 μV). Same patient as Fig. 6.4

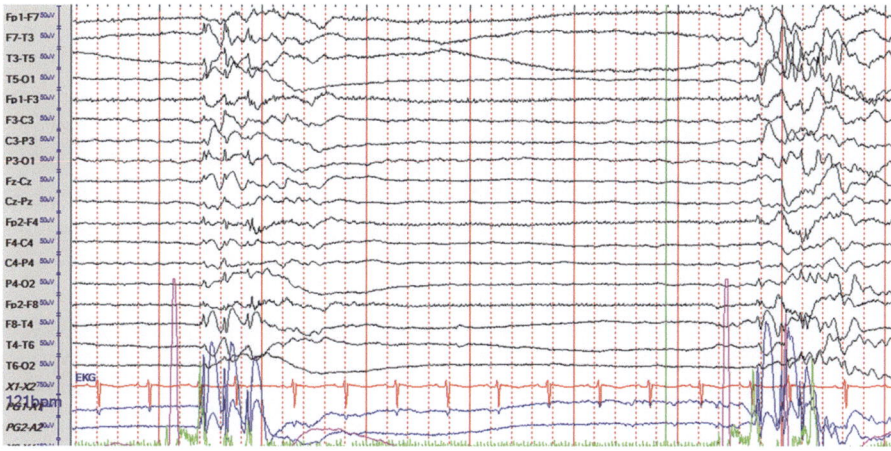

Fig. 6.7 Early myoclonic encephalopathy. Background activity is burst suppression and bursts are moderate-amplitude epileptiform spikes associated with several myoclonic movements (sensitivity = 7 μV)

Table 6.5 Characteristics of EIMFS

	EIMFS
Time of onset of seizures	Months 1–3
Interictal pattern	Normal, then burst suppression, slowing
	Multifocal discharges
Seizures—clinical typical	Focal, migrating pattern
Seizures—electrographic	Multifocal epileptiform discharges during one seizure
Seizures—clinical also seen	Status epilepticus
Etiology (genes)	KCNT1 most common, also SCN1A, SCN2A, SLC12A5, BRAT1, TBC1D24
Prognosis	Poor, developmental delay, epilepsy, encephalopathy

EIMFS epilepsy in infancy with migrating focal seizures

Table 6.6 Summarizing neonatal seizure types with associated background findings

Normal background	Abnormal background: nonspecific encephalopathy	Abnormal background: epileptic encephalopathies
SELNE/SELFNE	HIE—more severe	EME
SELFNIE	Use of AED or sedative meds	Ohtahara
HIE—mild	Focal seizures with other ongoing pathology to cause decreased alertness	Other DEE
Focal seizures of other etiologies	Focal seizures of other etiologies with high seizure burden to cause decreased alertness	EIMFS

Pina-Garza and James [7] and Pressler et al. [8]

AED anti-epileptic drugs, *DEE* developmental epileptic encephalopathy, *EIMFS* epilepsy in infancy with migrating focal seizures, *EME* early myoclonic encephalopathy, *HIE* hypoxic-ischemic encephalopathy, *SELFNE* self-limited familial neonatal epilepsy, *SELFNIE*, self-limited familial neonatal infantile epilepsy, *SELNE* self-limited nonfamilial neonatal epilepsy

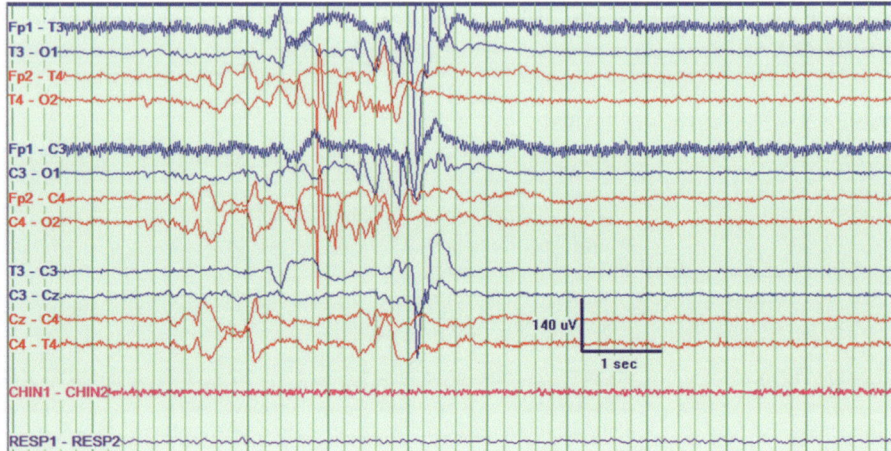

Fig. 6.8 Patient with migrating focal seizures in which the interictal background activity is burst suppression

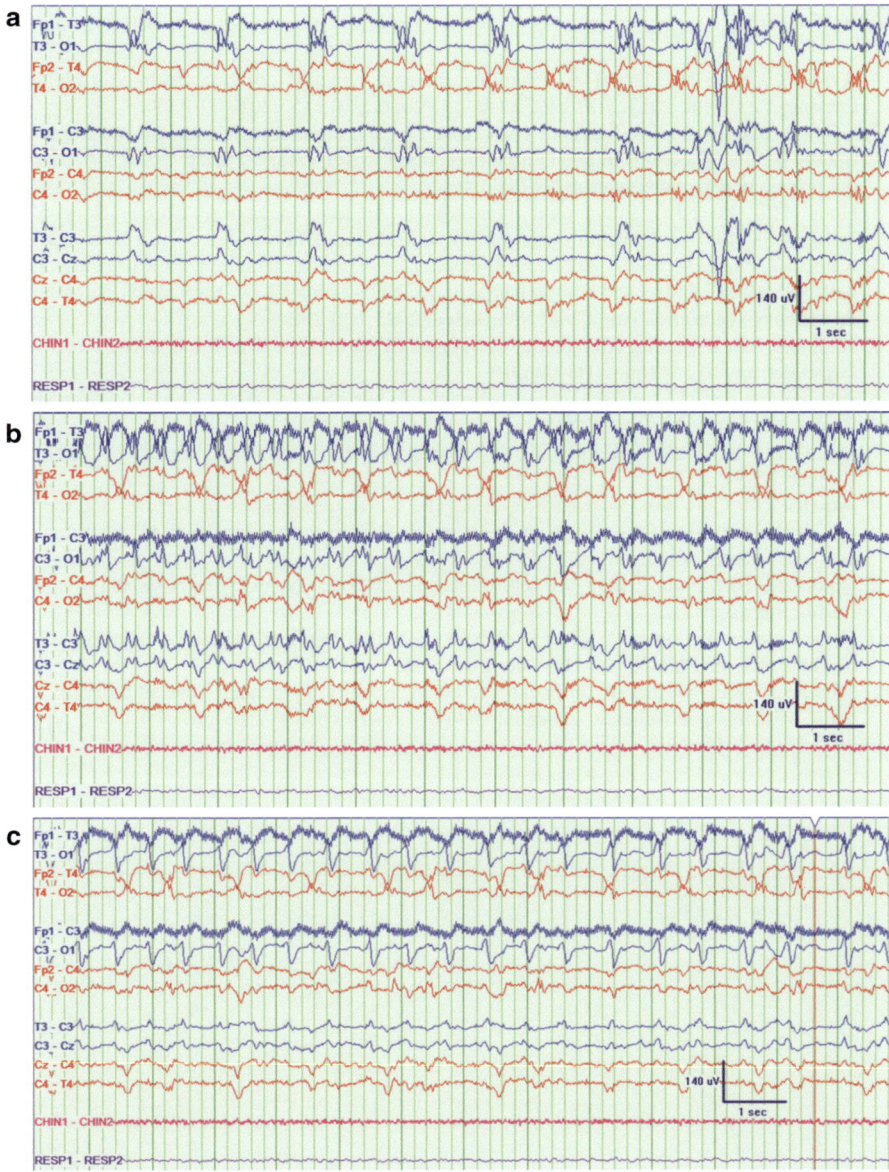

Fig. 6.9 (**a–c**) Patient with migrating focal seizures in which the ictal (seizure) activity consists of multiple focal seizures concurrently. Left hemisphere seizure (C3, T5, O1 leads) is at a different harmony than the right hemisphere seizure (C4, T4 leads), which suggests two distinct focal seizures. This figure depicts the first part of the seizure. (**b**) Patient with migrating focal seizures. Continuation of seizure. (**c**) Patient with migrating focal seizures. Further continuation of seizure

References

1. Agadi S, Quach M, Haneef Z. Vitamin responsive epileptic encephalopathies in children. Epilepsy Res Treat. 2013;2013:510529. https://doi.org/10.1155/2013/510529.
2. Glass HC, Shellhaas RA, Tsuchida TN, Chang T, et al. Epidemiological, diagnostic and evolutionary profile of seizures in young infants at Albert Royer. Open J Pediatr. 2024;14(6) https://doi.org/10.1016/j.pediatrneurol.2017.04.016.
3. Hong HS, Lee JY. Intracranial hemorrhage in term neonates. Childs Nerv Syst. 2018;34(6):1135–43. https://doi.org/10.1007/s00381-018-3788-8.
4. Kannan V, Pareek A, Das A, et al. "Fifth-day fits" revisited: a literature review of benign idiopathic neonatal seizures and comparison with KCNQ2- and KCNQ3-associated benign familial epilepsy syndromes. Ann Child Neurol Soc. 2023;1(3):202–8.
5. Karamian AG, DiGiovine MP, Massey SL. Neonatal seizures. Pediatr Rev. 2024;45(7):381–93. https://doi.org/10.1542/pir.2023-006016.
6. Panayiotopoulos CP. A clinical guide to epileptic syndromes and their treatment. Oxfordshire: Bladon Medical Publishing; 2002.
7. Pina-Garza JE, James KC. Fenichel's clinical pediatric neurology. 9th ed. Philadelphia: Elsevier; 2024.
8. Pressler RM, Cilio MR, Mizrahi EM, et al. The ILAE classification of seizures and the epilepsies: modification for seizures in the neonate. Position paper by the ILAE task force on neonatal seizures. Epilepsia. 2021;62(3):615–28.
9. Saudubray J-M, Baumgartner MR, et al. Inborn metabolic diseases: diagnosis and treatment. Berlin: Springer; 2022.
10. Volpe J, Inder T, Darras B, Vries L, Plessis A, Neil J, Perlman J. Volpe's neurology of the newborn. 6th ed. Philadelphia: Elsevier Inc; 2025.
11. Woodward KE, Murthy P, Mineyko A, et al. Identifying genetic susceptibility in neonates with hypoxic-ischemic encephalopathy: a restrosepctive case series. J Child Neurol. 2023;38(1–2):16–24.

Common Artifacts of Neonatal EEG Recordings

Mary Payne and Kristen Newcomer

7.1 Introduction

Artifacts can be mistaken for electrographic seizure activity because they may be rhythmic in nature. Some artifacts have typical patterns and can be identified rather confidently. However, causes of unusual artifact activity can sometimes be discerned through the use of video recording, witnessing the activity in person, or having the EEG technician or medical personnel document different movements at the bedside. Artifacts can occur from neonatal movements or external sources.

A. Movements of neonates causing artifacts:

 1. Stretch, startle, benign (not epileptic) myoclonus, which could be an exaggerated startle movement or benign sleep myoclonus (Figs. 7.1, 7.2, 7.3, 7.4, 7.5, and 7.6)
 2. Hiccoughs (Figs. 7.7 and 7.8)
 3. Sucking movements (Figs. 7.9, 7.10, 7.11 and 7.12)
 4. Jitteriness, tremor—these movements are usually faster than clonic seizures and stop when the shaking limb is touched or repositioned (Fig. 7.13)

B. Environmental/physiological artifacts

 1. Eye movement (Figs. 7.14, 7.15, 7.16, 7.17, 7.18 and 7.19)
 2. ECG lead (Figs. 7.20, 7.21 and 7.22)
 3. Pulse (Figs. 7.23 and 7.24)

M. Payne (✉)
Department of Pediatrics, Division of Pediatric Neurology, Joan C. Edwards School of Medicine, Hoops Family Children's Hospital, Marshall University, Huntington, WV, USA
e-mail: paynem@marshall.edu

K. Newcomer
WVU Medicine Children's Hospital, Neurodiagnostic Clinical Preceptor, Morgantown, WV, USA

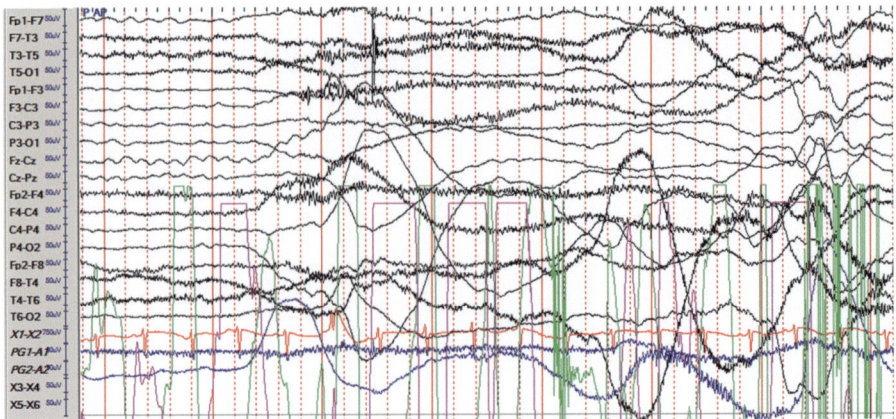

Fig. 7.1 Muscle artifact on EEG recording
Example of muscle and movement artifact occurring during an arousal. Movement artifact occurs with higher amplitude waveforms and overriding fast muscle activity. Muscles generate electrical potentials that are faster than cortical potentials, resulting in a superimposed fast activity. The larger waveforms correlate with big amplitude body movements and the smaller, lower amplitude fast activity correlates with the muscle artifact occurring under that particular electrode. The eye leads, respiratory and chin lead waveforms also show erratic high-amplitude signals, also indicating large whole-body movements

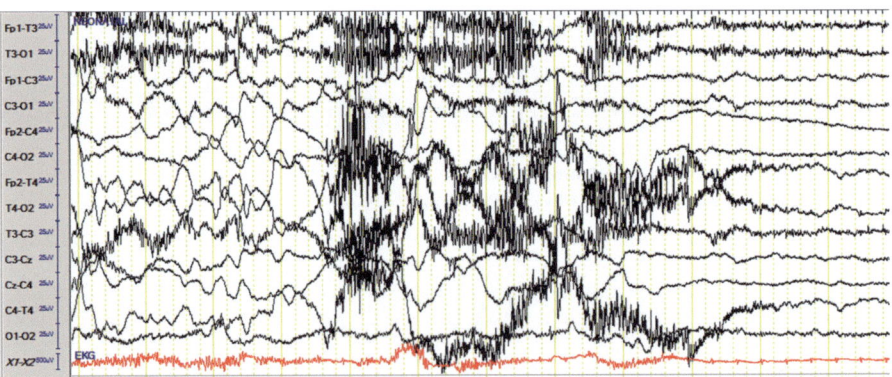

Fig. 7.2 Muscle artifact on EEG recording. This picture demonstrates another example of an arousal with muscle and movement artifact

4. Cardiac pacemaker device (Fig. 7.25)
5. Ventilator/oscillator (Figs. 7.25, 7.26, and 7.27)
6. Patting (Figs. 7.28, 7.29 and 7.30)
7. Rocking (Fig. 7.31)
8. Electrode "pop"—loose lead (Figs. 7.32 and 7.33)
9. Headbox (electrode) adjustment (Fig. 7.34)

7 Common Artifacts of Neonatal EEG Recordings

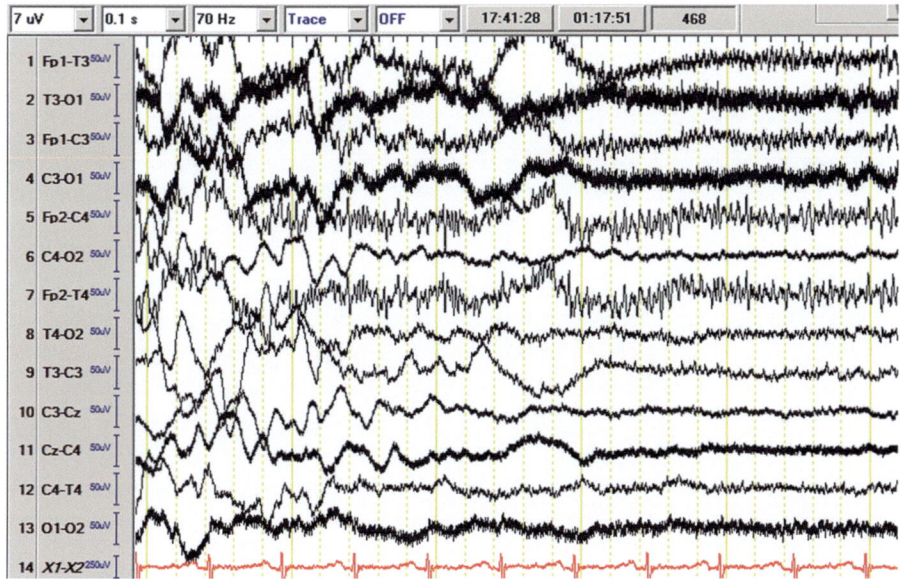

Fig. 7.3 Muscle artifact on EEG recording. Patient is arousing, which is causing attenuation of the background EEG activity. With the arousal, the patient moves, and frontalis muscles are activated, seen as low-amplitude fast activity in frontal leads bilaterally. Muscle activity is faster than 20 Hz and, therefore, is faster than cortical signals. In this image, the high-frequency filter is set at 70 Hz, so all frequencies below 70 Hz will be seen

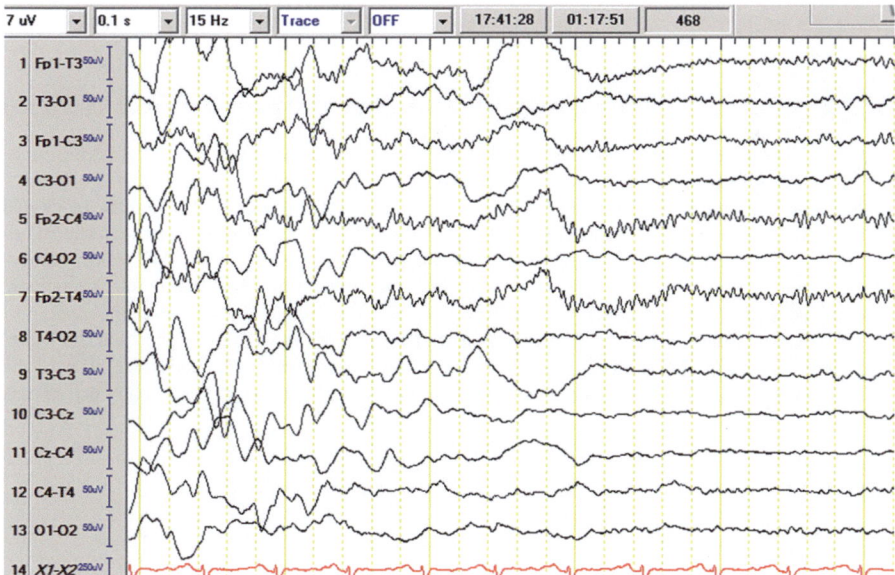

Fig. 7.4 Muscle artifact on EEG recording. Same epoch as in Fig. 7.3; however, the high-frequency filter is lowered to a setting of 15 Hz. This will filter out frequencies greater than 15 Hz, which in this case will eliminate most of the muscle artifact activity. Although beneficial, this can also mask higher frequency cortical potentials

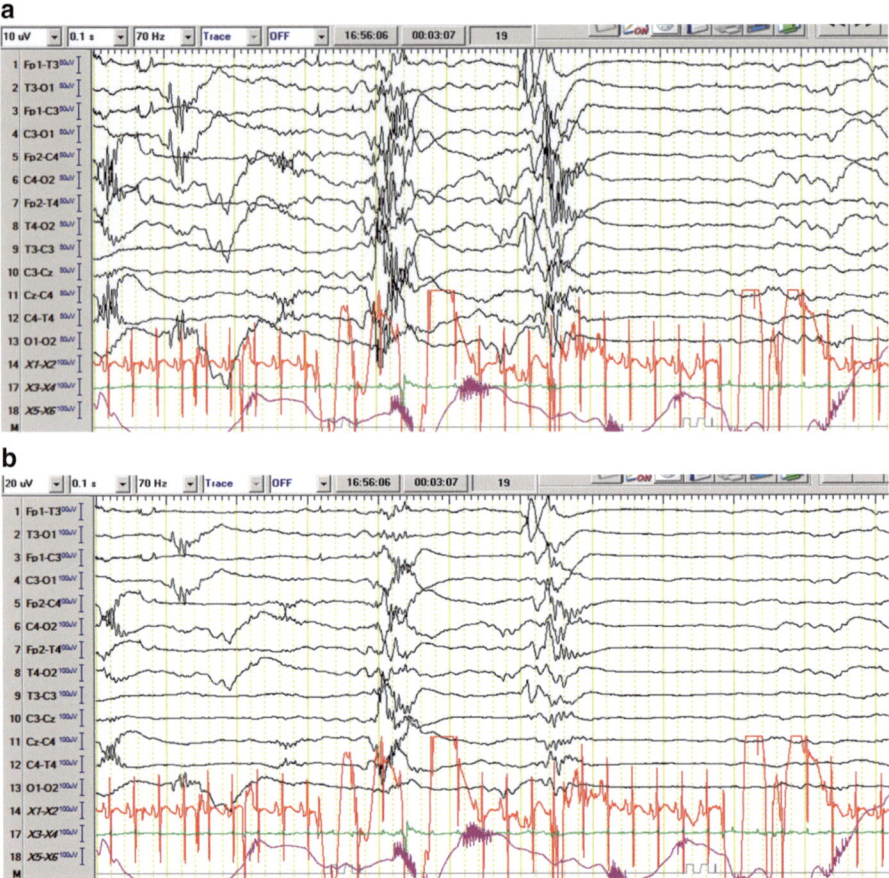

Fig. 7.5 (**a**) Nonepileptic myoclonic movements on EEG. This patient had nonepileptic myoclonic movements as a manifestation of withdrawal symptoms from in utero substance exposure. Meanwhile, the lower chin EMG lead (X5-X6) shows frequent chin movement, and the ECG lead shows artifact at the time of the jerking movements. In addition, the cortical electrodes show sudden high-amplitude movement artifact with superimposed fast muscle artifact. The jerking movements appear to then cause an arousal, as seen with EEG attenuation. (**b**) Nonepileptic myoclonic movements on EEG. Same epoch as Fig. 7.5a, but this view is at a higher sensitivity setting of 20 μV. Changing this setting lowers the waveform height and allows the reader to see the waveforms more distinctly. This can be helpful to decipher artifact from epileptic activity as both can be very high amplitude. However, decreasing the sensitivity setting can also obscure many waveforms

7 Common Artifacts of Neonatal EEG Recordings

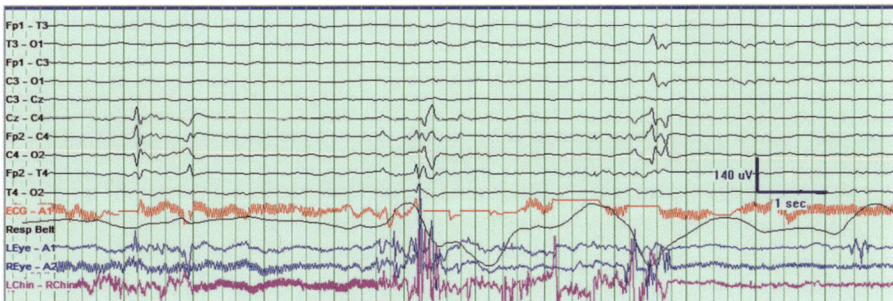

Fig. 7.6 Patient is lying with the right side of the head on the mattress. Nursing staff is pressing on the patient's body and causing artifact on the right side of the head as the head is pressed into the mattress. This would be very difficult to discern without video recording accompanying the study

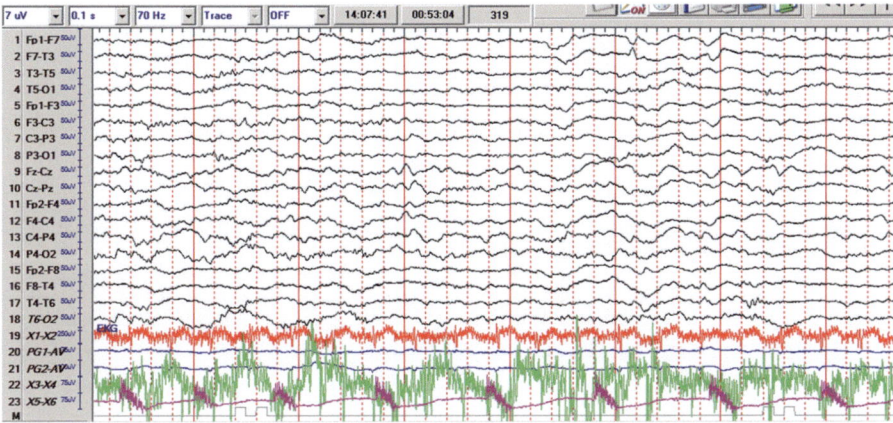

Fig. 7.7 Hiccough artifact on EEG tracing. The chest belt lead (X3-X4) hiccough artifact, corresponding to chest wall movement. Hiccough artifact in the chin EMG lead (X5-X6) follows each chest movement

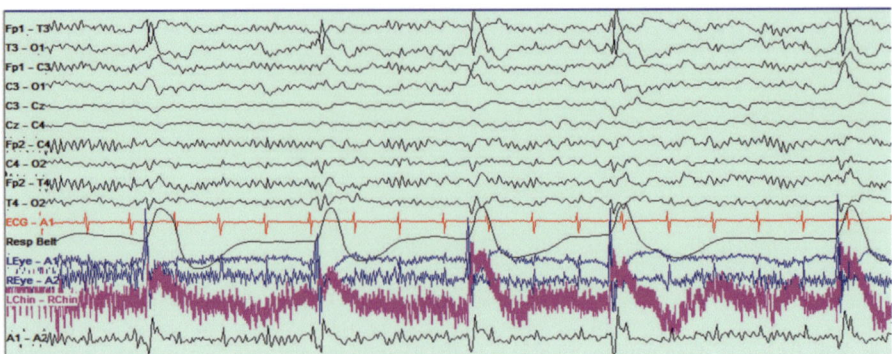

Fig. 7.8 Hiccough artifact on EEG tracing. The respiratory belt lead shows hiccough artifact with corresponding chest wall movement. In this case, the chin EMG lead (L Chin–R Chin) shows corresponding in-time movement artifact with the hiccough. Eye leads and left temporal (T3) lead also show corresponding time-locked movement artifact

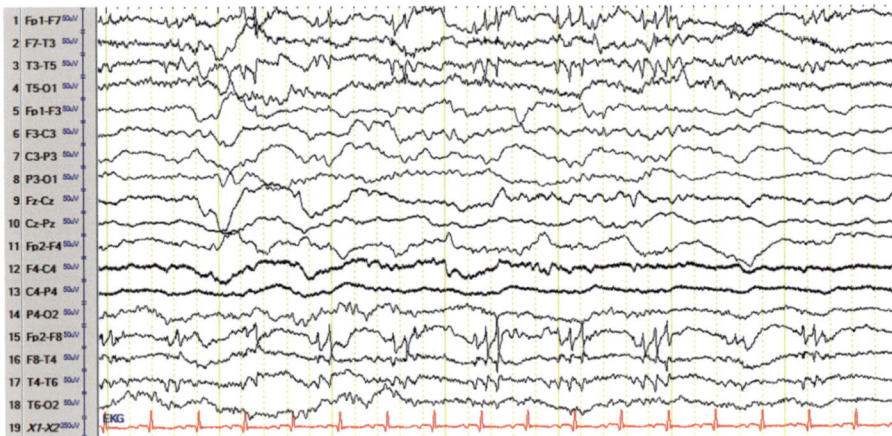

Fig. 7.9 Sucking artifact on EEG tracing. Patient sucking motion, seen as rhythmic muscle artifacts in the frontal and temporal leads

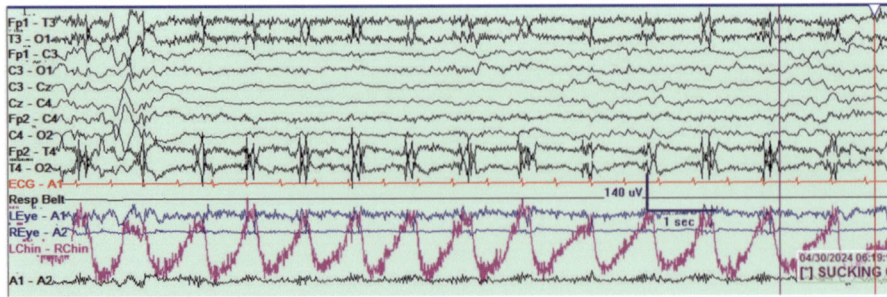

Fig. 7.10 Sucking artifact on EEG tracing in an intubated patient. Patient is intubated and sucking on the endotracheal tube. In this picture, muscle artifact occurs in temporal leads from the sucking movement and the chin also shows correlated movements. The temporal leads often show mouth movement artifacts (chewing, sucking) due to the placement of the temporal leads near the jaw muscles of mastication

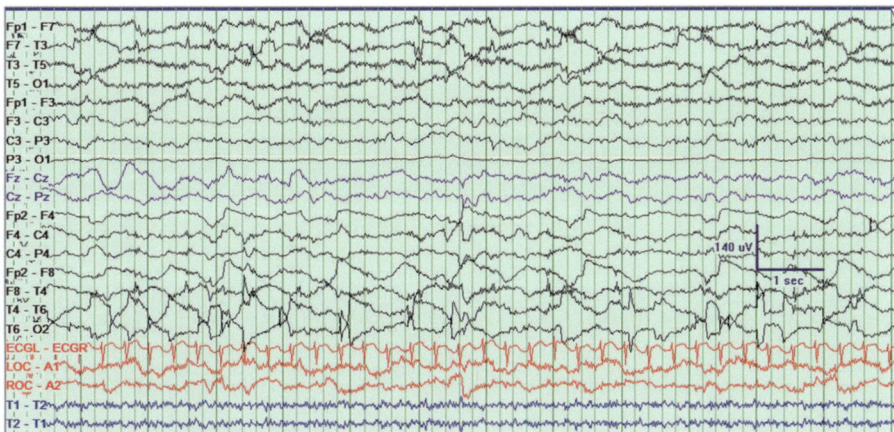

Fig. 7.11 Sucking artifact on EEG tracing. Suck artifact slightly asymmetrical with more movements seen in the right temporal region

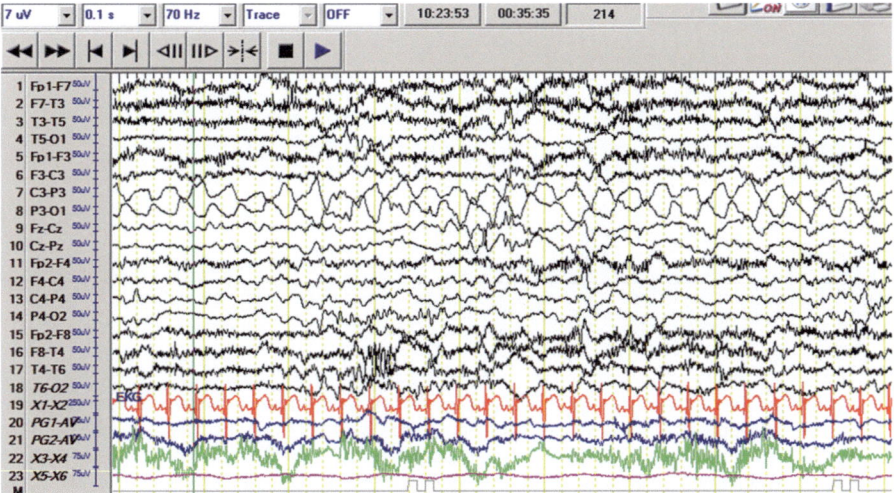

Fig. 7.12 Sucking artifact on EEG tracing. Artifact in one lead corresponding to sucking movements. P3 lead is likely loose and the sucking movements are exaggerating the movement in this lead

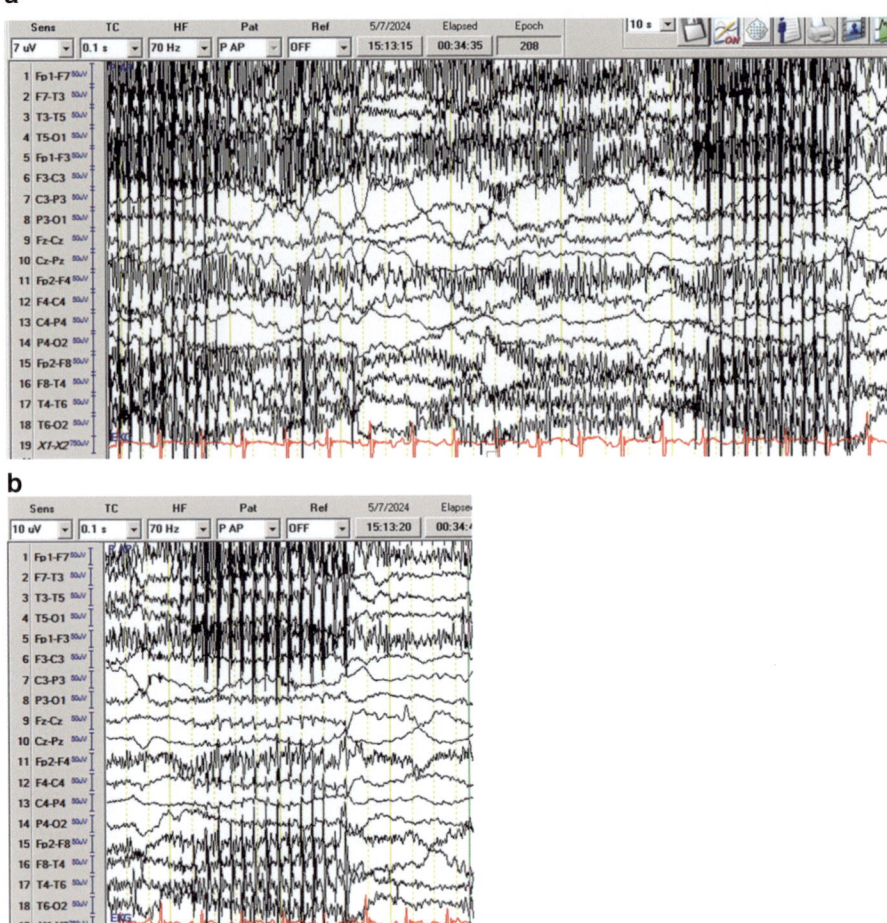

Fig. 7.13 (**a**) Tremor-like movements as an artifact on EEG tracing. Patient is having jittery, tremor-like movements. Frequency of these potentials is in the range of muscle (greater than 20 Hz). There is an abrupt start and end. Sensitivity is 7 µV. (**b**) Tremor-like movements as an artifact on EEG tracing. This is the same epoch as above, but the sensitivity is lowered to 10 µV. Changing this parameter lowers the height of the waveforms to ease in reviewing the entire waveform

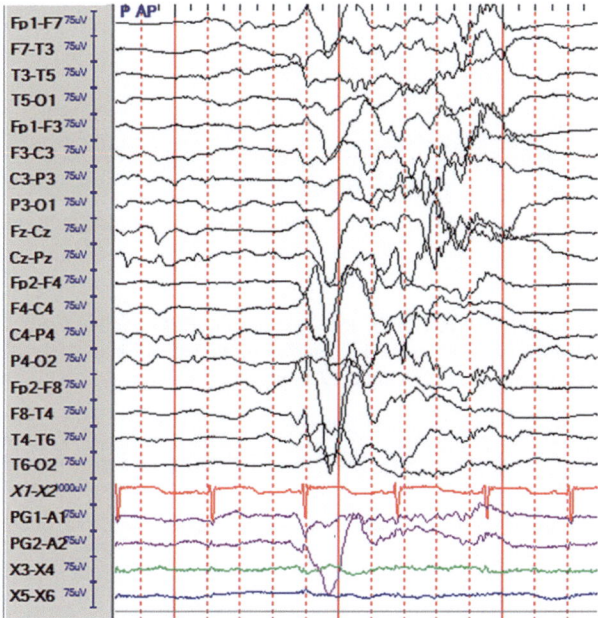

Fig. 7.14 Eye leads showing cortical signals in the EEG tracing. Eye leads are in purple and listed as PG1-A1 (left eye) and PG2-A2 (right eye). Cortical activity is being detected by the right eye lead, which is lateral and above the right eye. The left eye lead is below and lateral to the left eye, so is not detecting as much cortical activity

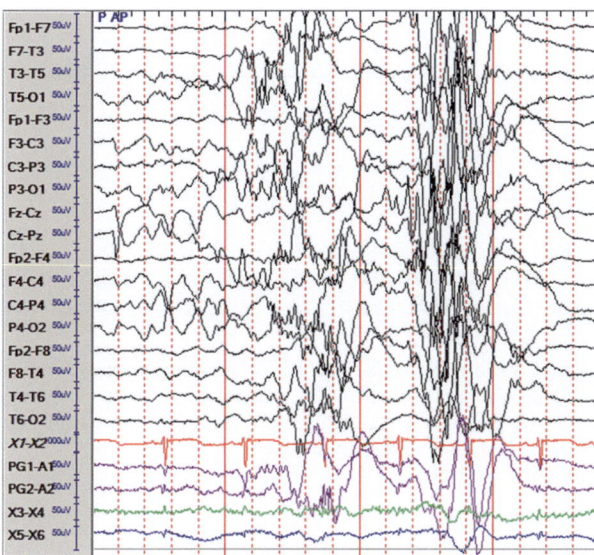

Fig. 7.15 Interpreting eye lead tracings. Eye leads showing cortical signals in the EEG tracing

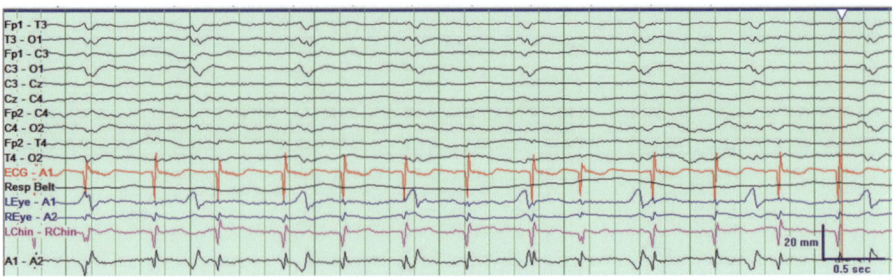

Fig. 7.16 Seizure creating artifact in the eye leads on the EEG tracing. Cortical signals show a seizure in the left hemisphere and are being detected in the left eye lead (Leye-A1). The right eye (Reye-A2) line is detecting artifact from the ECG signal

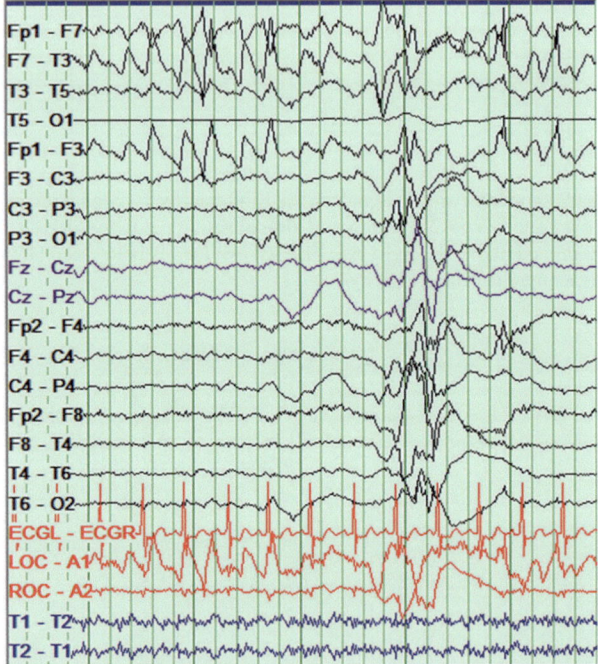

Fig. 7.17 Dysconjugate eye movements seen on EEG tracing. Left eye movement to the right direction (left eye looking toward the nose). The retina is negative so F7 shows a phase reversal. Meanwhile, the LOC-A1 lead shows correlating movements. Following this, the eye leads show cortical activity with the high-amplitude cortical wave

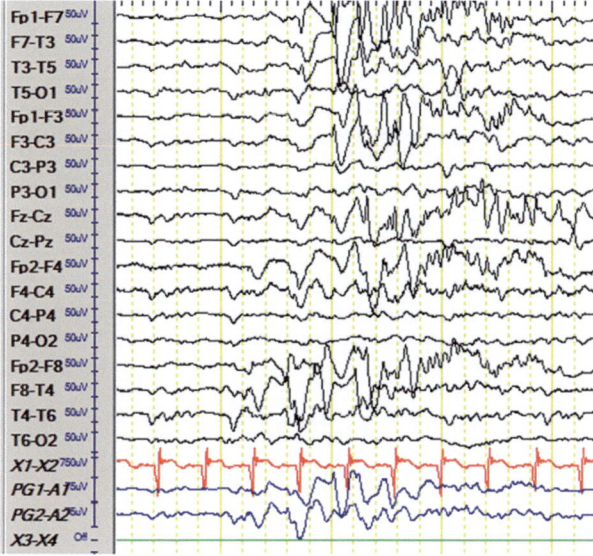

Fig. 7.18 High-amplitude frontal sharp activity is also seen in the eye leads since the eye leads are detecting frontal electrical activity

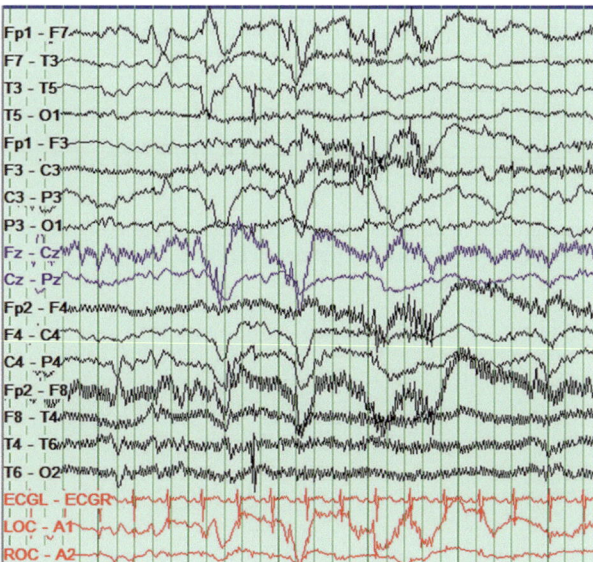

Fig. 7.19 Left eye lead detecting left frontal cortical waveforms. In this case, the left eye lead is above the left eye and the right eye lead is below the right eye

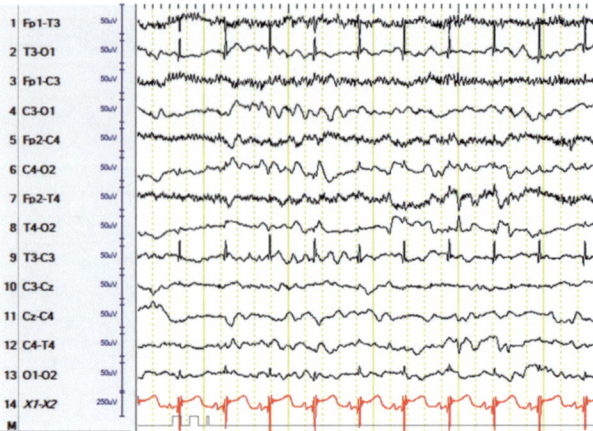

Fig. 7.20 ECG lead artifact in an EEG tracing. ECG lead signal is shown in the cortical leads

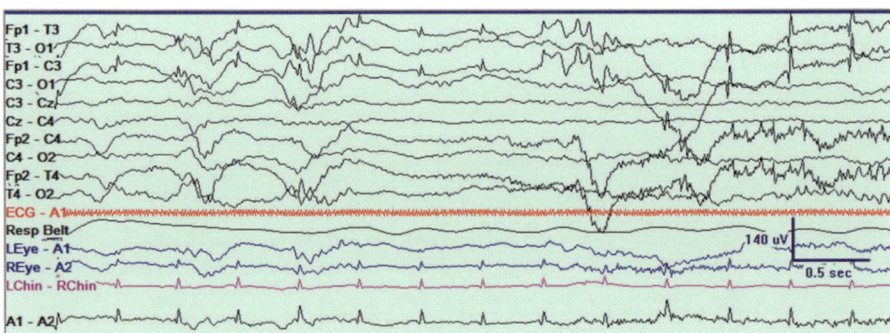

Fig. 7.21 ECG lead artifact in an EEG tracing. ECG lead signal is shown in the cortical leads, however, the actual ECG lead contains fast frequency artifact

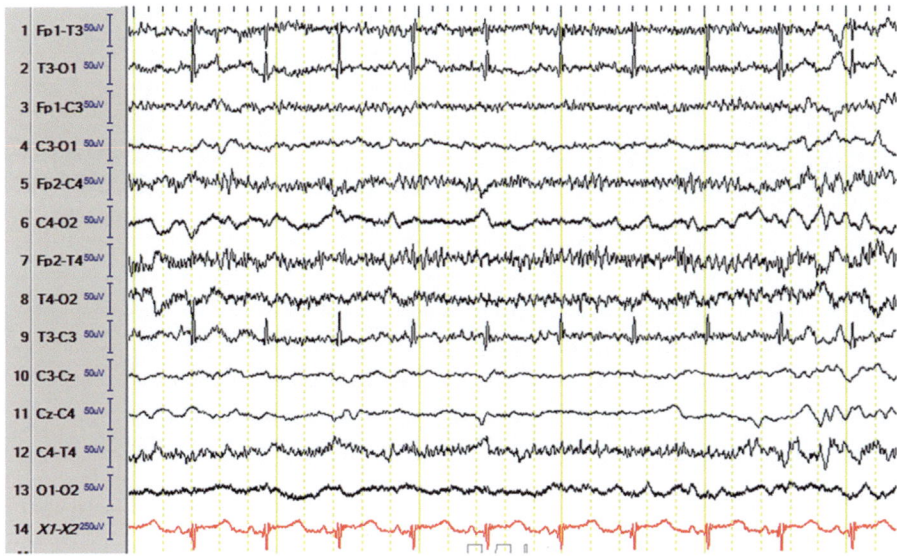

Fig. 7.22 ECG lead artifact in an EEG tracing. ECG lead signal is shown in the left cortical lead T3

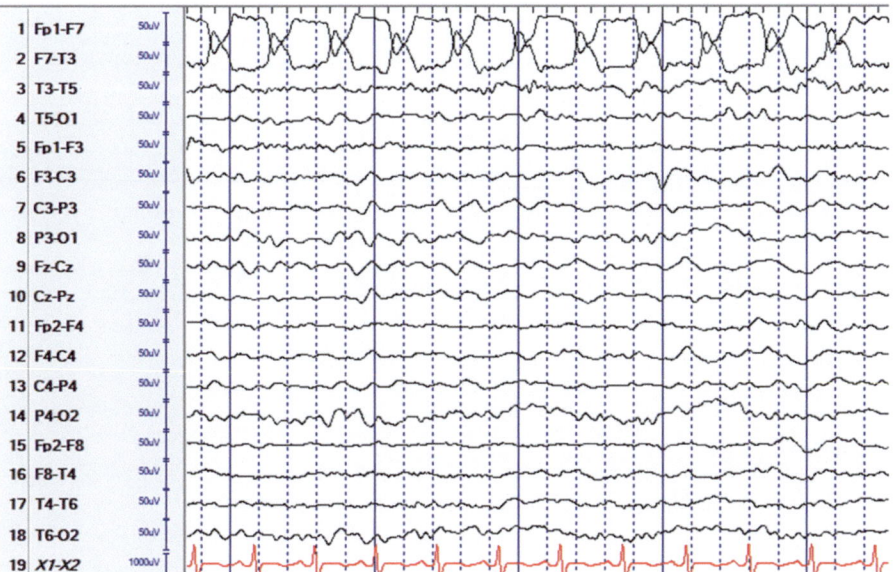

Fig. 7.23 EEG tracing showing pulse artifact. This pulse artifact in the left frontal region. These waveforms are in sync with and follow the ECG tracing heart rate

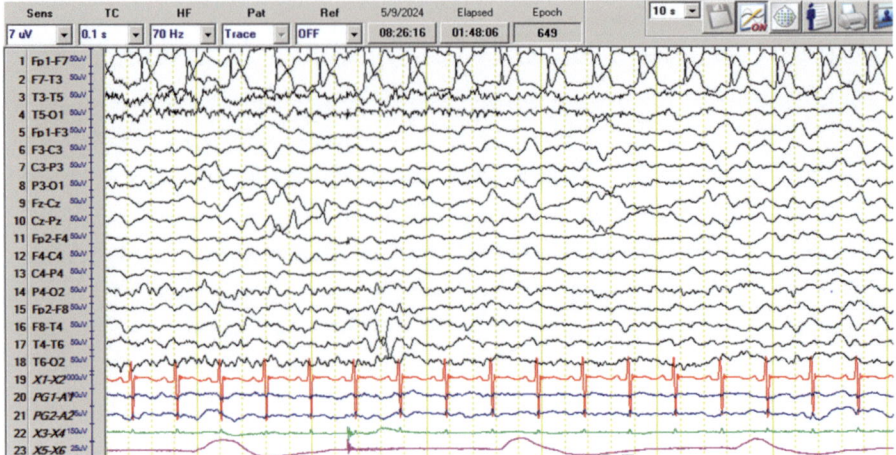

Fig. 7.24 EEG tracing showing pulse artifact. This pulse artifact shows rhythmic artifact in the F7 lead that is in synch with the ECG lead QRS complex

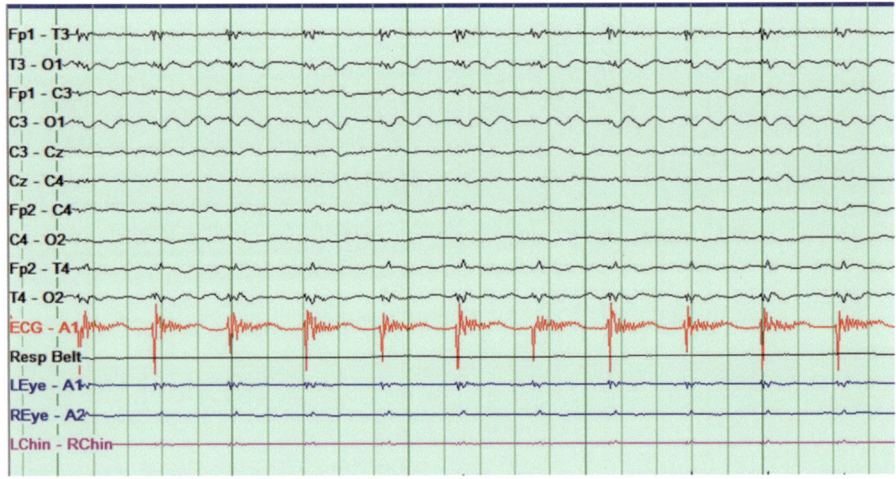

Fig. 7.25 Pacemaker and oscillator artifact in a neonate

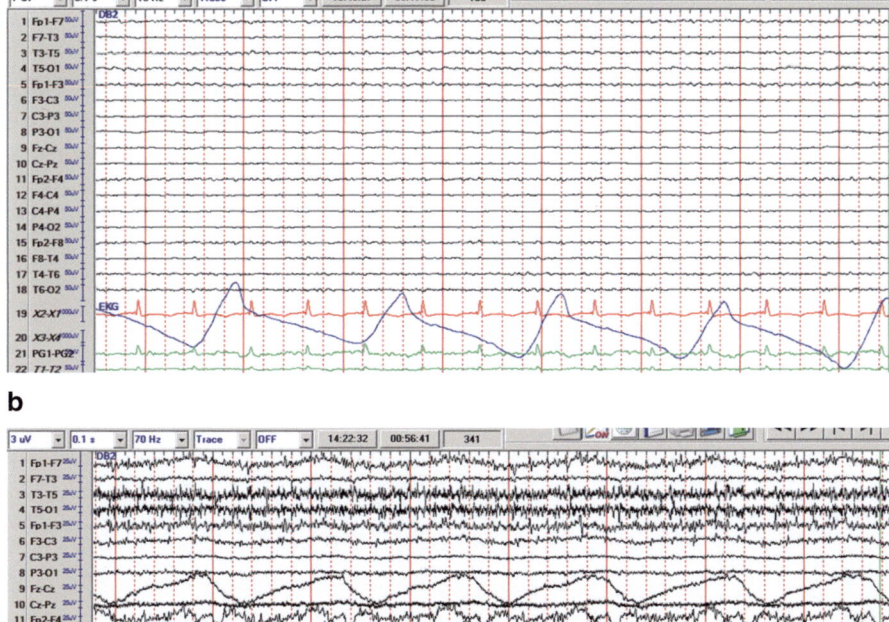

Fig. 7.26 (**a**) Ventilator artifact in a patient with electrocerebral inactivity. The background cortical activity is extremely suppressed. X3-X4 represents the respiratory belt lead, and the rate of chest wall movement can be seen. (**b**) Ventilator artifact in a patient with electrocerebral inactivity. Ventilator artifact is noted in the blue lead of the X3-X4 electrodes. In addition, corresponding artifact is detected in the right hemisphere leads. This patient was intubated with the head turned toward the right side and the right side of the head was resting on the bed. Each movement of the chest caused the head to move as well and pressed the electrodes into the bed

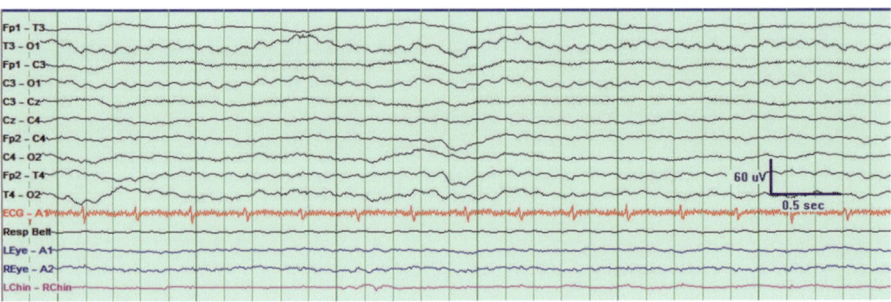

Fig. 7.27 Oscillator artifact

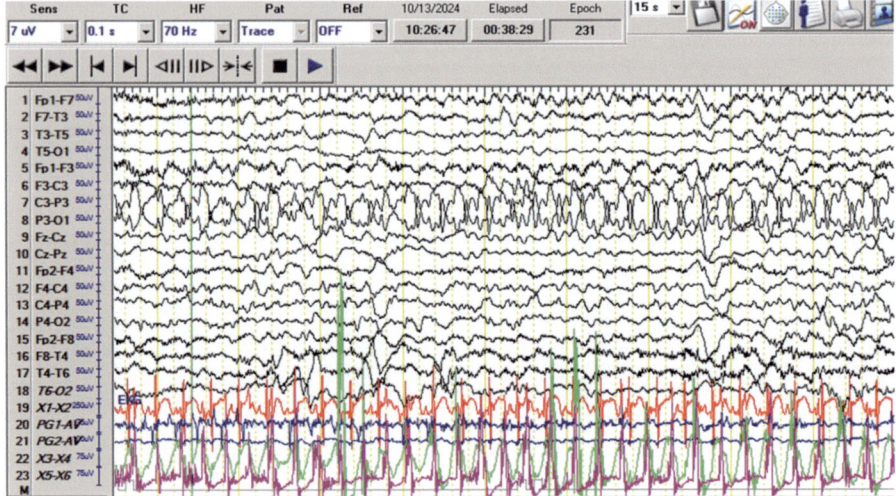

Fig. 7.28 EEG tracing showing patting artifact. Patting artifact creates rhythmic activity, in this case, seen in the P3 electrode

7 Common Artifacts of Neonatal EEG Recordings

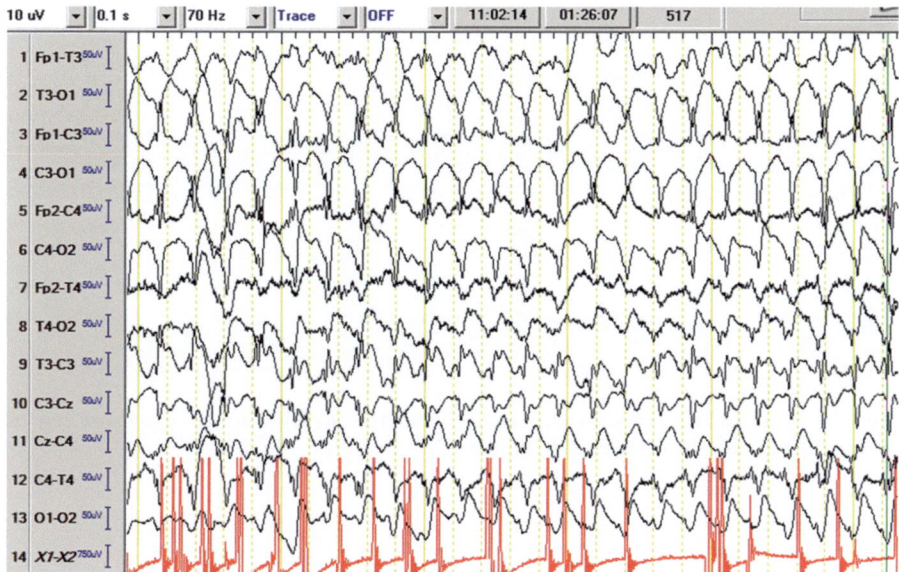

Fig. 7.29 EEG tracing showing patting artifact. Patting artifact causing diffuse rhythmic activity, maximal in the posterior head leads

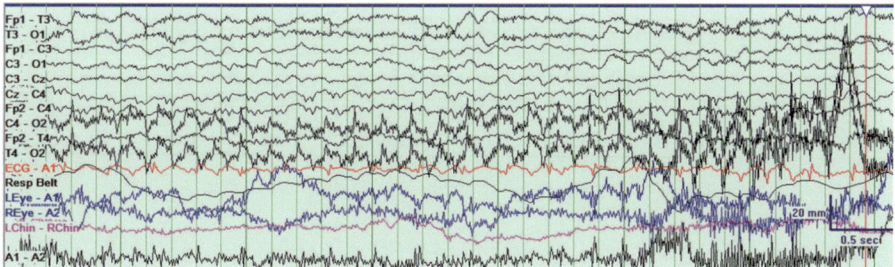

Fig. 7.30 EEG tracing showing patting artifact

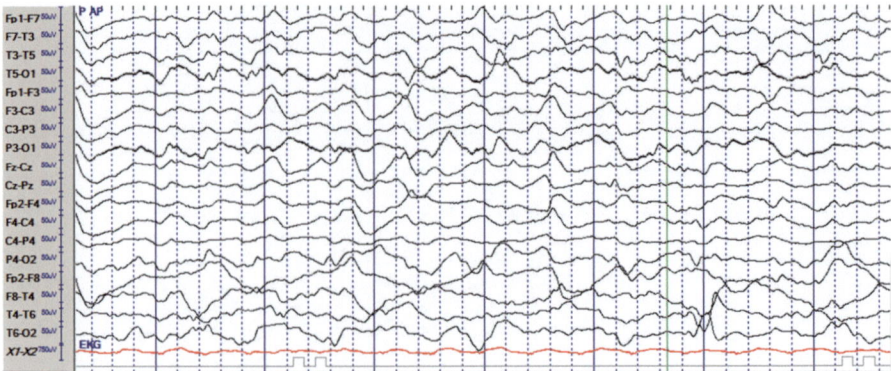

Fig. 7.31 EEG tracing showing rocking artifact. Baby is being rocked in a rocking chair. Occipital movements correlated with rocking movements

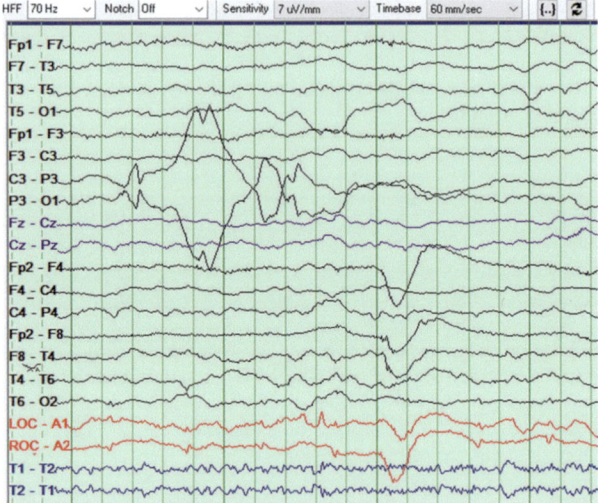

Fig. 7.32 Loose electrode artifact on EEG tracing. Loose electrode, also called electrode "pop" artifact. This causes a positive deflection in the loose lead (P3)

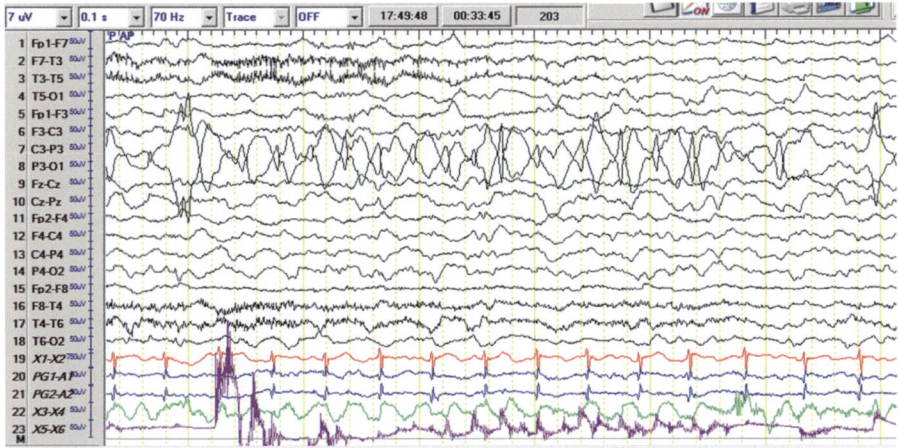

Fig. 7.33 Loose electrode artifact on EEG tracing. Electrode pop, or loose P3 lead

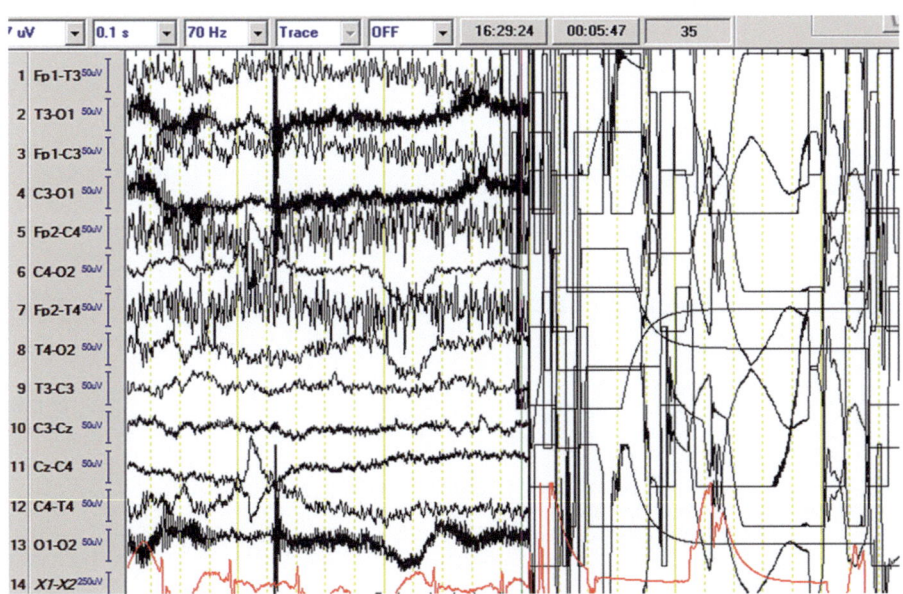

Fig. 7.34 Artifact due to technician adjusting EEG headset. The box that housed the electrodes is being adjusted. This causes an oversaturation of all the electrodes

Amplitude-Integrated EEG and Its Application for Neonates

8

Mary Payne, Rebecca Barnett, and Stefan R. Maxwell

8.1 Amplitude-Integrated Electroencephalogram

8.1.1 Introduction

Amplitude-integrated EEG (aEEG) is a type of abbreviated EEG recording. It was originally developed as a quick bedside monitor for adult intensive care patients since it uses only 3–5 electrodes and can be placed quickly by any medical personnel. The aEEG works by detecting changes in amplitude, which then interprets the background activity and detects seizures. This device does not require an EEG technician for electrode placement, so in urgent situations, especially after typical business hours, any trained medical provider can apply the electrodes in just a few minutes. The machine is portable and stays at the patient bedside for continuous review.

Acknowledgments for figures: Natus Medical Incorporated.

M. Payne (✉)
Department of Pediatrics, Division of Pediatric Neurology, Joan C. Edwards School of Medicine, Hoops Family Children's Hospital, Marshall University, Huntington, WV, USA
e-mail: paynem@marshall.edu

R. Barnett
Department of Pediatrics, Division of Neonatal-Perinatal Medicine, Joan C. Edwards School of Medicine, Hoops Family Children's Hospital, Marshall University, Huntington, WV, USA

S. R. Maxwell
Pediatrix Medical Group, WVU School of Medicine, WV Osteopathic School of Medicine, CAMC Women's and Children's Hospital, Charleston, WV, USA

© The Author(s), under exclusive license to Springer Nature Switzerland AG 2025
M. Payne, D. Gloss II (eds.), *Neonatal EEG*,
https://doi.org/10.1007/978-3-031-92556-6_8

8.2 Part 1: Basics of the aEEG

The aEEG is used often in term neonates to help identify a pattern suggestive of encephalopathy or presence of seizures. This finding can be a factor when deciding candidates for the hypoxic-ischemic hypothermia treatment protocol. The window of starting therapeutic hypothermia is 6 h post-delivery, so quick assessment ability is definitely advantageous for these patients and neonatal intensive care unit (NICU) staff. In addition to evaluating background activity, the aEEG can also detect seizures. This is especially helpful with subclinical seizures, which are not clinically apparent and then can be treated urgently. Eventual traditional complete EEG study is recommended in each of these scenarios, but using the aEEG setup quickly can facilitate prompt appropriate treatment, especially when traditional EEG access may be limited [1]. In addition, following hypothermia, the background activity can show improvement.

The aEEG has some limitations, however.

- For preterm infants, the data and normal/abnormal findings have not been well established. Recall that preterm infants can have a discontinuous background activity as a normal pattern for their gestational age. While the traditional EEG can detect minor changes and abnormal nuances about the degree of this discontinuity, the aEEG is unable to translate and display these subtle abnormalities.
- Seizure length must be at least 30 s to be detected by the aEEG algorithm. Electrodes used are in the parietal regions and perhaps central regions (depends on the customary procedure of the NICU), so seizures occurring outside of these cortical regions may be missed. Thus, a traditional EEG is recommended if any clinical seizure activity is detected or subclinical seizure activity is suspected or detected.
- Artifacts are common, just as in any EEG system. The aEEG logarithmic scale used for higher amplitude plotting and the aEEG frequency filters are designed to minimize artifacts being incorporated into the EEG signal. However, filtering out or attenuating all artifacts is impossible. Certain patterns to be aware of and mentioned below are liquid bridging showing a flat trace and electrical activity or movement artifacts showing a seizure-like pattern.

8.2.1 Placing the aEEG

Electrodes used are hydrogel, subdermal, or disposable gold.

Diagram of electrode placement. Reference electrode is placed midline as well.

The electrodes in purple circles represent the electrodes used in the aEEG study. If two electrodes are used (single channel mode), only the P3 and P4 electrodes are placed. If four electrodes are used (dual channel mode), C3 and C4 electrodes are also placed (Fig. 8.1).

8 Amplitude-Integrated EEG and Its Application for Neonates

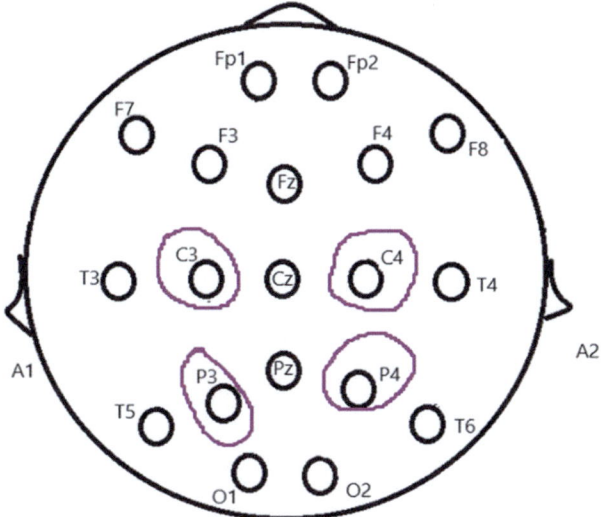

Fig. 8.1 Schematic of electrodes used in standard montage compared to the amplitude-integrated EEG

8.2.1.1 Two Modes for Gathering Data and Displaying Data

Single channel mode uses two electrodes placed in the left and right parietal regions (P3 and P4 electrodes). The parietal regions of the brain tend to be where watershed infarctions occur, such as that seen in HIE. The area of parietal electrodes also minimizes interference from nursing care.

Dual-channel mode uses electrodes in the bilateral parietal and central regions (C3 and C4 electrodes), thus enhancing detection for epileptic events as neonatal seizures are often in the central regions.

Guides are provided for accurate placement of electrodes. Impedance, which is measured as resistance to flow of current, is also a way to verify adequate contact of the electrode with the scalp. This is measured in ohms and should be less than 10 Ω. High impedance will increase the likelihood of artifacts contributing to the recording signal.

8.2.1.2 How the aEEG Works

The electrodes receive cortical potentials just as the traditional EEG does. The amplitude of these cortical potentials is then measured and plotted on the display graph on the cerebral function monitor (CFM).

Frequencies less than 2 Hz and greater than 15 Hz are attenuated. A bandpass filter shows the frequencies between 2 and 15 Hz at a greater weight. Less than 2 Hz activity is likely activity due to electrode artifact and activity greater than 15 Hz tends to be electrical artifact. Additional processing such as time and amplitude compression occurs to yield the final pattern on the CFM.

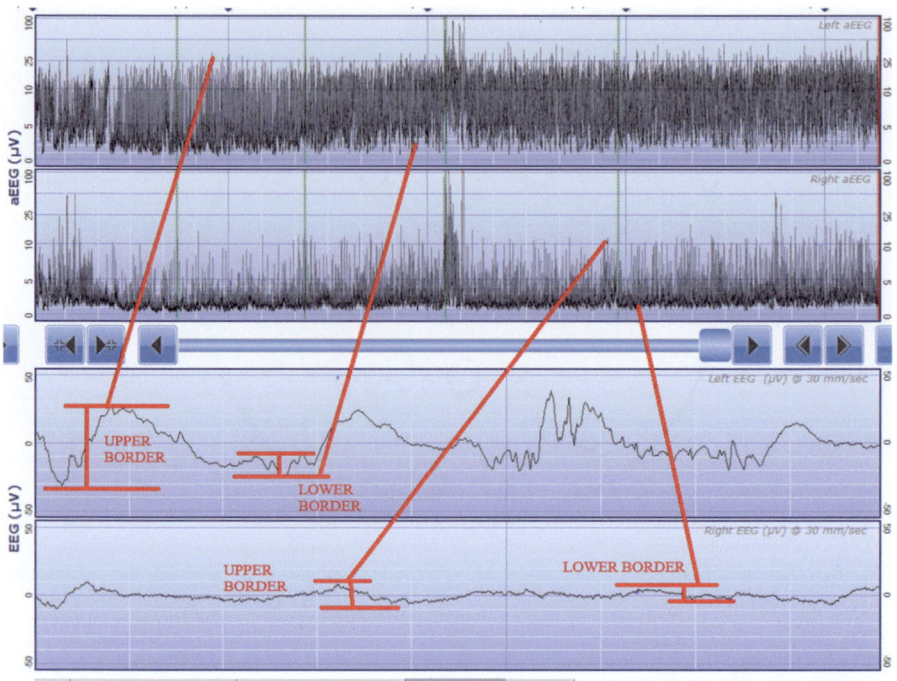

Fig. 8.2 Sample picture of a cerebral function monitor display showing the overall patterns and functions of an aEEG

Amplitudes less than 10 μV are translated to the CFM using a liner scale. However, amplitudes over 10 μV are displayed on a logarithmic scale. By doing so, the lower amplitudes (less than 10 μV) are depicted with greater weight than the amplitudes over 10 μV, also limiting higher amplitude artifact interference. The lower amplitude is the lower border and the highest amplitude is the upper border. These waveforms produce the pattern referred to as the bandwidth.

Data displayed on the CFM (Fig. 8.2):

5–6 cm on the time scale of CFM represents 1 h of recording.
X axis is time, measured in seconds.
Y axis is voltage, measured in microvolts.

Some displays also show the raw EEG data (keep in mind only raw data of 2–4 electrodes). This can help if artifacts are suspected. The raw data is displayed on a linear scale.

The amplitude-integrated EEG data is displayed on a semilogarithmic scale of the amplitude-integrated curve.

8.3 Part 2: Interpreting the aEEG Background Activity

- Five patterns of background activity
  1. Continuous = voltage between 5 and 50 μV
  2. Discontinuous = voltage less than 5 μV and greater than 10 μV
  3. Burst suppression = discontinuous periods of very low activity (<5 μV) intermixed with burst of higher amplitude (>25 μV)
  4. Continuous low voltage = all amplitudes less than 10 μV
  5. Flat or isoelectric = all amplitude less than 5 μV
- Note about sleep–wake cycling

Sleep–wake cycles can be seen in neonates as early as 30 WGA as they cycle through all 3 states (awake, active sleep, and quiet sleep) within every 60 min. *This pattern will be seen superimposed onto the continuous pattern (number 1) mentioned above.* Premature babies who have a baseline background activity of discontinuity (number 2) typically do not have this type of sleep–wake cycle since they predominately have indeterminate sleep (refer to chapter on maturation).

When a sleep–wake cycle pattern is present, the lower margin of the bandwidth shows a sinusoidal wave pattern over time as the quiet sleep amplitudes are a wider range than the awake state amplitudes. Cycling into quiet sleep, with its discontinuous background and broader range of amplitudes corresponds to a broad bandwidth. Wakefulness and active sleep show a narrower bandwidth and more continuous activity.

Absence of a sleep–wake cycle in a near-term or term infant may suggest encephalopathy as seen in hypoxic-ischemic encephalopathy, opiate use, sedative, or antiepileptic administration [3].

8.3.1 Pattern 1: Continuous

This pattern is considered to be continuous. All voltages are between 5 and 50 μV. Sleep–wake cycle is also recognized. Likely the infant is cycling between quiet sleep and active sleep/awake throughout this time frame. The larger bandwidths correspond to the trace alternant quiet sleep pattern seen in normal-term babies. This overall pattern suggests normal-term baby background activity (Figs. 8.3 and 8.4).

8.3.2 Pattern 2: Discontinuous

This is an example of discontinuity seen in normal preterm infants or in encephalopathic term infants. In this pattern, the background amplitudes vary: either less than 5 μV or greater than 10 μV. Recall that premature babies (typically less than 32 WGA) have a discontinuous pattern most of the time, as seen in quiet and indeterminate sleep. This bandwidth shows higher lines representing the periods of higher voltage and lower lines representing the periods of lower voltage. The slight cyclical variation of the bottom line may be seen in a cycle of arousals and indeterminate sleep (Fig. 8.5).

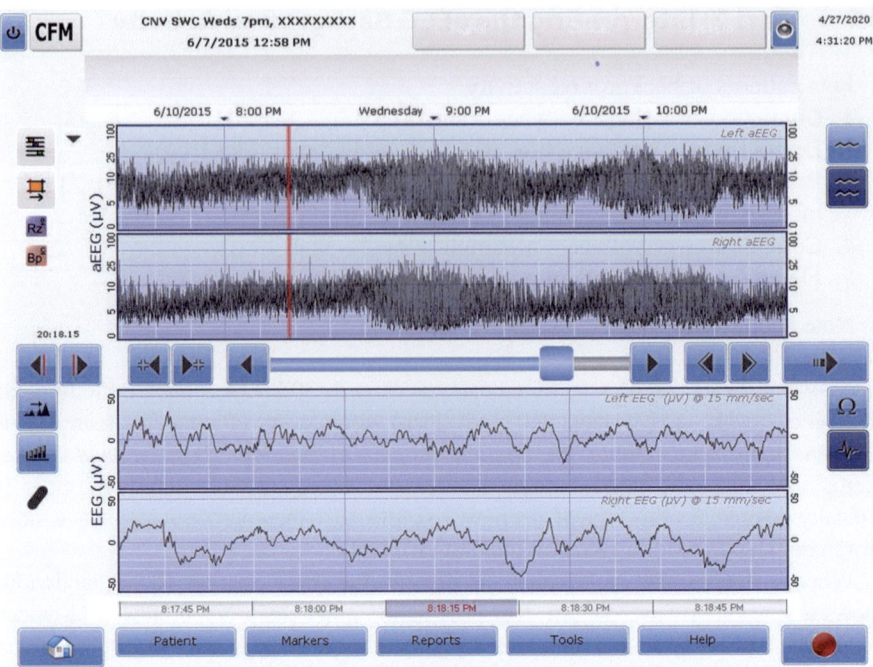

Fig. 8.3 Example of a continuous pattern in a dual-channel aEEG in a neonate

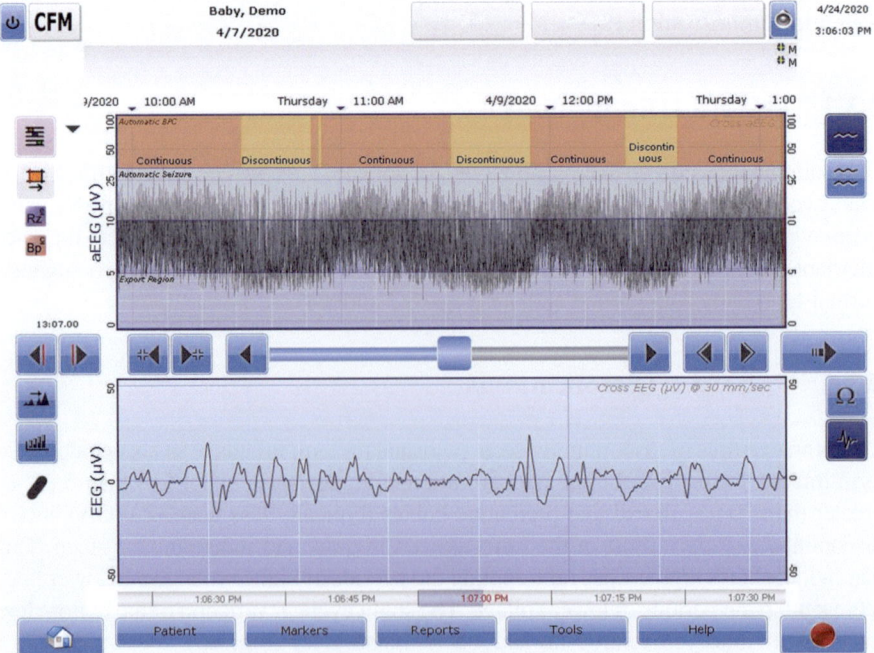

Fig. 8.4 Example of a continuous pattern in a single-channel aEEG in a neonate

8 Amplitude-Integrated EEG and Its Application for Neonates

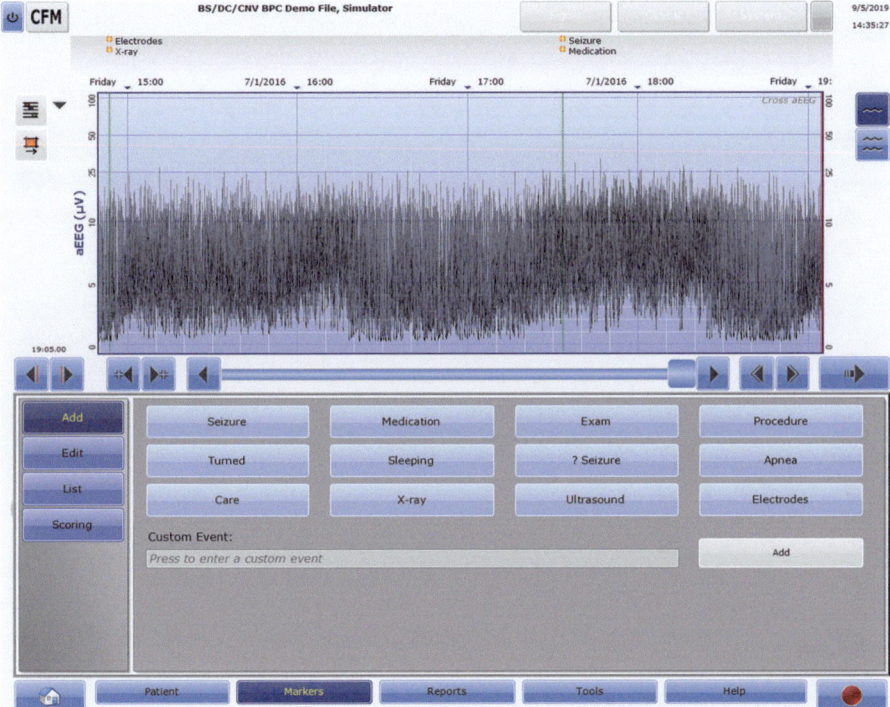

Fig. 8.5 Example of a discontinuous background pattern in a neonate as seen on an aEEG

8.3.3 Pattern 3: Burst Suppression

This bandwidth represents activity that is less than 5 µV and greater than 25 µV. In a pathological burst suppression pattern, such as seen with encephalopathy, the lower amplitudes are lower and higher amplitudes are higher than what is typically seen in the preterm age-appropriate discontinuous pattern. This bandwidth example shows the bottom line (lowest amplitude) hovers just above zero. Conversely, the top line (highest amplitude) is mostly equal to or above 25 µV (Fig. 8.6).

8.3.4 Pattern 4: Continuous Low-Voltage Activity

This bandwidth is seen in the setting of minimal cortical activity. In this example, amplitudes are under 10 µV. This would be a pattern seen in severe cortical dysfunction. The bandwidth is narrow because of the narrow range in amplitudes (all being under 10 µV) (Fig. 8.7).

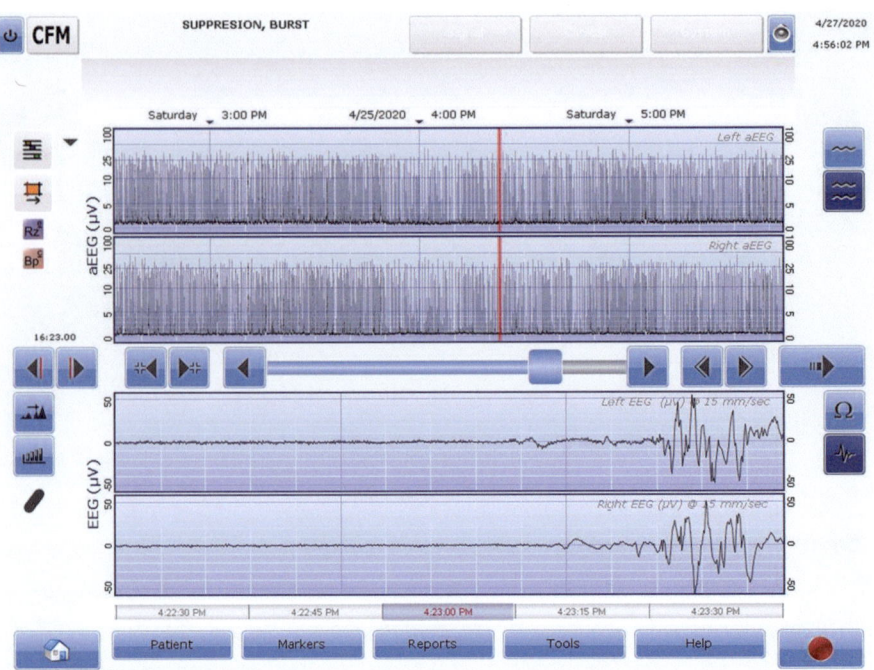

Fig. 8.6 Burst suppression pattern in a neonate as seen on an aEEG

8.3.5 Pattern 5: Flat Trace

The flat or isoelectric trace correlates with absent cortical activity (Fig. 8.8). In this example, amplitudes are under 5 μV. When cortical potentials are all so low, the EEG data acquisition often shows artifacts being higher in amplitude than the cortical potentials. In this bandwidth example, the narrow high lines likely represent artifact that otherwise would be mixed in with the normal background.

8.3.5.1 Seizure Characteristics on aEEG
Bandwidth shows a rapid rise in lower and upper margins followed by decreased amplitude section. During a seizure, cortical potentials are shifted higher; for example, a background of amplitudes 10–25 μV changes to a background of 15–50 μV (Figs. 8.9 and 8.10).

- Sz must be at least 30 s in length and at least 2 μV in amplitude to be seen on aEEG CFM.
- Repetitive seizures can yield a sawtooth pattern, in which there is repetitive narrowing with increased peak-to-peak amplitude.
- Artifacts tend to show a gradual, not sudden, increase, and decrease in the bandwidth.

8 Amplitude-Integrated EEG and Its Application for Neonates

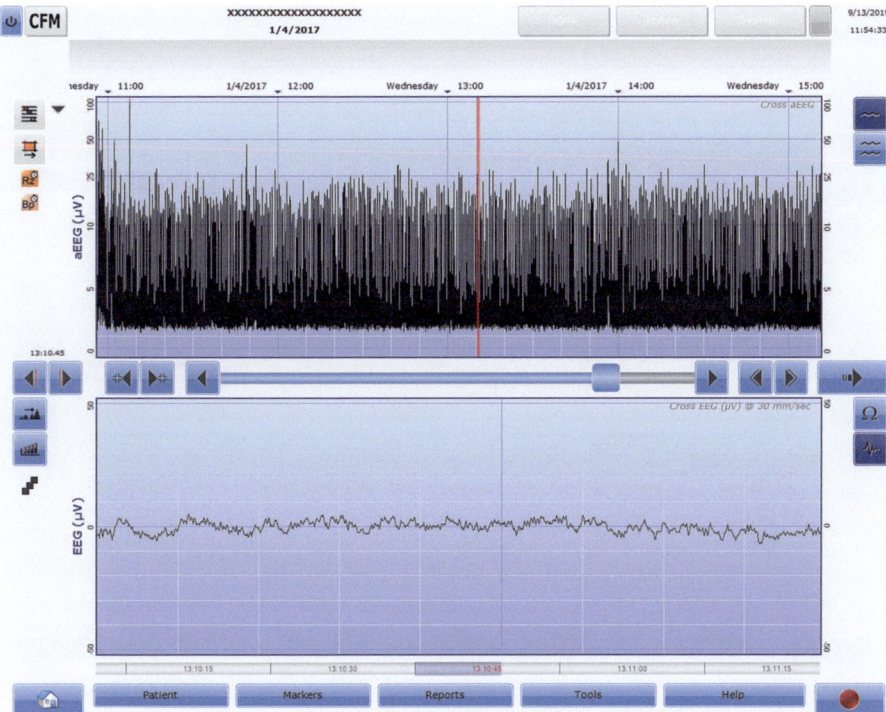

Fig. 8.7 Continuous low-voltage activity as seen on an aEEG in a neonate

- In preterm infants, however, seizures can be hidden and not stand out separate from the background activity by the discontinuous pattern and may only be detected by viewing the raw EEG. Not all systems will have the option to view the raw EEG data [2].

8.3.5.2 Artifacts

Liquid bridging can cause an apparent flat trace. Usually, this happens in the dual-channel aEEG (intraparietal curves where the central and parietal electrodes can either be too close to each other, connected to each other by sweat or gel). Settings can be changed to show left hemisphere electrodes compared to right hemisphere electrodes and by doing this, the flatness of the tracing disappears.

Electrical interference, movements, and handling can lead to an apparent seizure or even to an apparent status epilepticus. If this happens, impedance and the reference electrode should be checked, and the raw EEG should be compared (Fig. 8.11).

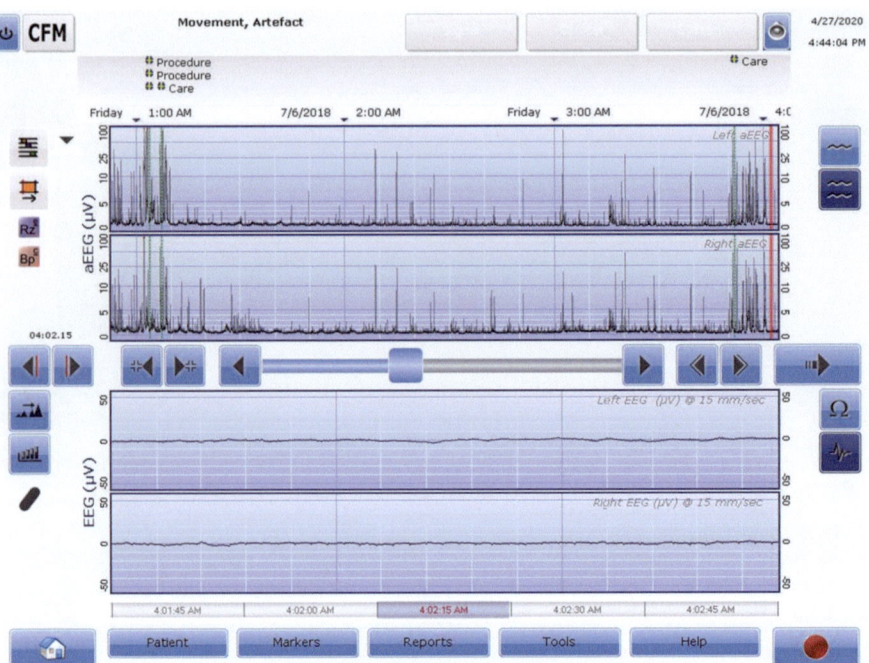

Fig. 8.8 Isoelectric tracing in a neonate as displayed with aEEG

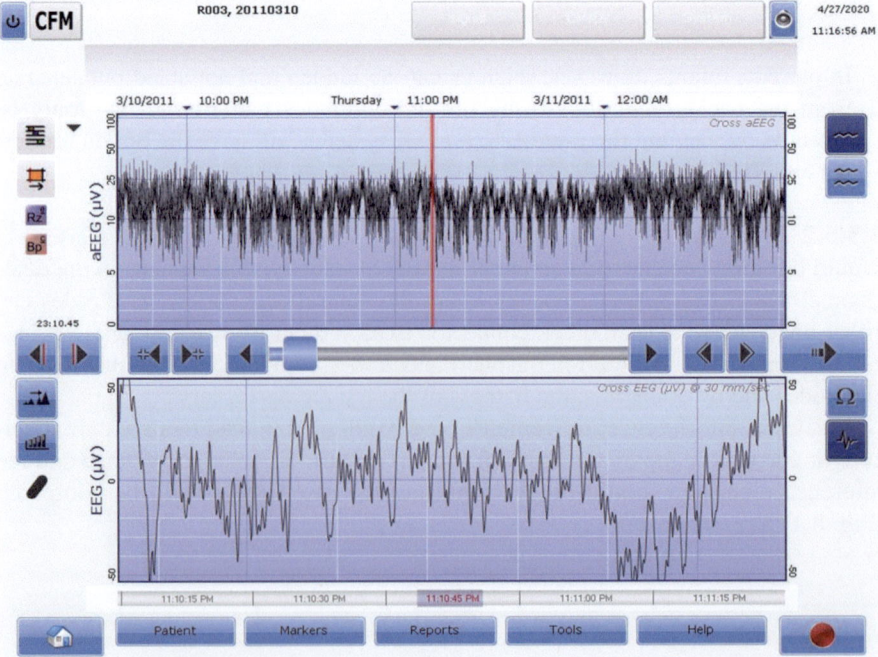

Fig. 8.9 Status epilepticus as seen on an aEEG in a neonate with continuous seizure activity

8 Amplitude-Integrated EEG and Its Application for Neonates

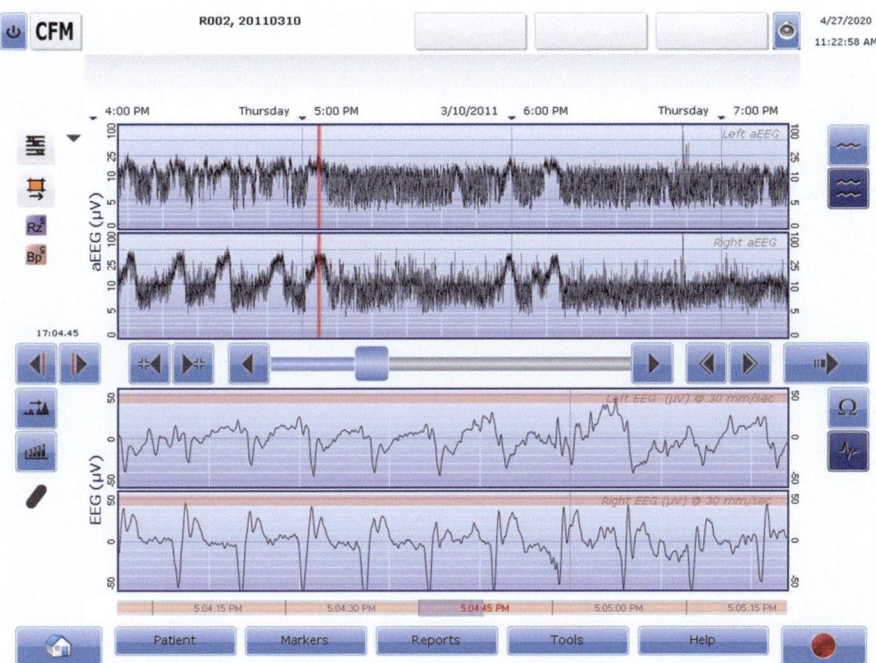

Fig. 8.10 Intermittent seizure activity displayed on an aEEG in a neonate. The red bar shows the raw EEG data at that time, which corresponds to seizure activity

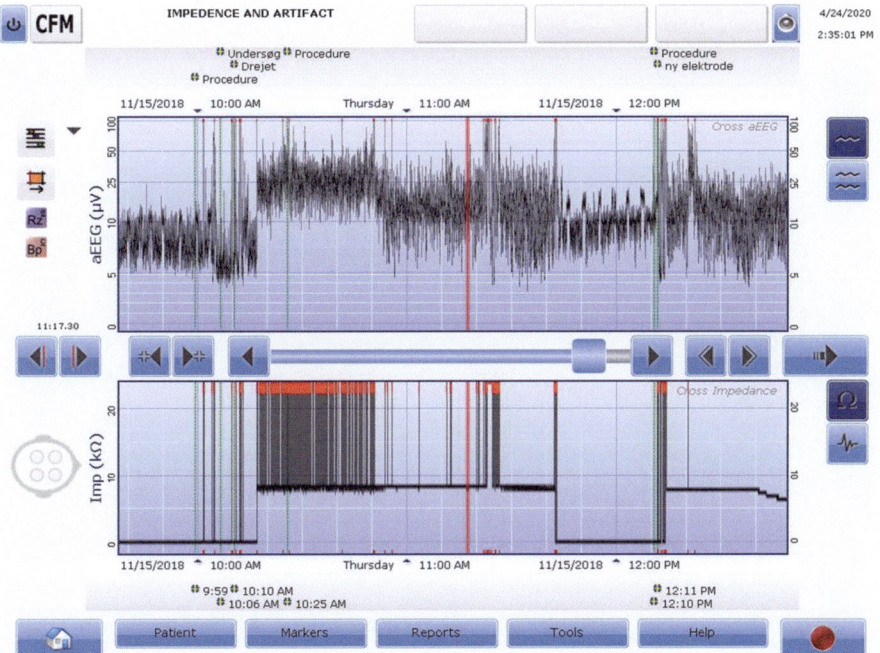

Fig. 8.11 Tracing showing artifact with movements in a neonatal aEEG recording

References

1. Bruns N, Blumenthal S, Meyer I, et al. Application of an amplitude-integrated EEG monitor (cerebral function monitor) to neonates. J Vis Exp. 2017;127:55985. https://doi.org/10.3791/55985.
2. Durrani N, Dinan M. Amplitude integrated EEG: a primer for neonatologists and practitioners in the NICU. NeoReviews. 2022;23(2):e96–e107.
3. Feldman K, Baisie J, Amr ES, et al. Introduction of amplitude-integrated electroencephalography (aEEG) monitoring in a level 2 NICU: improving the quality of care for neurologically at-risk newborns. Neonatal Netw. 2023;42(4) https://doi.org/10.1891/NN-2022-0056.

Case Examples in Neonates with Clinical Scenarios Using Electroencephalogram Recordings

9

Christopher Luke Damron, Rebekah Fabela,
Alicia Heyward, Cynthia Massey, Dustin Miller, Mary Payne,
and Lauren Thompson

Introduction This chapter presents case examples of hypoxia, apnea, and epilepsies with various etiologies. Our role as medical providers to evaluate, diagnose, and treat neonates is often complicated by genetic factors, in utero environment, and the delivery process.

9.1 Case 1: Hypothermia for Neonates with Hypoxic-ischemic Encephalopathy (HIE) and Use of EEG

This patient's mother arrived at labor and delivery at 37 weeks gestational age (WGA). She reported decreased fetal movements for the past 24 h. Ultrasound showed concern for absent end diastolic flow of the placental, so the decision was made to induce delivery. The baby was born with Apgar scores 2 and 5 at 1 and 5 min, respectively. Umbilical cord pH was 6.9, and the baby was intubated and resuscitated in the delivery room. Birth weight was 2500 g, and physical exam did not show any congenital malformations. She met the criteria for therapeutic hypothermia, and whole-body cooling was initiated. Her temperature was maintained around 34 °C for 72 h, and she required minimal dosing of sedative medications for

---

C. L. Damron · A. Heyward · C. Massey · L. Thompson ·R. Fabela · D. Miller
Department of Pediatrics, Division of Neonatal-Perinatal Medicine, Joan C. Edwards School of Medicine, Hoops Family Children's Hospital, Marshall University, Huntington, WV, USA

M. Payne (✉)
Department of Pediatrics, Division of Pediatric Neurology, Joan C. Edwards School of Medicine, Hoops Family Children's Hospital, Marshall University, Huntington, WV, USA
e-mail: paynem@marshall.edu

shivering and comfort. Continuous electroencephalogram (EEG) recording accompanied the hypothermia period and was then discontinued after she was rewarmed. The EEG background initially showed mild encephalopathy with diffusely low-amplitude activity (Fig. 9.1). However, around 48 h after cooling onset, the background activity improved. By the time of rewarming, background activity was considered normal for age (Fig. 9.2). The patient did not have any seizures. Magnetic resonance imaging (MRI) of the brain did not show any evidence of white matter or cortical abnormalities. Diffusion-weighted images, which detect water shifts seen in acute hypoxic injury, were also negative.

Hypoxic-ischemic encephalopathy is the most common cause of neonatal encephalopathy. In addition, it is a major factor in overall child disability and contributes to infant death worldwide. Determining the time and reason for hypoxic

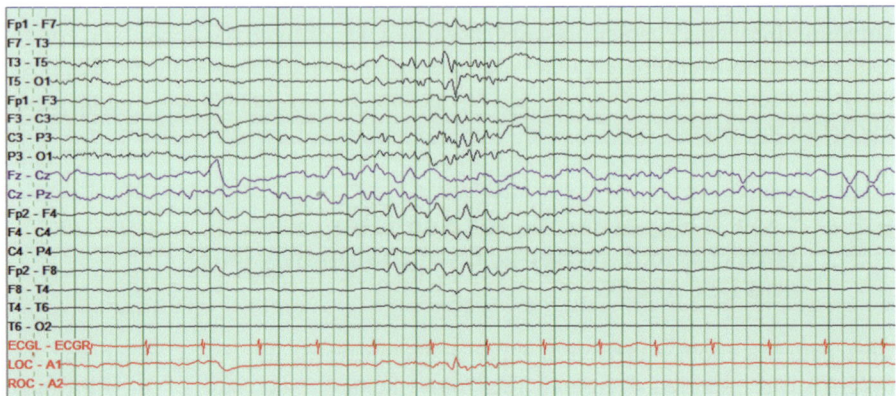

Fig. 9.1 Discontinuous background pattern showing mild encephalopathy in a full-term neonate with HIE

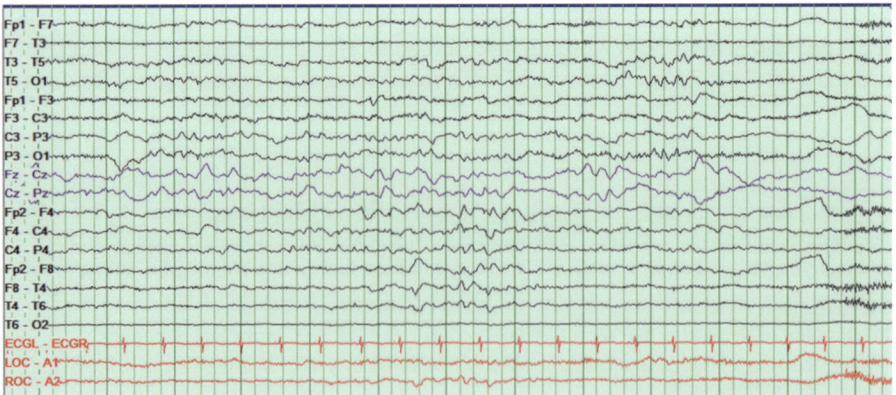

Fig. 9.2 Improvement of background activity in the neonate with HIE after being rewarmed, showing continuous background activity

insult is difficult as the insult may have occurred prior to labor onset or at an unknown point during the labor and delivery process. The causes are many, but in all cases, oxygen is depleted in the blood, which decreases cardiac output. Cerebral blood flow is then reduced. In this scenario, cranial blood flow is shunted to the brainstem and deeper brain structures, so that the cortex and watershed areas are first compromised. However, with further injury, the basal ganglia, thalami and brainstem can also be affected [24]. Fortunately, therapeutic hypothermia has been shown to reduce morbidity and mortality by 25% and is the only proven clinical therapy to lessen brain injury in moderate-to-severe HIE [7].

Several phases of hypoxic-ischemic encephalopathy occur based on cellular pathophysiology:

- Primary phase
  - Occurs within the *first hour post birth.*
  - Deprivation of oxygen and glucose causes a shift to anaerobic metabolism that increases serum lactate.
  - Cell membrane dysfunction is present, which causes depolarization and increase in intracellular glutamate, calcium, and oxygen-free radicals.
  - Cell death occurs.
- Latent phase
  - *1–6 h after birth* and occurs with medical intervention.
  - Cerebral reperfusion is reestablished with some improvement of cellular environment.
  - Metabolic derangements are still present and lead to further cell toxicity.
  - Note this is the time frame in which therapeutic hypothermia needs to begin.
- Secondary phase
  - *6–72 h* after birth.
  - Neuronal damage is further propagated with ongoing cytotoxic environment with intracellular hypercalcemia, mitochondrial malfunction, and presence of oxygen-free radicals.
  - Further neuronal injury and cell death.
  - Seizures can occur at this time.
  - Therapeutic hypothermia can hopefully minimize this effect on neuronal damage.
  - Cooling is thus 3performed for 72 h [6, 19].

Seizures in the setting of HIE and therapeutic hypothermia:

- Increase cellular demand and may impede cellular repair.
- Can occur with encephalopathy and acute injury.
- Typically begin within 6–35 h.
- Rare to occur in first 1–2 h. If this occurs, neonate likely had seizures in utero, which would suggest an earlier insult and likely additional confounding etiology.
- Incidence is over 50% and up to 80% can be subclinical.
- Can occur during the rewarming process.

Table 9.1 Inclusion and exclusion criteria for neonatal therapeutic hypothermia

Inclusion criteria	Exclusion criteria
Greater than or equal to 35 WGA	More than 6 h of age
Identified within 6 h of birth	Birth weight less than 2 kg
Moderate or severe encephalopathy or seizures	Life-threatening abnormalities of cardiovascular or respiratory systems
Evidence of intrapartum hypoxia (life-threatening coagulopathy or Apgar score less than or equal to 5 at 10 min of age)	Major congenital malformations or chromosome anomalies
Mechanical ventilation or resuscitation by 10 min of age	
Cord pH < 7 or arterial pH < 7 or base deficit greater than or equal to 12 mmol/L within 60 min of birth	

Mosalli [16]
kg kilogram, *L* liter, *mmol* millimole, *pH* potential of hydrogen (scale), *WGA* weeks gestational age

- Normal EEG background has been shown to have better outcomes [28].
  - Sedatives can cause diffuse amplitude attenuation and slowing.
  - Hypothermia can cause diffuse amplitude attenuation and slowing.
  - These factors need to be considered when making prognostic judgments about the patient's background activity.

Many institutions have their own criteria and protocols for therapeutic hypothermia. Below is an example of cooling inclusion and exclusion criteria from the *Journal of Clinical Neonatology*, 2012, Whole Body cooling for Infants with Hypoxic Ischemic Encephalopathy by Rafat Mosalli (Table 9.1).

Protocol also outlined by Mosalli [16]:

- Time needed to achieve cooling is at least 1 h (whole body or only head).
- Temperature goal is 33.5–34.5 °C for 72 h.
- When rewarming, increase temperature to 36.5–37 °C not faster than 0.5 °C/h.
- EEG monitoring is part of most protocols as either amplitude-integrated EEG (aEEG) or traditional EEG. The EEG is applied during or before the cooling process and continued until rewarming is complete.
- EEG valuable tool to evaluate for encephalopathy and seizures.
- MRI brain performed once the baby is rewarmed.
  Severely abnormal MRI is associated with at least 75% adverse outcomes.

9.2 Case 2: Neonatal Apnea as a Common Newborn Treatment Challenge

The patient was a 2-week-old infant born at 34 WGA with an uncomplicated delivery with Apgar scores of 7 at 1 min and 9 at 5 min. Her birth weight was 2600 g. Neonatal intensive care unit course consisted of mainly feeding and temperature support. Apneic and bradycardia events occurred and did not resolve as she matured. Laryngoscopy of the upper airway and MRI of the brain were normal. EEG did not show any seizure activity corresponding to these events; however, EEG showed

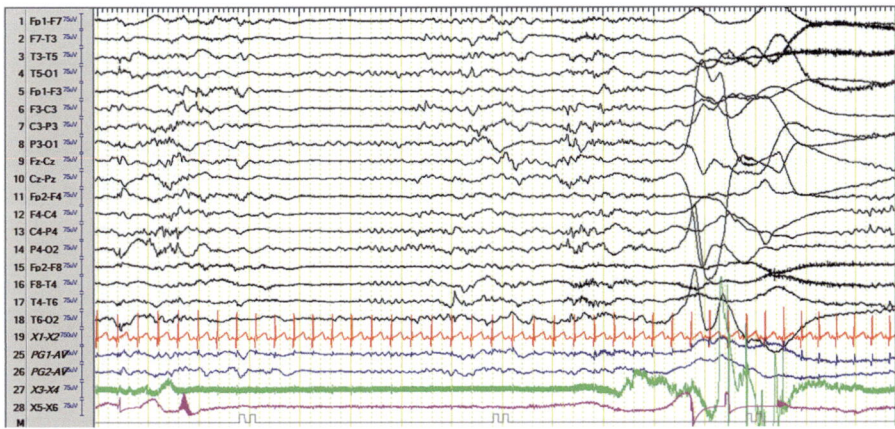

Fig. 9.3 Pause in chest wall movement in a neonate depicted on EEG. The patient is in quiet sleep when the brief 8-second event of no chest wall movement occurs. The patient arouses and resumes breathing, as seen by the chest wall movement lead (purple line)

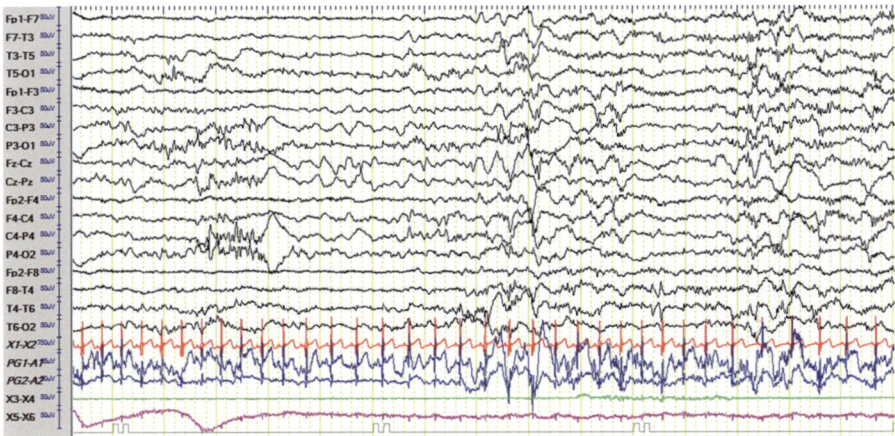

Fig. 9.4 EEG showing findings consistent with neonatal central apnea, in which the chest wall movement lead does not show movements during the apneic event. In this segment, the apneic event begins. The lower purple line represents the lead for the chest wall movement band. The patient is in quiet sleep

apneic events to occur in quiet sleep and were most consistent with central apnea. Alarm parameters were set for an apneic event of 20 seconds. Sometimes the patient was able to breathe again without external stimulation (Fig. 9.3). However, the EEG recording also revealed an instance in which the patient did not stimulate herself out of the event but did respond to the alarm noise (Figs. 9.4 and 9.5). The patient was treated with caffeine with improvement of events.

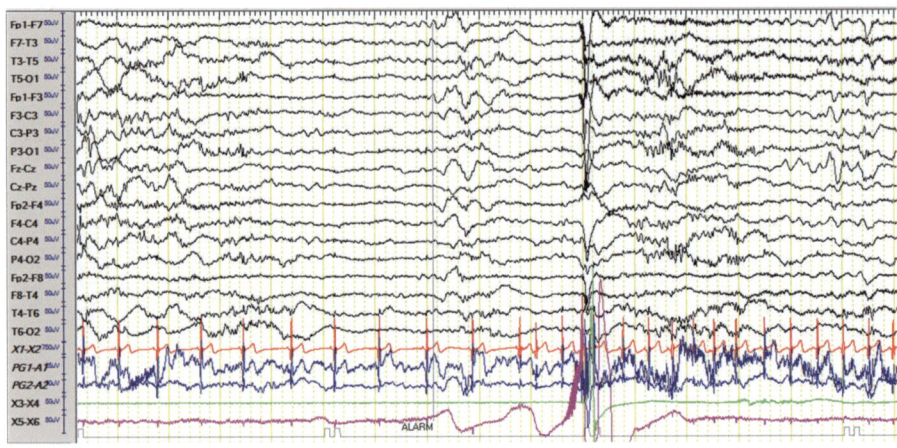

Fig. 9.5 EEG showing findings consistent with neonatal central apnea. The chest wall movement lead does not show movements during the apneic event. The lower purple line represents the lead for the chest wall movement band. Heart rate lead shows bradycardia. The patient is in quiet sleep when the apneic event occurs. The alarm noise stimulated the patient to breathe again, notation ALARM. Background activity shows continuous activity after the alarm, so the patient is either awake or in active sleep

Neonatal apnea, or apnea of prematurity, is defined by cessation of respirations for at least 20 s with an associated desaturation and/or bradycardia. Three types of neonatal apnea in order of most common to least common are

– Mixed (combination of central and obstructive apneas)
– Central
– Obstructive.

Prolonged apnea causing hypoxia can lead to diffuse electrographic attenuation.

The incidence of apnea lowers with increasing gestational age and thus likely represents a combined physiological and neurological immaturity rather than a pathological process. The maturation of the physiological processes that control breathing patterns are nearly complete by 42 weeks gestational age in both term and preterm infants.

Treatment is typically with continuous positive airway pressure (CPAP) or administration of xanthine medication, typically caffeine. Uncomplicated apnea of prematurity will usually resolve by 36–40 weeks corrected gestational age but can persist in more immature infants until approximately 43–44 weeks corrected gestational age. Prognosis with regards to apnea is difficult to assess as the most high-risk

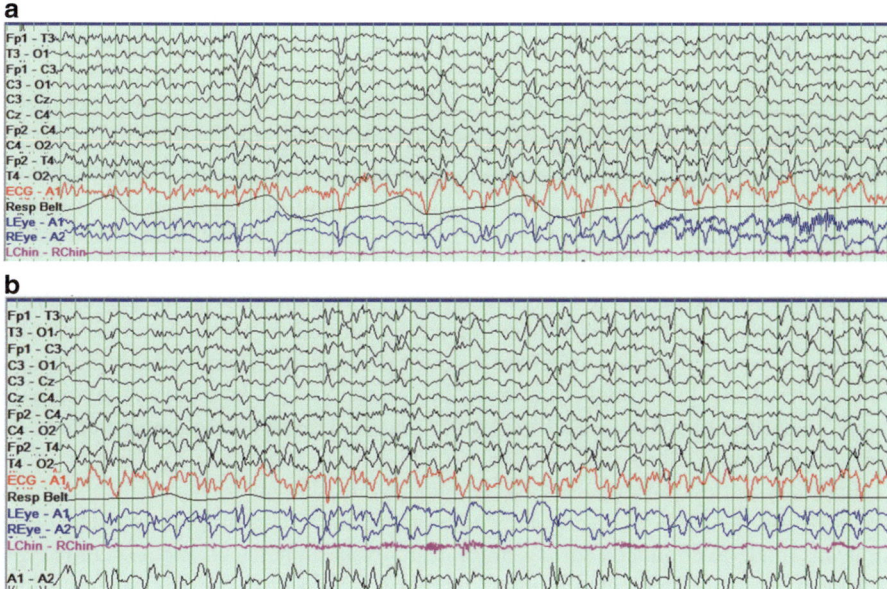

Fig. 9.6 (**a**, **b**) Apnea occurring during a seizure in a neonate. The seizure begins with left hemisphere discharges, then becomes bilateral. Apnea is present during the seizure

infants typically have additional risk factors that also factor into the clinical prognosis. It is suspected, however, that persistent apnea and bradycardia beyond 36 weeks corrected gestational age are associated with a higher incidence of suboptimal neurodevelopmental outcomes, likely resulting from recurrent hypoxia with resultant effect on neural plasticity.

Differential diagnoses of persistent apnea are broad and can include [15]

- Genetic abnormality (PHOX2B)
- Intraventricular hemorrhage
- Hypoxic-ischemic encephalopathy
- Congenital malformations
- Sepsis
- Anemia
- Gastroesophageal reflux
- Sedating medications
- Viral infection
- Seizures
- Seizures are a very important cause of apnea, and this occurrence can be determined by continuous video EEG monitoring (Fig. 9.6) [11].

9.3 Case 3: Intricacies of Brain Death Diagnosis in Preterm and Term Neonates

This patient was a male born at 36 WGA. Pregnancy and delivery were uncomplicated, and the baby was discharged from the nursery with the family. At 3 weeks of age, the baby presented emergently to the hospital due to lethargy. The patient was intubated and not placed on sedative medications. Neuroimaging showed evidence of acute diffuse hypoxic injury. Continuous EEG was begun, and background activity was extremely low voltage with no reactivity. The pattern was not quite isoelectric but was concerning for diffuse cortical dysfunction. 36 h after presentation, focal subclinical electrographic seizures were captured on the EEG. Antiepileptic medication was started and subclinical seizures resolved. Meanwhile, background activity remained low voltage and over the following 3–4 days became extremely suppressed (less than 5 µV). The baby was continued on an antiepileptic medication for seizure control.

Five days after presentation, the clinical exam did not reveal any brainstem reflexes, and the EEG recording showed extreme amplitude suppression. The decision was made to conduct a formal brain death exam, apnea test, and a specific type of EEG to evaluate for electrocerebral inactivity. As expected, the EEG did not show any significant cortical activity at the sensitivity of 2 µV, which confirmed electrocerebral silence (Fig. 9.7a, b). Even though the baby was treated with an antiepileptic medication, with its potential effect of EEG depression, it was felt that the clinical exam and EEG study were both accurate indicators of the baby's functioning. A repeat clinical exam, apnea test, and electrocerebral silence EEG were done 24 h later and revealed the same results. The decision was made to extubate and provide comfort care.

EEG Tidbit
A sensitivity setting of 2 µV will display low-voltage activity as a higher wave on the screen, showing very small amplitudes clearly. In the intensive care unit, there are multiple electronic and mechanical artifact sources. A setting of 2 µV, with a patient in electrocerebral silence, may only show the artifactual waveforms. It also is common to have confusion of whether the waves seen are truly cerebral in origin or artifactual.

In older children and adults, a brain death exam and apnea test are performed to help determine the presence of irreversible injury that would help lead to the decision for withdrawal of care. Ancillary studies, such as cerebral blood flow (CBF) testing or EEG, can also be helpful in determining brain death [1]. However, there are no set guidelines for term or preterm infants in determining brain death. Often times, performing repeat brain death and apnea exams showing similar findings may be helpful to confirm that the patient's state is not transient, and chance of significant recovery is low [3]. In 1987, a task force suggested that for term neonates, two exams 48 h apart are sufficient to evaluate brain death [26]. A more recent recommendation in 2011 stated that a 24-h separation is sufficient to determine brain death if both exams are consistent with brain death [17].

9 Case Examples in Neonates with Clinical Scenarios Using Electroencephalogram…   213

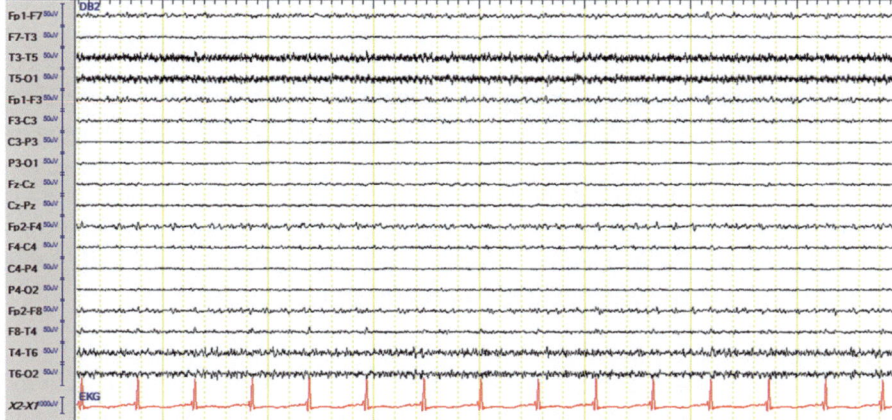

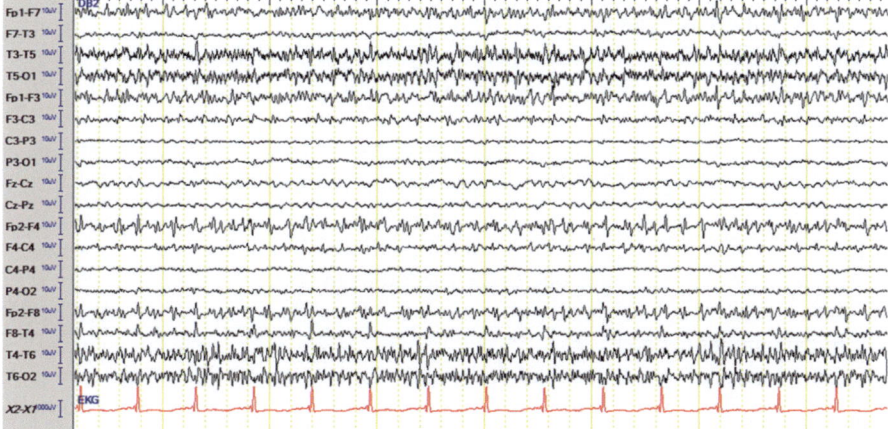

Fig. 9.7 (**a, b**) Neonatal EEG showing electrocerebral inactivity. Recording is at a sensitivity of 7 µV (**a**), and no cortical activity is observed. (**b**) Neonatal EEG showing electrocerebral inactivity. Recording is at a sensitivity of 2 µV and no cortical activity is observed. Low-amplitude 1 Hz activity in the left occipital electrode is from artifact from patient's head moving with each respiration

Preterm neonates are difficult to evaluate for brain death, and there are no standard criteria or guidelines for this population. In these scenarios, the infant is likely very ill, perhaps sedated and intubated. Thus, alertness is difficult to discern and an EEG background would likely be abnormal due to the sedation and the critically ill nature of the neonate. In addition, preterm neonates may not have developed complete brain stem reflexes, thus limiting the clinical exam for brainstem evaluation. The decision for continuation of care is often challenging and prognosis may be a factor in the decision-making process. Based on the Report of the AAN Guidelines

Subcommittee, AAP, CNS, SCCM. Pediatric and Adult Brain Death/Death by Neurologic Criteria Consensus Guideline, 2023 [23], the AAN states that the brain death exam for brain death determination in neonates less than 37 WGA is not reliable.

Ancillary studies, such as EEG and radiographs for the presence of cerebral blood flow, in a term neonate less than 30 days of age may not have the reliable impact as they do in older children and adults with only 40–60% sensitivity. However, the use of EEG as an ancillary study in the determination of brain death is described below, based on the *American Clinical Neurophysiology Society Guideline 3: Minimum Technical Standards for EEG Recording in Suspected Cerebral Death.* 2006 American Clinical Neurophysiology Update [2].

Neurology Tidbit

EEG can only detect cortical activity and does not assess brainstem activity. Brainstem functioning is determined by the clinical exam. The definition of brain death varies across states and facilities but the presence of cortical (EEG) activity excludes the diagnosis of brain death. However, the absence of cortical activity can still occur with preserved brainstem activity.

EEG criteria when used as ancillary study in brain death determination is a specific EEG protocol to evaluate for electrocerebral silence, defined as no cortical activity ABOVE 2 µV.

Guidelines (*American Clinical Neurophysiology Society Guideline 3: Minimum Technical Standards for EEG Recording in Suspected Cerebral Death* [2]):

1. A full set of scalp electrodes should be utilized (this may not be possible in preterm or term neonates due to their small head size).
2. Interelectrode distances should be at least 10 centimeters (may not be possible in the smaller neonate).
3. Interelectrode impedances should be between 100 and 10,000 Ohms.
4. The integrity of the entire recording system should be tested; this is usually done with the technician tapping each electrode and verifying its placement and signal changes.
5. Sensitivity must be increased from 7 µV to at least 2 µV for at least 30 min of the recording.
6. Filter settings should be set to allow for interpretation of low-voltage slow or fast activity. The high-frequency filter should be at least 30 Hz and the low-frequency filter at the most a setting of 1 Hertz (Hz). This will allow for a range of 1–30 Hz activity.
7. Additional monitoring techniques should be employed when necessary.
8. No EEG reactivity is present to stimulation.
9. Recordings only done by a qualified technologist and tap test completed (Fig. 9.8).
10. Repeat EEG performed if electrocerebral inactivity criteria are not met.

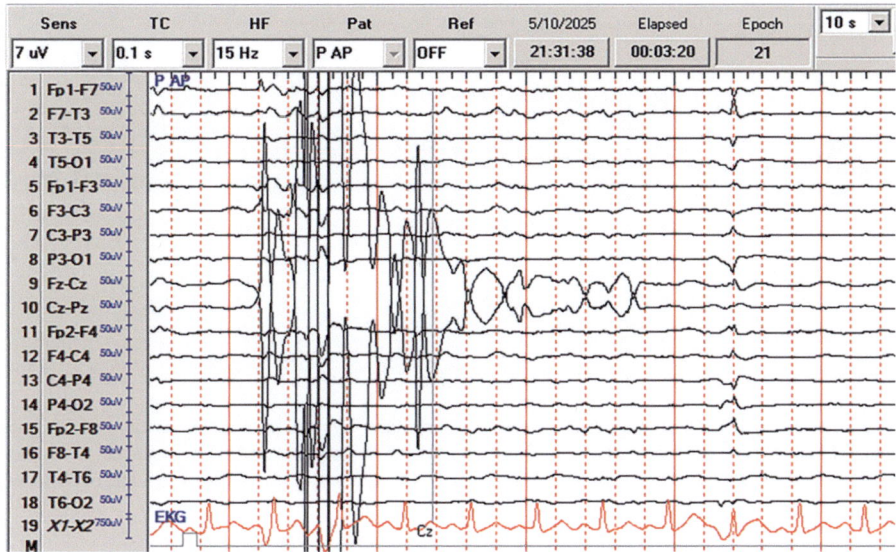

Fig. 9.8 Example of an electrode tapping test in a neonate. The vertex electrode (Cz electrode) is being tapped, a way that the technician can verify that the location of the electrode on the scalp correlates correctly with the location on the patient's scalp

Brain death determination in a neonate less than 37 WGA is unable to be made. The clinical exam and ancillary studies may help guide the medical team and family to make the best decision for care. In a term neonate, the clinical brain death exam may be somewhat more reliable but is still limited based on the presence of immature brainstem reflexes and inability to accurately assess brain function in an ill neonate. Ancillary studies may be helpful to show lack of cerebral blood flow or lack of cortical activity; however, neither of these tests can replace the clinical cranial nerve exam and apnea test. The decision to withdraw care of any patient is challenging, and in a neonate requires many difficult discussions and overall care plan for the family and patient.

9.4 Case 4: Hyperekplexia/Startle Disease

A term newborn male was delivered via spontaneous vaginal delivery to a healthy mother after an uneventful pregnancy. Shortly after birth, the infant exhibited exaggerated startle responses to minimal stimuli, increased muscle stiffness, and episodic apnea (Figs. 9.9 and 9.10). Physical examination revealed hypertonia with a persistently flexed posture, and clonus was absent. Neurological assessment showed intact reflexes but excessive jerking movements in response to touch and sound.

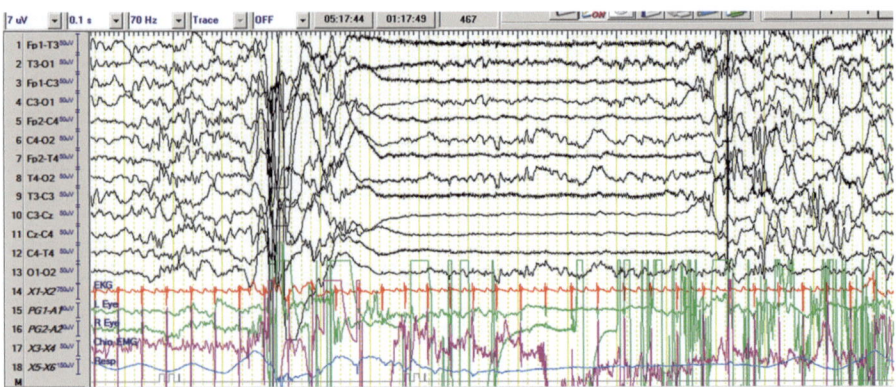

Fig. 9.9 Neonatal startle response leading to apnea and hyperekplexia. The patient is in quiet sleep, then startles (as seen by high-amplitude waveform signifying movement artifact). An attenuation occurs corresponding to the arousal. Meanwhile, the respiratory lead (blue line) shows no chest wall movement

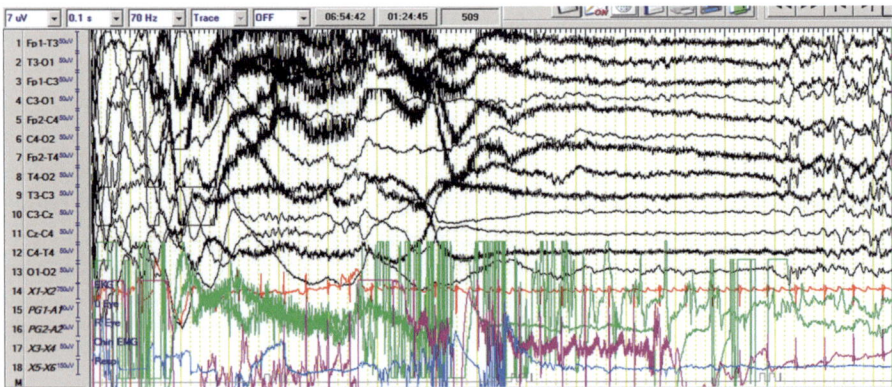

Fig. 9.10 Neonatal startle response leading to apnea and hyperekplexia. The patient startles (as seen by high-amplitude waveform signifying movement artifact) and attenuation occurs corresponding to the arousal. Meanwhile, the respiratory lead (blue line) shows no chest wall movement, leading to the apneic response

A clinical suspicion of hyperekplexia (HK) was raised, and genetic testing confirmed a mutation in the GLRA1 gene, which encodes the glycine receptor. Supportive care, including swaddling and reducing external stimuli, was initiated. The patient responded well to clonazepam, which helped decrease startle episodes and muscle rigidity. He was discharged home on clonazepam, and the events resolved by 18 months of age.

Hyperekplexia is also known as startle disease or congenital stiff-person syndrome. It is a rare condition characterized by a pathogenic overactivity of the physiological startle response as well as generalized muscle stiffness [18]. In some subtle cases, the presentation may only include an exaggerated startle response. In the more severe form, the triad occurs of exaggerated startle, nocturnal myoclonus, and generalized stiffness with an increased risk of sudden infant death syndrome (SIDS) [4]. The startle response is thought to be a protective reflex that involves a motor response following sudden, unexpected stimuli (usually auditory or tactile). In hyperekplexia, the excessive startle response leads to prolonged stiffening following the stimulus. The stiffening may lead to sustained tonic spasms and interfere with feeding, motor development, and even cause apnea leading to respiratory failure and death [10].

The exaggerated startle response can be elicited by nose tapping. Usually, serum electrolytes, neuroimaging, EEG, and other biochemical tests are normal. Continuous video EEG monitoring can be helpful to exclude the presence of epileptic activity as the cause. Attacks of hypertonicity with cyanosis can be stopped by a simple intervention called the Vigevano maneuver, which consists of flexion of the head and legs toward the trunk. This maneuver employs forced flexion of the head and legs toward the trunk and has been used in newborn to terminate cyanotic startle attacks [27].

Hyperekplexia may be caused by genetic mutations affecting the glycine receptor (GlyR), and more specifically, the alpha-1 subunit of the receptor. There are some reported cases affecting the beta-subunit [22]. Most cases are inherited in an autosomal-dominant pattern but may be autosomal-recessive or X-linked. Mutations in affected patients have been reported in the following genes: GLRA1, SLC6A5, GLRB, GPHN, and ARHGEF9. Genetic markers have been found for the major forms but are only unusually present in the minor forms.

Clonazepam is the treatment of choice for hyperekplexia. An intermediate- to long-acting benzodiazepine, clonazepam enhances the activity of GABA-A receptors by increasing the frequency of chloride channel opening, leading to neuronal cellular hyperpolarization and CNS depression. Infants often require relatively high doses (0.1–0.2 mg/kg/day) of clonazepam to maintain symptom control. Other medications have been mentioned, mostly in case reports, with variable efficacy. These include other benzodiazepines (clobazam, diazepam), antiepileptic medications (phenobarbital, carbamazepine, phenytoin, valproate), levetiracetam, and serotonergic medications (fluoxetine, 5-hydroxytryptophan). Events resolve by 1 year of age and there is no known effect on neurodevelopmental outcomes, although delay is mentioned in some cases [5, 12, 14].

9.5 Case 5: Pyridoxine-Dependent Epilepsy

The patient was a female born at 39 WGA. Mother had prenatal care and did not use any tobacco, alcohol or medications. However, mom recalls baby having frequent "hiccups" during her last trimester. Delivery was difficult with the complication of shoulder dystocia, and Apgar scores were 5 and 8 at 1 and 5 min, respectively. Soon after birth, the baby received positive pressure ventilation, which improved her respiratory status. She was admitted to the neonatal intensive care unit for observation.

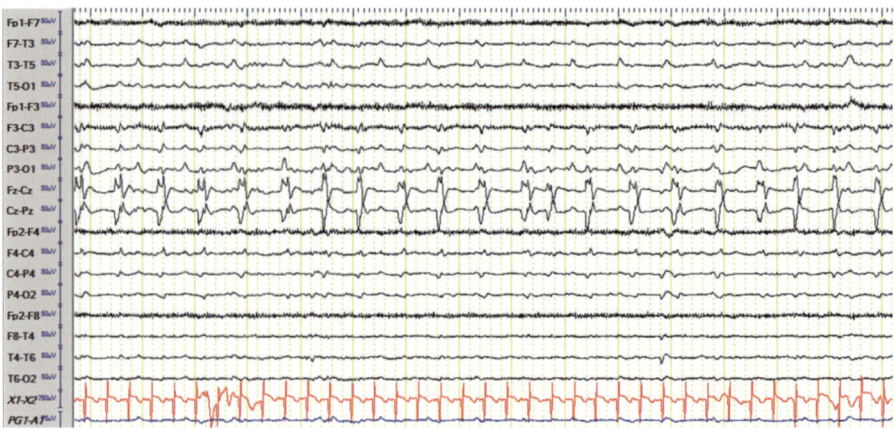

Fig. 9.11 Focal neonatal seizure in a patient with pyridoxine-dependent epilepsy. Seizure in the vertex region with spread to the left, more than right, hemisphere

About 24 h later, oral feeds were attempted but the baby struggled to take in adequate nutrition due to a poor latch and tiring easily while feeding. She was then gavage-fed most of her feeds. Around 36 h of life, focal clonic seizure activity began and continuous electroencephalography (EEG) monitoring was initiated. Seizures manifested as left or right arm or bilateral leg jerking with nystagmus. Seizures lasted approximately 2–3 min, and the EEG showed independent bilateral focal seizures (Figs. 9.11, 9.12, and 9.13). Antiepileptic medications (AEMs) were started with initial mild improvement. Background activity was discontinuous and showed an encephalopathic pattern (Fig. 9.14). However, as the next few days progressed, she required higher doses of antiepileptic medications and additional antiepileptic medications due to an increase in seizure activity. She was eventually intubated and given a continuous midazolam infusion to control seizures. Clinical seizures abated; however, subclinical (electrographic-only) seizures persisted. Magnetic resonance imaging (MRI) of the brain was obtained, which showed no anatomical abnormalities or evidence of hypoxic-ischemic encephalopathy.

Family history was negative for seizures or developmental delays. Metabolic evaluation was performed, including lumbar puncture for cerebrospinal fluid studies. All testing was negative, and there were no other etiologies found to cause seizures. Given the frequency of seizures, poor response to antiepileptic medications, and no identifiable etiology for the seizures, it was decided to try pyridoxine.

On day of life seven, 100 mg of intravenous (IV) pyridoxine was given. EEG showed mild improvement of background slowing and epileptic burden. She was discharged home on 10 mg/k) three times a day of oral pyridoxine. A repeat EEG study 1 month later revealed that her background activity was much improved with occasional interictal epileptiform discharges and no seizures (Fig. 9.5). Family reported only brief clinical seizures occurring one to two times daily. By this time, serum α-AASA and pipecolic acid obtained prior to starting pyridoxine resulted and elevated. Genetic testing, which was also performed the first week of life, was

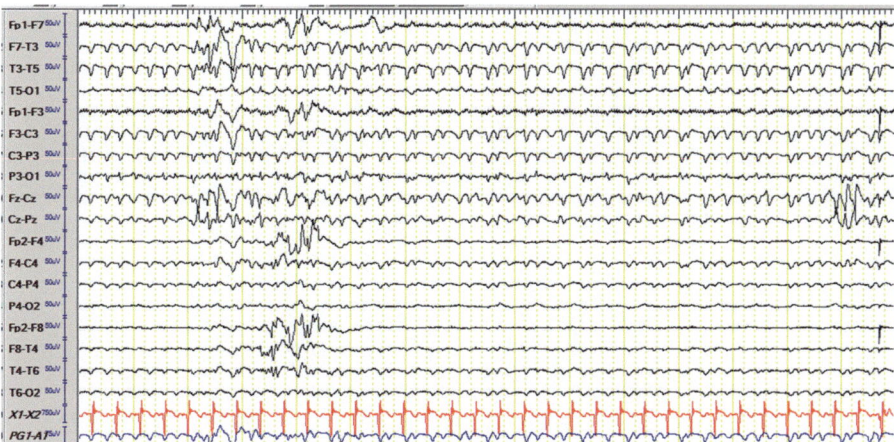

Fig. 9.12 Focal neonatal seizure in a patient with pyridoxine-dependent epilepsy. This seizure is located in the left hemisphere

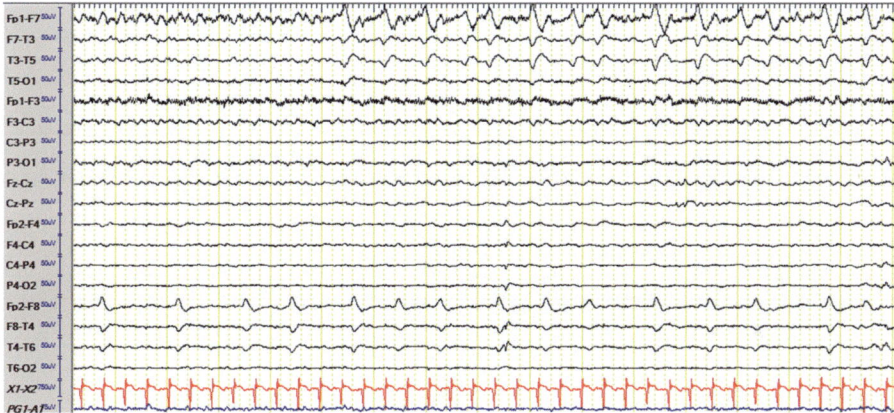

Fig. 9.13 Focal neonatal seizures in a patient with pyridoxine-dependent epilepsy. In this segment, two different focal seizures are occurring, one in each hemisphere

positive for a mutation of the ALDH7A1 gene. Over the next few months, clinical seizure frequency lessened, and the patient was able to be moderately controlled with pyridoxine and two other antiepileptic medications (Fig. 9.15). She has had developmental delays, for which she has been enrolled in early intervention services.

Pyridoxine-dependent epilepsy (PDE) is a rare, inborn error of pyridoxine metabolism with an estimated incidence of 1:65000 to 1:250000 live births. It is characterized by developmental delays with severe, refractory seizures that respond moderately to pyridoxine. PDE has also been referred to as pyridoxine dependency,

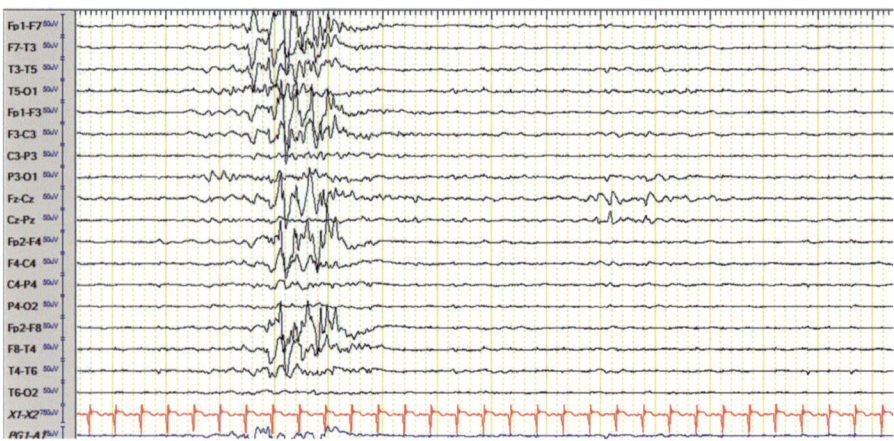

Fig. 9.14 Abnormal background activity in a patient with pyridoxine-dependent epilepsy. The background pattern shows excessive discontinuity with high-amplitude sharp waves, suggestive of encephalopathy

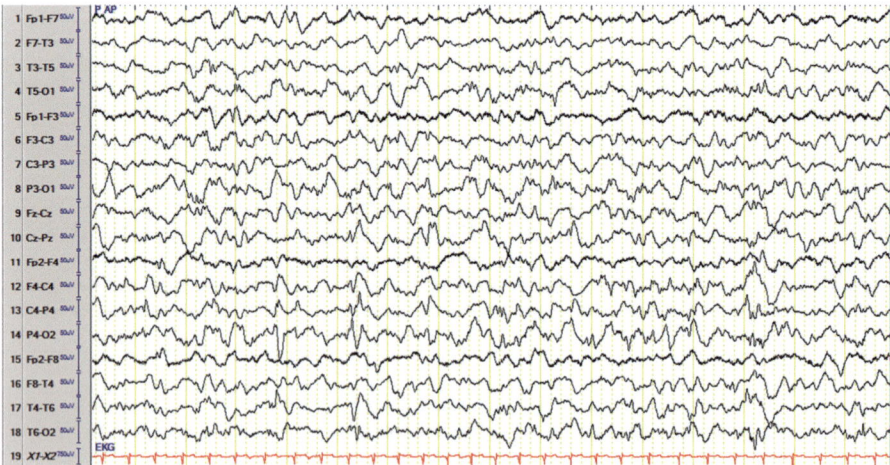

Fig. 9.15 Repeat EEG at 6 months of age in a patient with pyridoxine-dependent epilepsy. Background activity shows diffuse slowing with predominance of delta and theta frequencies. The presence of a slow background pattern suggests persistence of encephalopathy. Right hemisphere interictal epileptiform discharges are present

pyridoxine-dependent seizures, pyridoxine-responsive seizure disorders, as well as AASA dehydrogenase deficiency.

PDE is an autosomal-recessive condition with the most frequent mutation demonstrated in the ALDH7A1 gene. This mutation results in decreased α-aminoadipic semialdehyde dehydrogenase (ALDH7A1) activity, also known as antiquitin, which is involved in cerebral lysine catabolism and leads to the accumulation of multiple metabolites, including α-aminoadipic semialdehyde dehydrogenase (α-AASA), Δ1-piperideine-6-carboxylate (Δ1-P6C), and pipecolic acid. This accumulation of α-AASA leads to reduced activity of several enzymes in the brain that regulate transmission between neurons and brain development. It is important to note that affected individuals are metabolically dependent on pyridoxine, rather than pyridoxine deficient, therefore, requiring substantially more than normal amounts of pyridoxine. Pyridoxal phosphate (PLP), the biologically active form of vitamin B6, is often used to assess vitamin B6 status. This reflects liver concentration and is minimally influenced by dietary fluctuation. However, the assay is not always widely available, and results may be delayed. Greater than 30 nmol/L is considered sufficient, 20–30 nmol/L marginal, and less than 20 nm/L insufficient. A similar disorder is pyridoxamine 5′-phosphate oxidase deficiency, which requires treatment with pyridoxal phosphate (PLP).

Refractory seizures typically present within hours or days of birth. In some instances, seizures have been reported to occur intrauterine, with onset at the end of the last trimester. In fact, this may have been the case with our patient; the hiccup movements that mom detected may have actually been seizure activity. The classic case of an EEG normalizing with the administration of IV pyridoxine is very rare. Often, high-dose pyridoxine treatment overtime shows mild clinical improvement. Late-onset and other atypical forms of PDE can begin in late infancy and sometimes do not present until 3 years of age or later. These atypical forms can have an initial response to AEMs that subsequently become refractory with a suboptimal response initially to pyridoxine [25].

The standard treatment of PDE includes lifelong pyridoxine supplementation in pharmacological doses. The International PDE Consortium currently recommends "triple therapy," which includes pyridoxine supplementation as the mainstay for seizure control in addition to lysine reduction therapies, aiming to improve neurocognitive outcomes.

1. Pyridoxine supplementation
   (a) During initial acute seizures, administer 100 mg of pyridoxine intravenously and repeated up to four times (maximal dose 500 mg). Given the risk of apnea and hypotension, cardiorespiratory monitoring is important.
   (b) Newborns: 100–200 mg/day of pyridoxine (vitamin B6) supplementation.
   (c) Infants: 15–30 mg/kg/day of pyridoxine, max dose of 300 mg/day.
   (d) Children and adolescents: average of 20 mg/kg/day (range 5–30 mg/kg/day) of pyridoxine with a maximum dose of 500 mg/day.
   (e) Patients who are treated with greater than 500 mg/day of pyridoxine may be at higher risk of peripheral neuropathy.
   (f) Emergency treatment: in times of seizure relapse, for example, during a febrile illness, the dose of pyridoxine may be doubled up to a maximum of 60 mg/kg/day (in children) or 500 mg/day (adolescents and adults) for up to 3 days.
2. Lysine-restricted medical diet.
3. L-arginine supplementation.

The early consideration of pyridoxine therapy remains important in a newborn or in a child with refractory early-onset seizures. This patient likely had in utero seizures, which resulted in difficult delivery and early poor feeding. Testing for PDE is not able to result immediately, so a differential diagnosis including PDE is beneficial in which to begin early treatment with pyridoxine [8].

9.6 Case 6: A Unique and Treatable Etiology for Early Infantile Developmental and Epileptic Encephalopathy

A male neonate was born at 37 weeks of gestation by induction due to maternal preeclampsia. Prenatal screens were unremarkable, and there was no history of maternal tobacco, alcohol, or illicit drug use. Apgar scores were 7 and 7 at 1 and 5 min, respectively. Neonatal intensive care medical team was called to evaluate the infant at 12 min of life due to pallor, cyanosis, and increased work of breathing. The infant was intubated and his respiratory status improved. At 24 h of life, the infant developed clinical seizure activity consisting of truncal myoclonus. Continuous EEG recording was initiated. EEG background activity revealed a burst suppression pattern with associated epileptic myoclonic seizures. Consideration of post-anoxic myoclonus or epileptic myoclonic encephalopathy was debated (Figs. 9.16, 9.17, 9.18, and 9.19). The infant was then treated with antiepileptic medications. Over the next few days, clinical seizure activity subsided and the background activity gradually improved (Fig. 9.20). With this improvement, the diagnosis of epileptic myoclonic encephalopathy was favored.

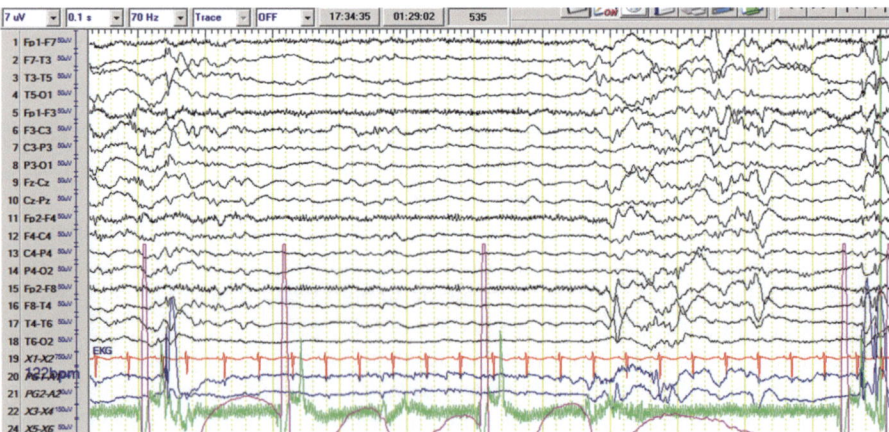

Fig. 9.16 Initial segment of EEG recording showing a burst suppression background pattern in the neonate with myoclonic events. The pink line shows artifact from the respiratory lead, which correlates with the truncal myoclonic movements. The movements do not correlate with an electrographic epileptic change on the EEG and were felt to be hiccoughs

9 Case Examples in Neonates with Clinical Scenarios Using Electroencephalogram... 223

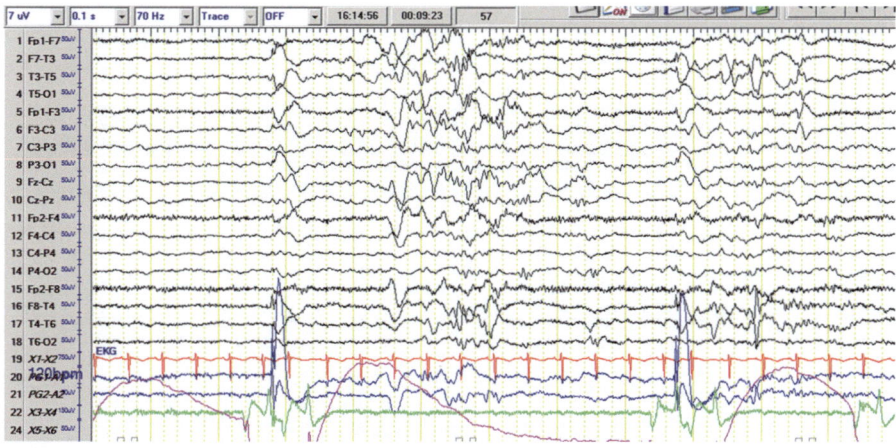

Fig. 9.17 Myoclonus in a neonate with burst suppression pattern in EEG recording. In this segment, the myoclonic movements are beginning to correlate with a sharp wave. However, it is not clear if the sharp wave is indeed cortical or is due to movement artifact as the baby is lying on the left side of his head

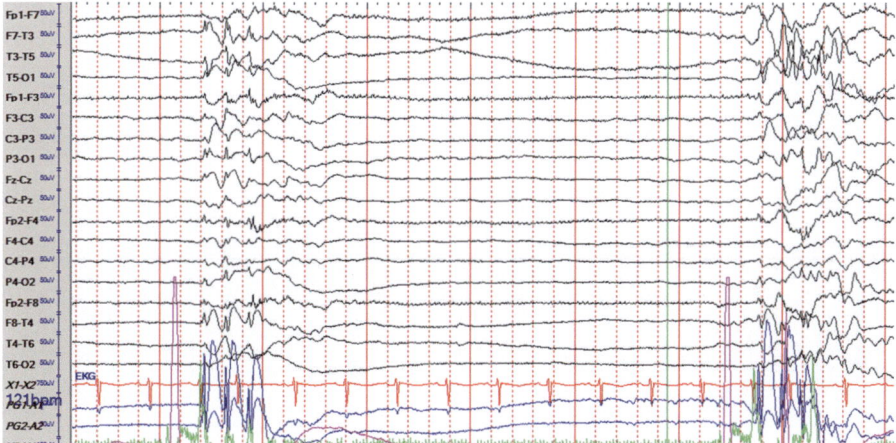

Fig. 9.18 Burst suppression background pattern in a neonate with myoclonic seizures. As the recording continues, the high-amplitude burst activity correlates with clinical myoclonic seizure. The additional eye, chin, and respiratory leads show movement, indicative of patient's myoclonic movements

Metabolic and genetic evaluations were negative. MRI of the brain showed scattered areas of hypoxia and a magnetic resonance venogram (MRV) of the head revealed small thrombi in the posterior aspect of the superior sagittal, right transverse and sigmoid dural venous sinuses and the straight sinus. Enoxaparin therapy was initiated, and coagulopathic evaluation revealed heterozygous mutation of

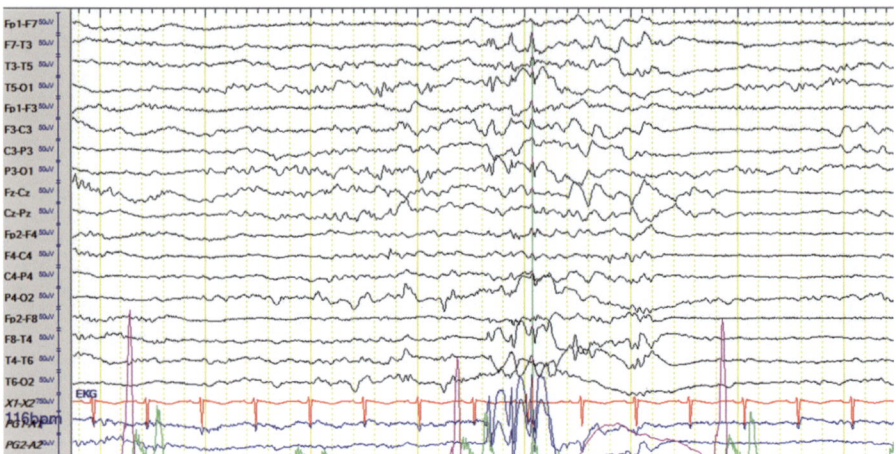

Fig. 9.19 EEG in a neonate with myoclonic seizures. Background activity is burst suppression but compared to initial segment, burst activity is longer lasting and periods of attenuation demonstrate higher amplitude. Myoclonic event correlated with burst activity

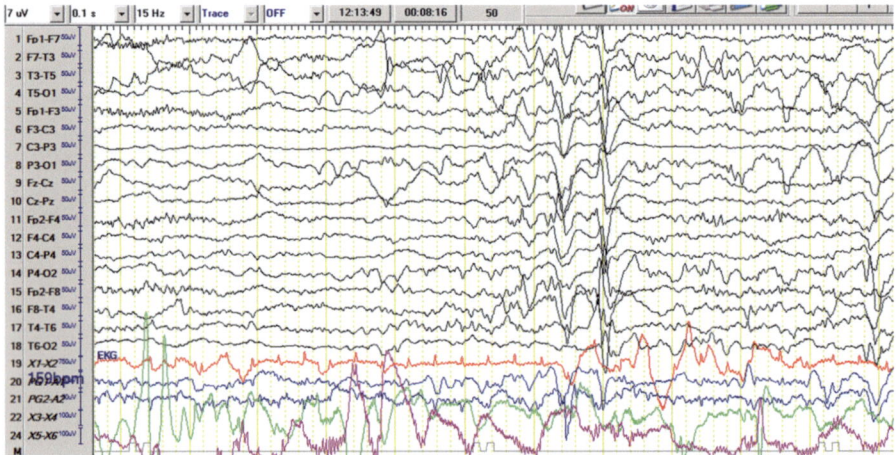

Fig. 9.20 Neonate with myoclonic seizures and burst suppression background activity, post treatment with antiepileptic medications. He was also found to have venous thromboses and was started on anticoagulant therapy. The EEG shows high-amplitude epileptiform discharge, but a clinical event does not occur at this time. The pink line does not show movement artifact

Factor V Leiden. EEG done on day of life 11 prior to discharge showed the presence of bilateral, independent sharp activity during quiet sleep (Figs. 9.21 and 9.22). Antiepileptic medications and heparin were continued after discharge. At 6 months of age, a routine EEG was normal and the infant was then weaned off antiepileptic medications (Fig. 9.23). Repeat MRI and MRV with and without contrast at

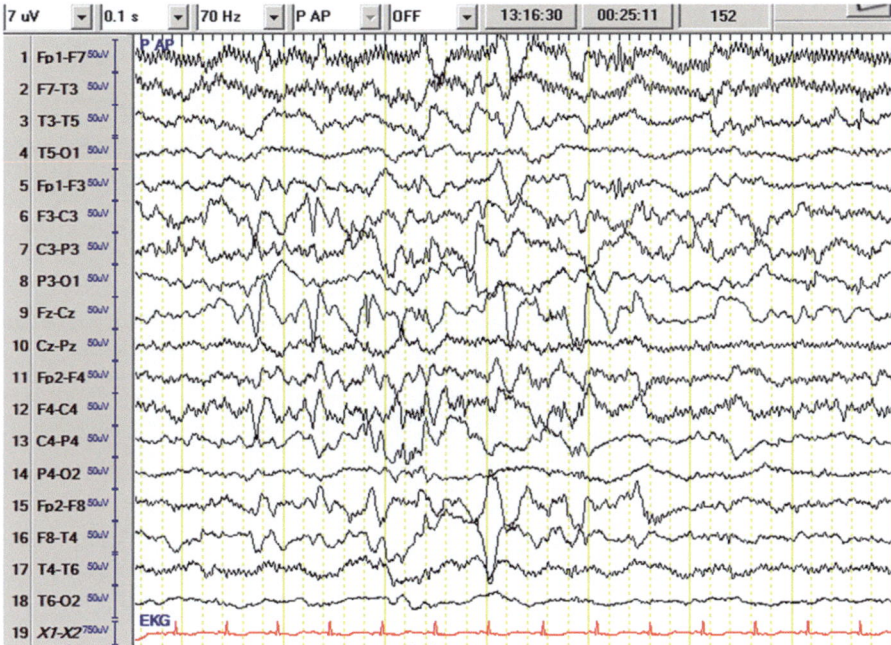

Fig. 9.21 EEG in a neonate with myoclonic seizures, burst suppression pattern, and venous thromboses. This EEG is done at 11 days of age and shows multifocal sharp waves in quiet sleep. Overall background activity is improved from birth showing continuity. In addition, bilateral frontal epileptiform sharp waves are present. No clinical events are occurring

4 months of age demonstrated patency of sinuses, so enoxaparin was discontinued. The patient has been developmentally appropriate and has had no further clinical seizure activity. He currently remains off antiepileptics and anticoagulants.

Early infantile developmental and epileptic encephalopathy (EIDEE) is characterized by encephalopathy with a burst suppression background, myoclonic or tonic seizures, and developmental delays. Prior label of early myoclonic encephalopathy (EME) was also characterized clinically by focal myoclonus, usually of the face or extremities and electroencephalographically consisting of a burst suppression pattern that is often more distinct during quiet sleep. EIDEE is a broader category incorporating the features of EME and Ohtahara syndrome, thus including myoclonic and tonic seizure types. EIDEE presents during the first 3 months of life, and sometimes within a few hours after birth. Focal seizures occur in about 80% of cases but may be subtle, involving only autonomic signs such as flushing or apnea. This neonatal seizure syndrome is typically genetic in etiology and is unresponsive to antiepileptic medications with a poor prognosis [27] However, in our case, the patient's encephalopathy and myoclonic seizures were thought to be due to the acute onset of multifocal infarctions and their associated neuronal injury. This patient's seizures fortunately resolved, and his neurodevelopmental outcome was

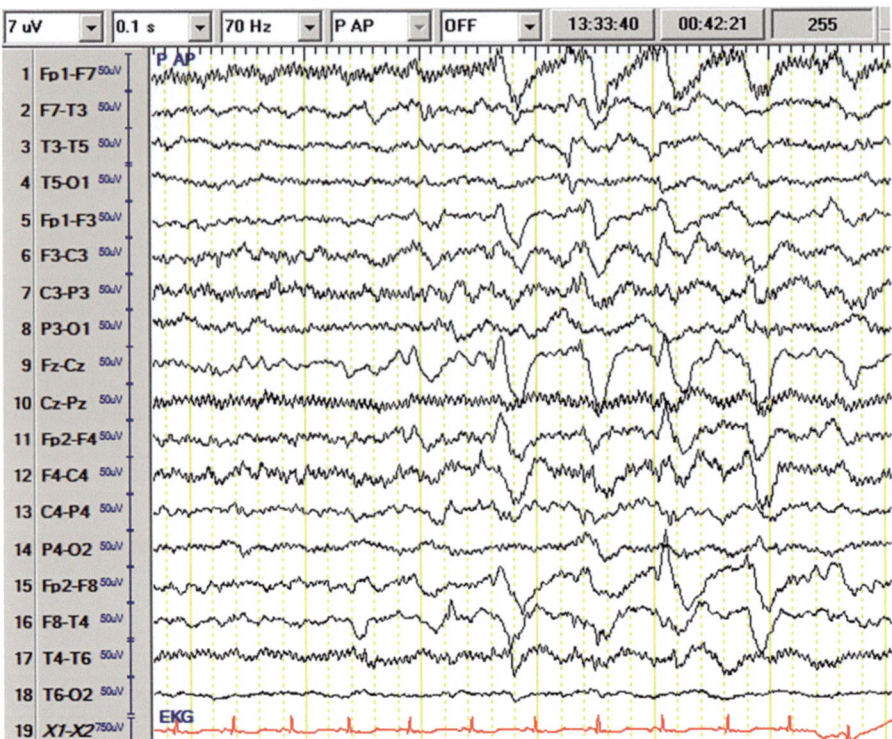

Fig. 9.22 EEG in a neonate with myoclonic seizures, burst suppression pattern, and venous thromboses. This EEG is done at 11 days of age, and background is improved with continuous activity. In addition, rhythmic frontal delta occurs, suggestive of typical for age anterior dysrhythmia

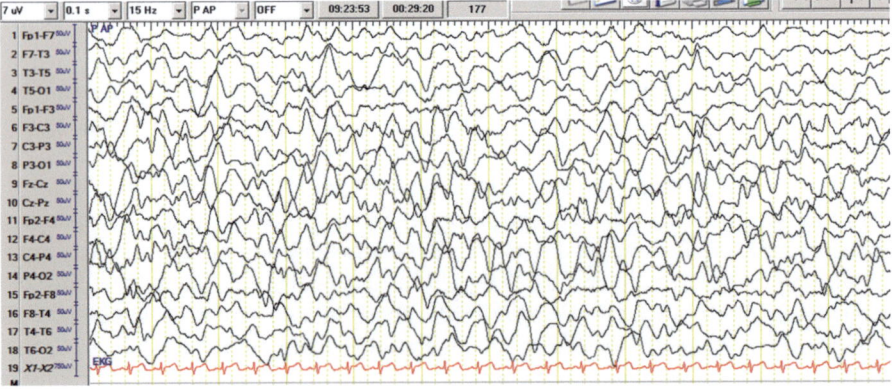

Fig. 9.23 Repeat EEG in a patient with myoclonic seizures showing improvement of background activity. At 6 months of age, this recording capturing stage 2 sleep was normal for age

favorable as cellular healing occurred and sinuses restored normal blood flow. This nonprogressive coagulopathic etiology proved treatable, although he does remain at increased risk for subsequent stroke and other thrombotic events given his diagnosis of Factor V Leiden.

The severe outcome typically seen with these myoclonic epileptic encephalopathies makes discussion with caregivers regarding this diagnosis quite delicate. Families should be referred to support groups if they exist in the area in which they live. This case highlights the importance of neurological evaluation to possibly detect more favorable outcome cases. It also serves as a reminder that seizures in neonates often have atypical, subtle presentations and should be considered in the differential for apnea, particularly in a term neonate.

9.7   Case 7: Holoprosencephaly and Its Unique EEG Findings

A male neonate was born at 40 WGA exposed to opiates, amphetamines, and gabapentin in utero. At delivery, he had respiratory distress, so he was admitted to the NICU for observation. Growth parameters revealed microcephaly. Head circumference was 32 centimeters (cm), 10% for age and length was 50 cm, 50% for age. MRI brain was performed, which showed partially fused thalami, fusion of frontal lobes, and absence of septum pellucidum. These findings were consistent with semilobar holoprosencephaly.

Within 3 days of life, the patient showed significant tremors and startles with autonomic dysfunction. EEG was abnormal with the presence of asymmetry of amplitudes and frequencies with frequent high-amplitude sharp transients (Figs. 9.24 and 9.25). Seizures were not captured. He was started on clonidine, which initially improved the withdrawal symptoms. However, about 7 days later, withdrawal symptoms worsened with excessive irritability and shaking. Phenobarbital was added to

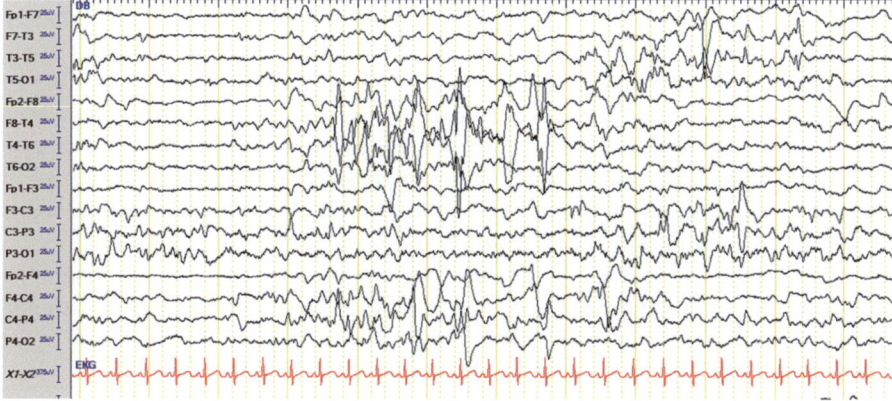

Fig. 9.24 EEG in a neonate with holoprosencephaly. Note the multifocal spikes, hemispheric asynchrony, intermittent low-voltage activity, and lack of normal organization

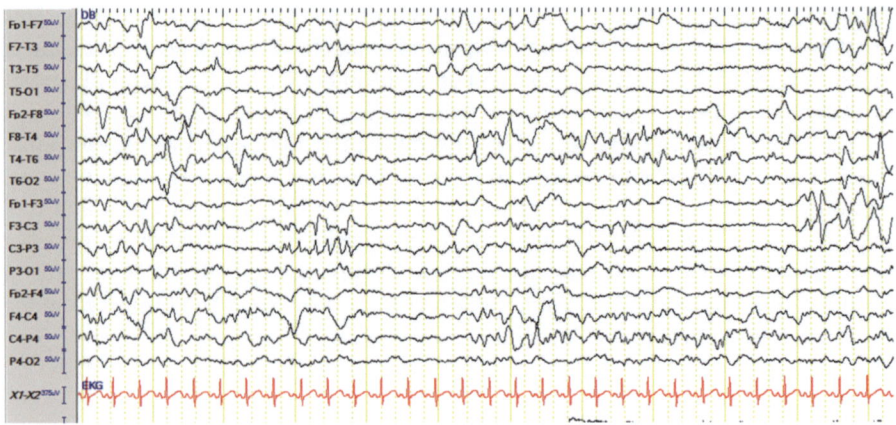

Fig. 9.25 EEG in a neonate with holoprosencephaly. Note the multifocal spikes, hemispheric asynchrony, intermittent low-voltage activity, and lack of normal organization. Monorhythmic theta and alpha frequencies are also noted in this segment

his regimen, and he improved, allowing him to be discharged 3 weeks later on no medications.

About 1 month later, he presented to the hospital with seizure-like activity. These new types of events were different than the typical jitteriness and exaggerated startles he had with withdrawal symptoms. Guardian reported event of head version to the right with associated right-side clonic activity. EEG was repeated and captured this clinical event (Fig. 9.26) and subclinical epileptic activity in bilateral hemispheres (Fig. 9.27). Antiepileptic medications were restarted. However, the patient has continued to have focal seizures refractory to medications and severe global developmental delays (Fig. 9.28).

Holoprosencephaly is defined as failure of the prosencephalon to separate into hemispheres.

This separation normally takes place between days 18–28 days of gestation. Estimates suggest it occurs in about 1 in 250 fetuses but often results in fetal death. Live birth occurs in roughly 1 in 8000 and represents a spectrum consisting of alobar, semilobar, and lobar holoprosencephaly, listed as most severe to least severe. Holoprosencephaly results from failure of the interhemispheric fissure to form with lack of separation of the prosencephalic vesicle around 5–6 weeks of gestation. Appropriate cleavage of the prosencephalon results in two separate hemispheres and development of the bilateral ventricular system, which patients with holoprosencephaly do not achieve. This leads to abnormal cortex generating frequent seizures, global developmental delays, and poor prognosis. In addition, patients with holoprosencephaly often have midline defects, such as cleft lip or palate, malformed pituitary, or abnormal tracts of the visual system [20].

EEG in a patient with holoprosencephaly has specific findings [9, 13]

- Multifocal spikes and polyspikes mixed with slow waves
- Periods of monorhythmic beta, alpha, theta, or delta frequencies

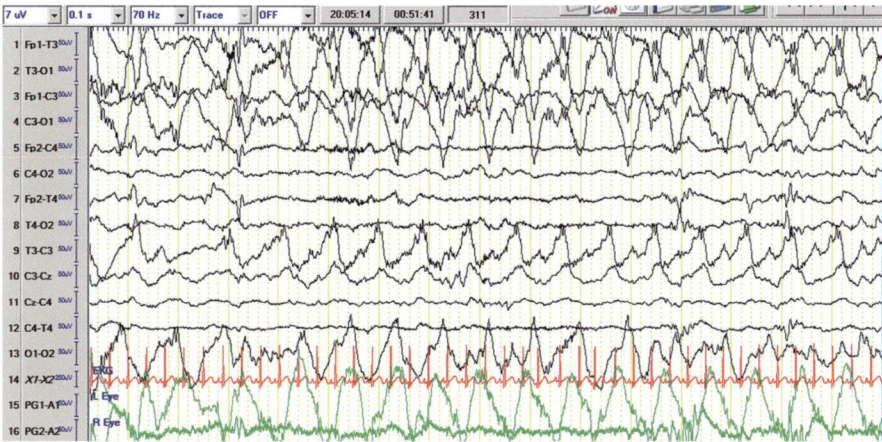

Fig. 9.26 Left centrotemporal seizure in a patient with holoprosencephaly. Seizure activity is occurring in the left hemisphere while the remainder of the background activity is suppressed. The left eye lead waveforms (PG1-A1) are detecting the left cortical activity and do not represent eye movement

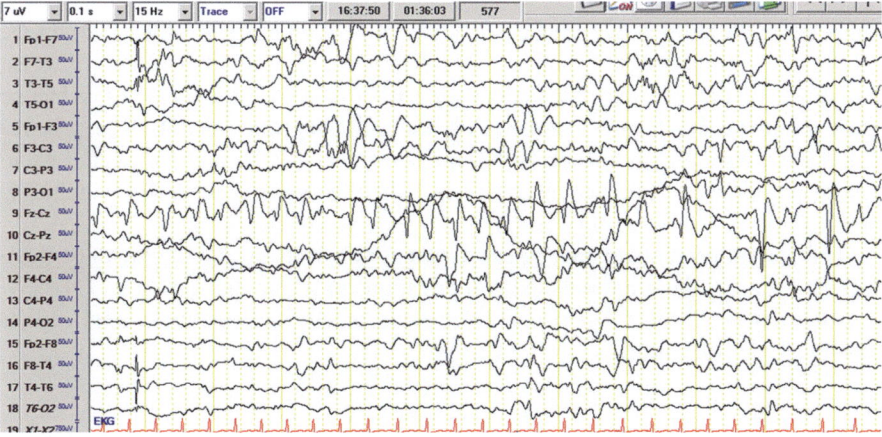

Fig. 9.27 EEG in a neonate with holoprosencephaly. Note the multifocal spikes, intermittent low-voltage activity and lack of normal organization. In addition, rhythmic frontal epileptiform spikes occur, suggestive of subclinical epileptic event. The patient does not show any clinical change at this time

- Hemisphere asynchrony
- Low-voltage activity
- Periodic patterns
- Lack of normal organization
- Poor correlation of clinical seizure-like events with electrographic EEG change

This patient likely had seizures during the withdrawal period, which may be why phenobarbital was more effective than clonidine alone treating her symptoms.

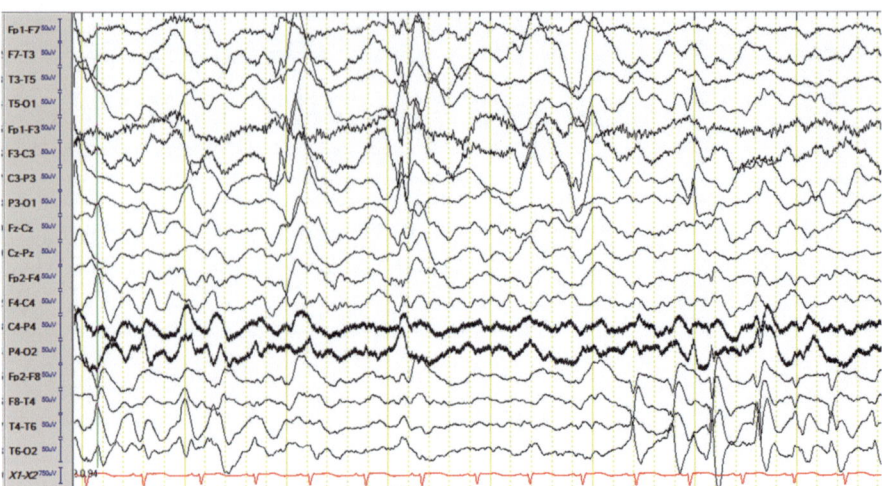

Fig. 9.28 EEG in an infant with holoprosencephaly. This EEG is performed at 2 months of age. Note the continued interhemispheric asynchrony and bilateral epileptiform spikes with regions of attenuation

However, with multiple substance exposures, it is often difficult to know when the timeline of withdrawal of certain substances may occur as substances have different half-lives and thus present at different ages post birth. An additional factor is that the baby was exposed to gabapentin, which has antiepileptic properties. The seizures could have been a combination of holoprosencephalic abnormal cortex and gabapentin withdrawal. Holoprosencephaly is linked to many gene defects, including trisomy 13.

The patient presented here represents the common diagnostic dilemma of treating patients with multiple medical complications in the neonatal period. The newborn is a constellation of genetics, in utero environment, and potential complications during the delivery process.

9.8 Case 8: Infantile Spasms

Although infantile spasms usually present beyond the neonatal age, this clinical scenario is presented here for awareness of this very important constellation of EEG abnormalities, seizures, and developmental delays. Prompt treatment is felt to greatly improve neurodevelopmental outcomes.

The patient was a 5-month-old female born at 36 WGA and presented with new-onset shaking events. Pregnancy and delivery were uneventful, and development was reported to be normal thus far. Several days prior to admission, parents noticed new occurrence of brief, rapid jerking movements of the arms and legs. These episodes occurred in succession, so in a 1-min period the baby had about 5–10 events. Sometimes her eyes rolled upward during the jerking. She was fussy afterward. There was no family history of seizures, no recent illness, or changes in medical history.

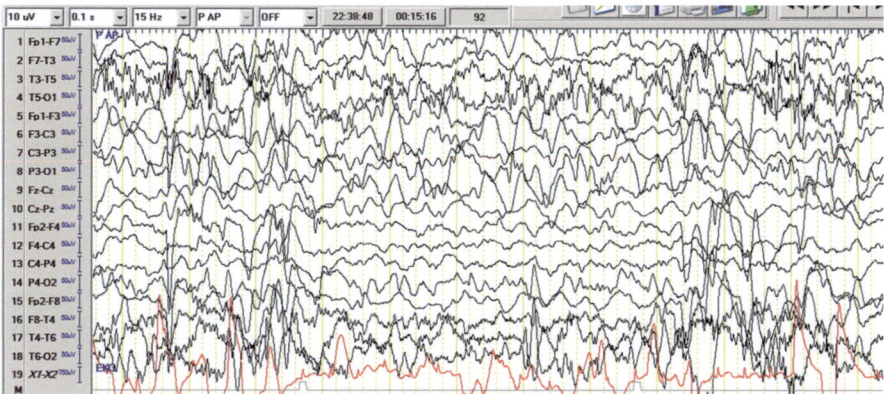

Fig. 9.29 Hypsarrhythmia EEG pattern. This segment shows high-amplitude background activity, multifocal spikes, and no normal background organization. In addition, the right frontocentral region shows suppression of amplitude, which correlates with the region of the porencephalic cyst. Sensitivity is 10 μV

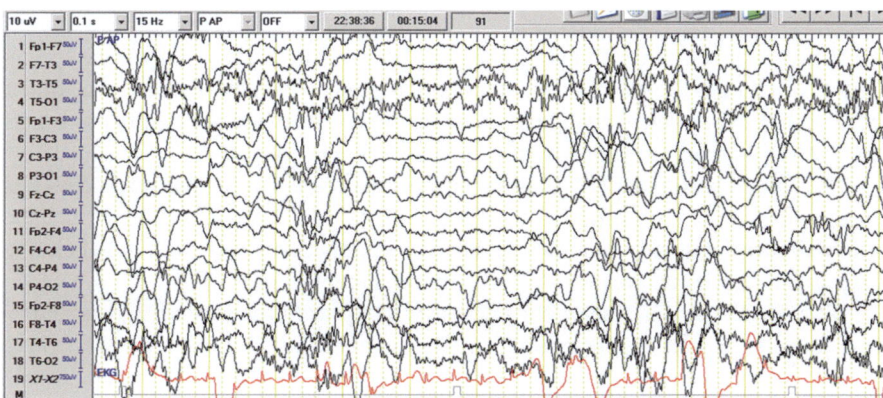

Fig. 9.30 Hypsarrhythmia EEG pattern with electrodecrement. This segment shows generalized electrodecrement that is seen as an interictal occurrence. Note that despite the patient having a focal area of dysfunction, the EEG abnormalities are bilateral and generalized at times. Sensitivity is 10 μV

Examination revealed left-hand fisting, but she did reach for objects equally with both hands when presented. Head circumference, height, and other findings were normal.

EEG showed a hypsarrhythmia pattern; high-amplitude slowing with multifocal epileptiform spikes. In addition, amplitude suppression occurred in the right hemisphere, maximal over the right centralparietal region. Intermittent electrodecrements occurred (Figs. 9.29, 9.30, and 9.31). Clinical events were captured, and these correlated with high-amplitude sharp waves followed by brief electrodecrements (Fig. 9.32a, b). Events were consistent clinically and electrographically with

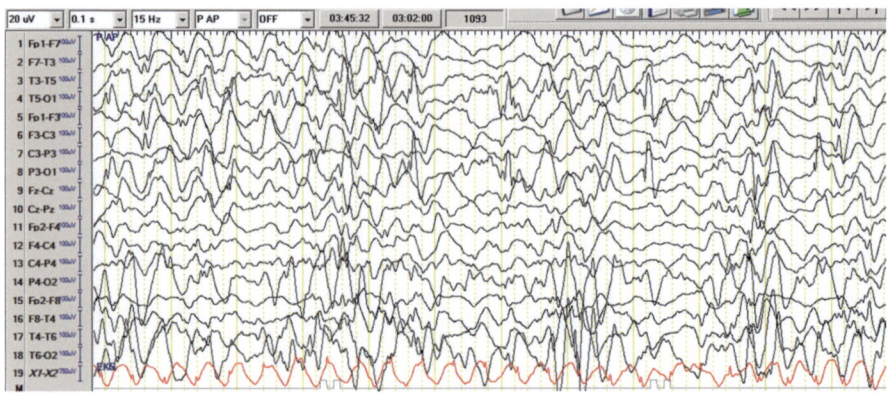

Fig. 9.31 Hypsarrhythmia EEG pattern. This segment shows high-amplitude background activity, multifocal spikes, and no normal background organization. In addition, the right frontocentral region shows suppression of amplitude, which correlates with the region of the porencephalic cyst. Epileptiform spikes are bilateral, despite the patient having a right hemisphere focal region of dysfunction. Sensitivity is 20 µV

infantile spasms. Also noted during the study were frequent runs of rhythmic epileptiform discharges in the right frontotemporal region showing evolution at times, with no apparent clinical change in the patient (per video and per family as observers). MRI brain demonstrated right hemisphere porencephaly.

The patient was treated with oral prednisone using a 6-week protocol. Epileptic spasms abated but focal clinical seizures began. An additional antiepileptic medication was added with a good response. She is currently doing well with mild hemiparesis and rare seizures treated with AED monotherapy (Fig. 9.33).

West syndrome is a triad of clinical spasms, hypsarrhythmia on EEG, and developmental regression that begins when the spasms begin. Etiology can be from a focal in lesion, such as epileptogenicity from prior insult, or a tuber in a patient with tuberous sclerosis. Genetic causes are also common, including Down syndrome and SCNA2. Infantile spasms may be seen in patients with a history of seizures or neonatal neurological conditions. These patients may already have developmental delay, which often worsens following the start of infantile spasms [27].

Currently, treatment protocols consist of hormone-based monotherapy, oral prednisolone, or vigabatrin [21]. The choice of specific treatment depends on each individual patient case. Prognosis can be poor, especially with cases of underlying brain dysfunction, delayed treatment, and history of neonatal seizures. As seen in our case patient, other seizure types can co-occur. Hypsarrhythmia interestingly is a specific background pattern that is only seen in this age group, identified as early as 4 months and as old as 18 months. As the child matures, the background pattern changes into high-amplitude slowing, as seen in Lennox–Gastaut syndrome, or a suppression with focal epileptiform discharges. Some babies return to normal EEG background activity. Clinical seizures will also change as the baby ages; the epileptic infantile spasms may alter to tonic spasms, atypical absence, myoclonic seizures, focal seizures, or generalized tonic-clonic activity.

a

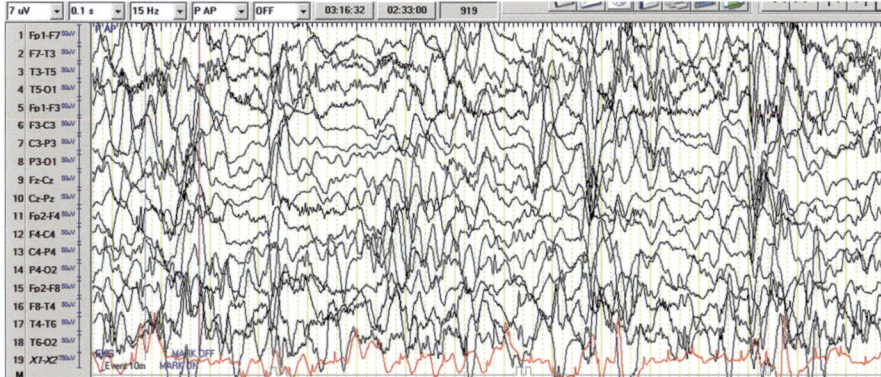

b

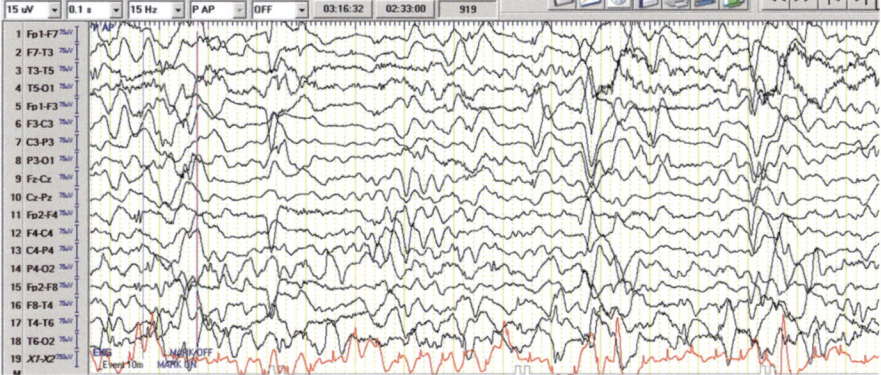

Fig. 9.32 (**a**, **b**) Hypsarrhythmia EEG pattern and clinical infantile spasm events captured. This segment shows the electrographic correlation with the patient's clinical events. The vertical pink line on the left is the patient event marker. She has a spasm movement correlating with each high-amplitude sharp wave followed by brief relative amplitude attenuation (electrodecrement). (**a**) This view is at a setting of 7 µV sensitivity. (**b**) Hypsarrhythmia EEG pattern and clinical infantile spasm events captured. This segment shows the electrographic correlation with the patient's clinical events. The vertical pink line on the left is the patient event marker. She has a spasm movement correlating with each high-amplitude sharp wave followed by brief relative amplitude attenuation (electrodecrement). This view is at a setting of 15 µV sensitivity, so the high-amplitude waveforms can be better viewed within the screen size

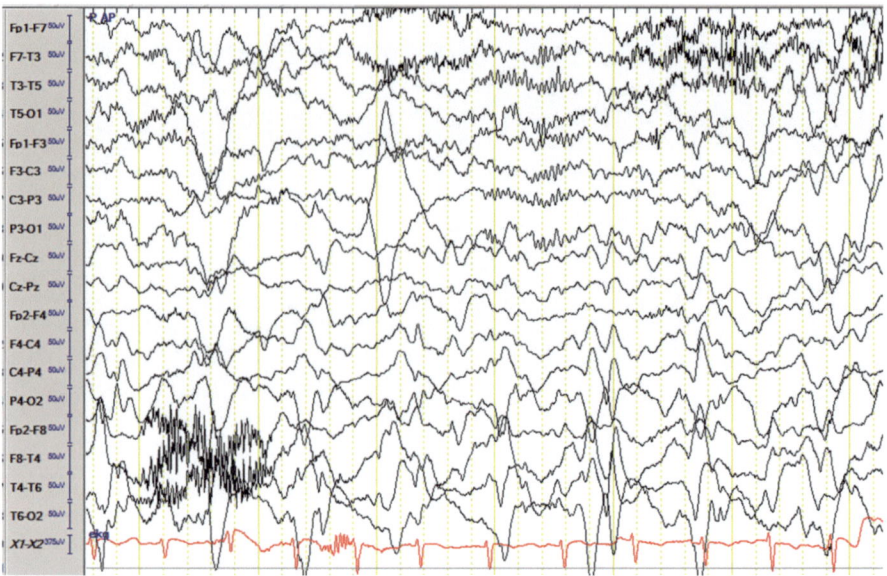

Fig. 9.33 Repeat EEG in a patient with a history of infantile spasms and right porencephalic cyst. This study was performed at 4 months of age. Epileptiform discharges are present in the right hemisphere with admixed focal slowing

References

1. Alvarez LA, Moshe SL, Belman AL, et al. EEG and brain death determination in children. Neurology. 1988;38(2):227. https://doi.org/10.1212/wnl.38.2.227.
2. American Clinical Neurophysiology Society. Guideline 3: minimum technical standards for EEG recording in suspected cerebral death. Bloomfield: American Clinical Neurophysiology Update; 2006.
3. Ashwal S. Brain death in the newborn. Current perspectives. Clin Perinatol. 1997;24(4):859–82.
4. Bakker MJ, van Dijk JG, van den Maagdenberg AMJM, et al. Startle syndromes. Lancet Neurol. 2006;5(6):513–24.
5. Balint B, Thomas R (2007) Hereditary hyperekplexia overview. GeneReviews [Internet], July 31. https://www.ncbi.nlm.nih.gov/books/NBK1260/
6. Cizmeci MN, Wilson D, Singhal M, et al. Neonatal hypoxic-ischemic encephalopathy spectrum: severity-stratified analysis of neuroimaging modalities and association with neurodevelopmental outcomes. J Pediatr. 2024;266 https://doi.org/10.1016/j.jpeds.2023.113866.
7. Committee on Fetus and Newborn. Hypothermia and neonatal encephalopathy. Pediatrics. 2014;133(6):1146–50. https://doi.org/10.1542/peds.2014-0899.
8. Coughlin C, Tseng L, Abdenur J, et al. Consensus guidelines for the diagnosis and management of pyridoxine-dependent epilepsy due to alpha-aminoadipic semialdehyde dehydrogenase deficiency. J Inherit Metab Dis. 2020;44:1–15.
9. Demyer W, White PT. EEG in holoprosencephaly. Arch Neurol. 1964;11:507–20. https://doi.org/10.1001/archneur.1964.00460230057005.
10. Dudipala S, Reddy R, Shankar R. Hyperekplexia: a treatable seizure mimicker in infants. Cureus. 2023;15(4):e38082. https://doi.org/10.7759/cerueus.38082.

11. Falsaperla R, Consentino MC, Vitaliti G, et al. Isolated ictal apnea in neonatal age. Clinical features and treatment options. A systematic review. Pediatr Neurol. 2007;37(5):366–70.
12. Gomella T, Eyal F, Bany-Mohammed F. Gomella's neonatology: management, procedures, on-call problems, diseases, and drugs. New York: 8th Edition, McGraw Hill Education; 2020.
13. Hahn JS, Delgado MR, Clegg NJ. Electroencephalography in holoprosencephaly: findings in children without epilepsy. Clin Neurophysiol. 2003;114(10):1908–17.
14. Lim T, Por C, Beh Y, Schee J, Tan A. Treatment of startle and related disorders. Clin Park Relat Disord. 2023; https://doi.org/10.1016/j.prdoa.2023.100218.
15. Martin RJ, Fanaroff AA. Fanaroff and Martin's neonatal-perinatal medicine disease of the fetus and infant. 12th ed. Philadelphia: Elsevier; 2025.
16. Mosalli R. Whole body cooling for infants with hypoxic-ischemic encephalopathy. J Clin Neonatol. 2012;1(2):101–6. https://doi.org/10.4103/2249-4847.96777.
17. Nakagawa TA, Ashwal S, Mathur M, et al. Guidelines for the determination of brain death in infants and children: an update of the 1987 Task Force recommendations. The Society of Critical Care Medicine, Section on Critical Care and Section on Neurology of the American Academy of Pediatrics, and the Child Neurology Society. Pediatrics. 2011;128(3):e720–40. https://doi.org/10.1542/peds.2011-1511.
18. National Organization for Rare Diseases (2013) Hyperekplexia. https://rarediseases.org/rare-diseases/hyperekplexia/#complete-report
19. Pekeles H, Amrani FA, Morgui MP, et al. Characteristics of children with cerebral palsy in the post-therapietic hypothermia era. J Child Neurol. 2023;38(3–4):130–6. https://doi.org/10.1177/08830738231159162.
20. Raam M, Solomon B, Muenke M. Holoprosencephaly: a guide to diagnosis and clinical management. Ind Pediatr. 2011;48(6):457–66.
21. Ramantani G, Bolsterli B, Alber M, et al. Treatment of infantile spasm syndrome: update from the interdisciplinary guideline committee coordinated by the German-speaking society of neuropediatrics. Neuropediatrics. 2022;53(6):389–401. https://doi.org/10.1055/a-1909-2977.
22. Rees MI, Lewis TM, Kwok JB, et al. Hyperekplexia associated with compound heterozygote mutations in the beta-subunit of the human inhibitory glycine receptor (GLRB). Hum Mol Genet. 2002;11(7):853–60.
23. Report of the AAN Guidelines Subcommittee, AAP, CNS, SCCM. Pediatric and adult brain death/death by neurologic criteria consensus guideline. Neurology. 2023;101(24):1112–32.
24. Shankaran S, Laptook A, Ehrenkranz R. Whole-body hypothermia for neonates with hypoxic-ischemic encephalopathy. N Engl J Med. 2005;353(15):1574–84. https://doi.org/10.1056/NEJMcps050929.
25. Stockler S, Plecko B, Gospe SM. Pyridoxine dependent epilepsy and antiquitin deficiency. Clinical and molecular characteristics and recommendations for diagnosis, treatment and follow-up. Mol Genet Metab. 2011; https://doi.org/10.1016/j.ymgme.2011.05.014.
26. Task Force for the Determination of Brain Death in Children. Guidelines for the determination of brain death in children. Neurology. 1987;37(6):1077. https://doi.org/10.1212/WNL.37.6.1077.
27. Volpe J, Inder T, Darras B, Vries L, Plessis A, Neil J, Perlman J. Volpe's neurology of the Newborn. 6th ed. Philadelphia: Elsevier; 2025.
28. Walsh BH, Murray DM, Boylan GB. The use of conventional EEG for the assessment of hypoxic ischemic encephalopathy in the newborn: a review. Clin Neurophysiol. 2011;122:1284–94.

Glossary: Terminology Used in Describing Neonatal EEG's[1]

Active sleep   Also known as REM sleep, this stage is characterized by closed eyes with irregular eye movements, irregular respirations, and small muscle twitches. This specific sleep state can be determined with eye leads, respiratory leads, and EEG data.

Activité moyenne   This term is used to describe the continuous activity in wakefulness after 35 WGA. EEG is characterized by continuous, low-voltage, irregular delta theta activity with intermittent overriding beta activity pattern. Theta activity is typically 25–50 µV, and delta frequencies may be lower voltage. This term means "medium activity" and is synonymous with trace continu.

Adjusted age   A term used when discussing premature babies. The adjusted age is also referred to as the corrected age. This is the age based on the initial due date, so at 40 WGA would be birth and the age is adjusted for that. For example, a 6-month-old infant born at 24 WGA would have an adjusted or corrected age of 2 months.

Alpha frequency   Frequencies at 8–12 Hz (cycles per second).

Amplitude   The amplitude of the EEG is measured in voltage, in the measurement unit of volts (V). Most cortical activity is in the microvolt (µV) range. The voltage value is measured from peak to peak (pp) of the waveform.

Anterior dysrhythmia   Anterior dysrhythmia (AD) is a similar pattern and qualifies as runs of frontal sharp waves with a frequency of 5–9 Hz that last a few seconds with an amplitude of 50–150 µV. They are seen best between 38–42 WGA during transitional or quiet sleep.

Asymmetry   Term used when the left and right hemispheres do not display the same activity on each side. This could include asymmetry of amplitude, frequency, and/or morphology. Amplitude asymmetry is typically noted when the ratio of amplitude is greater than 50% (ratio 2:1) difference. Small variations may occur, so reporting would be for anything that is persistent.

---

[1] This chapter describes the common terms used in neonatal EEG recordings.

© The Author(s), under exclusive license to Springer Nature Switzerland AG 2025
M. Payne, D. Gloss II (eds.), *Neonatal EEG*,
https://doi.org/10.1007/978-3-031-92556-6

Asynchrony When the left and right hemispheres do not display bursts within 1.5 s of each other.

Attenuation Activity that is low voltage relative to the remainder of the background activity.

Automatism An involuntary movement that is usually repetitive. These movements can occur as part of a seizure. It may be difficult to distinguish between epileptic and nonepileptic automatisms without an EEG. Automatisms seen in neonates: lip smacking, sucking/tongue thrusting, and bicycling movements of the legs.

Axon The long threadlike portion of a nerve cell where electrical impulses are conducted away from the cell body toward other neuron cell bodies.

Beta frequency Frequencies greater than 12 Hz (12 cycles per second).

Bilateral independent Usually referring to epileptiform discharges or epileptic (seizure) activity with activity occurring simultaneously in two regions but that begin, evolve, and behave independently of each other.

Brief rhythmic discharges (BRDs)/brief potentially ictal rhythmic discharges (BIRDs) Brief, less than 10 s rhythmic often epileptiform activity that has an amplitude greater than 2 µV without a clinical correlate. This activity can have some evolution similar to a seizure but does not meet the criteria for a seizure due to its short duration and lack of clinical correlation. BRDs are part of the interictal–ictal continuum.

Brush Beta activity superimposed on other frequency waveforms. This creates a "brush-like" effect.

Burst suppression Pattern of high-amplitude slow activity (burst) alternating with extremely low-amplitude (interburst) activity. Interburst amplitude is less than 5 µV to be considered burst suppression.

Central Referring to the central electrode that is placed over the central head region (Cz). This region most often represents primary motor cortex involving the face and arm (see homunculus). This is also the area where sleep architecture originates. Often there are supporting electrodes on the left (C3) and right (C4) to evaluate laterality of central cerebral activity.

Chronological age Time since birth of a neonate, also known as the age of the patient.

Conceptional age The age of the baby measured beginning at the time of conception. Conception is usually 2 weeks after the first day of the last menstrual period. A full-term infant born at 40 weeks gestational age is born at 38 weeks conceptional age.

Continuity Background activity with minimal variations in amplitude, giving the appearance of waveforms without interruption. Neonates can have subtle mild breaks in continuity, so the American Clinical Neurophysiology Society (ACNS) parameter states that a background can be considered continuous if activity less than 25 µV only occur at most for 2 s.

Corrected age A term used when discussing premature babies and is also referred to as the adjusted age. This is the age based on birth being at 40 WGA. For example, a 6-month-old infant born at 24 WGA would have an adjusted or corrected age of 2 months.

Delta brush A waveform consisting of a delta (slow wave) with superimposed beta (fast activity). Delta brushes are seen in early premature infants maximally in the central regions in active sleep. Around 32 WGA, delta brush location changes to be maximal in the temporal and occipital regions and most often in quiet sleep. This waveform continues to 40 WGA. Other terms used to describe this waveform are ripples of prematurity, spindle-delta bursts, spindle-like fast waves, beta-delta complexes, and rapid bursts.

Delta frequency Frequencies less than 4 Hz.

Diffuse Refers to a pattern that is seen in both hemispheres at the same time. This does not imply exact symmetry or synchrony, however.

Discontinuity Pattern during which there are periods of relatively higher amplitude bursts that alternate with periods of lower amplitude activity. The period of lower amplitude activity interrupting the burst is termed interburst interval (IBI) and measured in seconds. Two different sources state that for discontinuity to be present, the interburst interval amplitude is between 25 and 50 μV for at least 2 s or less than 25 μV for 3 s [6].

Dysmaturity Inconsistency between postmenstrual age (PMA) and expected EEG background for that age. If there is confidence that calculated PMA is correct, dysmaturity can be representative of a generalized encephalopathy and depending on the degree of dysmaturity may be associated with poor neonatal outcomes. However, if the PMA was incorrectly calculated, there may be inconsistency among the PMA and expected EEG background due to using the incorrectly calculated PMA as a point of reference.

Electro-oculographic Eye leads used in EEG recordings. Placement of these leads are at the outer corner of the eyes (lateral canthus) and often one lead is placed slightly above the lateral cantus and the contralateral side slightly below the lateral canthus. However, placement can vary and one should verify placement with the neurodiagnostic technician. Activity recorded from these leads can be helpful in identifying awake and sleep states as well as deciphering possible artifacts.

Electrode Small metal discs affixed to the scalp used to measure electrical potentials from brain cells. These may be made of stainless steel, tin, or silver. There are platinum electrodes that are non-ferromagnetic making them more compatible with magnetic resonance imaging (MRI) scans.

Electroencephalogram A graphical representation of brain waves obtained using a machine that records electrical activity from electrodes affixed to the scalp.

Encoches frontales Frontal predominant, synchronous, broad sharply contoured transients that are most prevalent and most abundant in the transition from active to quiet sleep. These transients are a normal finding in neonates and are typically seen between 34 and 44 WGA. Presence of persistent asynchronous encoches frontales usually suggests a pathological process.

Epilepsy Tendency to have unprovoked seizures. This diagnosis can be difficult to ascertain and certainly varies based on the age, seizure character, and EEG findings.

Epileptic Term used to describe seizures electrographically.

Epileptiform Term used to describe electrographic abnormalities that are indicative of potential epileptic activity. Other terms may be used such as seizure tendency, tendency to generate seizure, and epileptogenic potential.

Evolution Term used to describe the typical characteristics of an electrographic seizure in which the amplitude, frequency, and morphology change, and there is spread to adjacent cortical regions. The change in frequency is generally considered to be more than 1 Hz to qualify for evidence for a seizure. Presence of this evolution process can help discern electrographic epileptic activity in children and adults and is not as frequent in neonatal seizures.

Filter: high-frequency (low pass) Filter that allows lower frequency activity to pass through to the recording.

Filter: low-frequency (high pass) Filter that allows higher frequency activity to pass through to the recording.

Frequency Measure of cycles per second, unit is Hertz. This is used to describe the frequency of waveforms seen in a given time unit (second). Typical frequency ranges may include delta, theta, alpha, beta, and gamma activity.

Frontal Frontal cortex, anterior portion of the brain and represented by frontal electrodes, corresponding to the motor cortex involving the contralateral head, trunk, and lower extremities.

Gestational age The age that a neonate is born measured by the time from first day of last menstrual period to the day of delivery. Gestational age plus time since birth is postmenstrual age.

Graphoelements Transient sharp waves, which are often normal in neonates. Characteristics such as morphological appearance, prevalence, symmetry, asynchrony, and presence or absence at a given gestational age range may be utilized to distinguish transients from pathological waveforms. Examples may include encoches frontales, anterior dysrhythmia, and delta brush, among others.

Gray matter Neurons in the cortex (outer surface of the brain) or nuclei (deeper structures of the brain) associated with cognition and other brain functions. Cortical gray matter and presence of gray matter in inappropriate brain regions (such as periventricular nodular heterotopia) are responsible for seizure generation.

Humunculous (motor) The cartoon figure used in anatomical pictures of the brain to demonstrate the relationship between the motor cortex and regions of the body.

Ictus Seizure.

Indeterminate sleep Sleep state in neonates that is characterized by closed eyes, but lack of other clinical and EEG features associated with definite periods of quiet, or active sleep. Indeterminate sleep is prevalent in preterm and younger gestational age neonates.

Interburst interval The periods of lower amplitude activity interrupting burst of higher amplitude activity within a discontinuous EEG pattern measured in seconds.

Interictal Occurring in between seizures. This term is general and refers to any time between any type of events. Most of the time, the ictus is a seizure so this term implies epileptiform abnormalities that occur in the background when the patient is not in a seizure.

Isoelectric Background activity showing a lack of electrical potential difference between electrode channels. Graphically, this appears as a flat line with no upward or downward deflection. If isolated to a single or small group of channels, this may be secondary to technical issues such as too small a distance between electrodes or a salt bridge. This finding typically suggests minimal cortical function.

Lateralized Refers to a seizure or interictal epileptiform abnormality that is more often seen in one hemisphere. Used to describe periodic and rhythmic patterns [lateralized periodic discharges (LPDs)] for example.

Migrating Description for a type of seizure that begins in one hemisphere and spreads to the other hemisphere.

Montage How the electrodes are linked together and displayed on the software page.

Multifocal Presence of three different regions of abnormality and involves both hemispheres.

Neuron Brain cell.

Non-REM sleep Develops from quiet sleep, around the age of 2 months. At this time, sleep spindles are present and there is a discernible progression from waking to stage 2, non-REM sleep.

Occipital Region of the brain that is posterior. The occipital cortex is responsible for vision and processing of visual input. Occipital electrodes represent the occipital cortex. Occipital electrodes (O1, O2) represent the occipital cortex.

Paper speed Despite being in the digital age, where actual paper is not used, this term is still used and refers to how many seconds are displayed on a digital screen. The standard is 10 s per page, as if there are 10 s per paper page in the paper era. Neonatal standard is typically 20 s per page. However, this setting can be easily changed with computer software recordings.

Parietal Parietal cortex and represented by parietal electrodes. Potentially represented by P3, P4 electrodes but dedicated parietal electrodes may not be standard for a given EEG neonatal protocol.

Periodic An EEG pattern (often used to describe epileptiform discharges including sharps and spikes) characterized by discharges that have at least six waveforms with at least 50% consistency of similar morphology and duration (can predict the next discharge with at least 50% confidence) with periods of intervening background EEG. Waves with a periodicity are reported in terms of cycles per second (cps) to describe the peak-to-peak frequency between discharges. Periodic discharges are not common in neonates but can occur in acute destructive processes such as HSV encephalitis, stroke, and global hypoxic-ischemic encephalopathy.

Postmenstrual age (PMA) Gestational age plus chronological age.

Quiet sleep Sleep that is a precursor to non-REM sleep. This sleep state is characterized by eye closure, absent rapid eye movement (REM), and limited body movements aside from occasional startles or suckling.

Reactivity Term that refers to how the EEG background changes with stimulation. First appears at 30–32 weeks WGA but may not be seen with every stimulus. The EEG background can change from sleep to awake, or even as minor changes of frequency, amplitude, or increase in continuity.

REM sleep Develops from active sleep. During REM sleep, eye movement is rapid. This sleep state is present in about 50% of total sleep time in full-term infants.

Rhythmic An EEG pattern characterized by discharges that have at least six waveforms with at least 50% consistency of similar morphology and duration (can predict the next discharge with at least 50% confidence) but without intervening periods of background EEG. These are reported in Hertz (Hz) to describe the peak-to-peak frequency between discharges. In neonates, rhythmic activity may be normal with some graphoelements as rhythmic occipital delta activity and/or anterior dysrhythmia (symmetric rhythmic delta activity in the frontal leads seen most often in periods of transitional sleep).

Ripple Typically beta activity between 16 and 20 Hz superimposed on delta frequency waveforms. This creates a "brush-like" effect.

Seizure Electrical activity with evolution in time, space, frequency, and amplitude. Clinical activity accompanying this electrographic change indicates a clinical seizure. Lack of clinical accompaniment indicates subclinical seizure. ACNS defines a minimum of 10 s (less than 10 s is BRD). ILAE does not specify a minimum time for seizure activity. Both ACNS and ILAE define seizures electrographically.

Tsuchuda [7] defined a neonatal seizure as "a sudden abnormal EEG event, defined by a repetitive and evolving pattern with a minimum of 2 μV (microvolt) peak-to-peak voltage and duration of at least 10 seconds."

ILAE [4]: Neonatal seizures are defined by their EEG findings rather than their semiology. "An electrographic event with a pattern characterized by sudden, repetitive, evolving stereotyped waveforms with a beginning and end. The duration is not defined but has to be sufficient to demonstrate evolution in frequency and morphology of the discharges and needs to be long enough to allow recognition of onset, evolution, and resolution of an abnormal discharge."

Semiology Term used for clinical manifestation of what the patient seizure looks like.

Sensitivity A modifier of the amplitude displayed on the screen and unit is μV/mm. This setting can be easily changed with digital recordings. A higher sensitivity (less sensitive) makes the waveform lower and a lower sensitivity (more sensitive) makes the waveform higher. Standard sensitivity setting is 7 μV/mm.

Sharp wave Isolated polyphasic discharge lasting 70–200 ms followed by a slow wave or other disruption of the background. May be indicative of epileptiform potential or region of dysfunction. Some sharp waves are normal graphoelements, and determination of normal or abnormal is based on morphology, location, state, and gestational age.

Sleep spindle A characteristic of stage II sleep. Sleep spindles are 11–16 Hz and appear around 48 weeks gestational age in central head regions.

Spike wave Similar morphological characteristics and disruption of the background as a sharp wave but with a duration of 20–70 ms. Indicative of epileptic potential in older children and adults. In neonates, highly favors epileptic potential but may also indicate a region of dysfunction.

Spindle Typically beta activity between 11 and 16 Hz superimposed on delta frequency waveforms. This creates a "brush-like" effect.

Status epilepticus Historically, neonatal status epilepticus has been defined as a single continuous seizure (regardless of electrographic only, electro-clinical, or clinical only) lasting more than 30 min or a series of seizures over at least 30 min in which baseline brain function has not normalized. However, ACNS and ILAE have provided an additional definition as the summed duration of seizure activity of an arbitrarily defined 1 h epoch of the EEG that equals or exceeds 50%.

Symmetry Symmetry in neonatal EEG refers to symmetrical activity. This term can refer to the amplitude, frequency, or sharp activity. In addition, symmetry should be measured over a set period of time, for example, in a 60-min study, the amount of activity in one hemisphere should equal the same amount of activity in the other hemisphere.

Synchrony When activity is seen in both hemispheres and at the same time. Considered to be less than 1.5 s difference between the onset of EEG burst between hemispheres. Synchrony is well developed until 27 weeks GA, declines around 34 weeks GA, then increases to 100% around term.

Temporal Region of the brain associated with the temporal lobes. Temporal electrodes represent the temporal cortex. Some institutions may have variable naming conventions and/or add additional electrodes so one should clarify hookup protocols with the neurodiagnostic technician. In neonates, this region can produce seizures with contralateral motor movements.

Theta frequencies Frequencies in the 5–7 Hz range.

Tracé alternant Pattern seen after 32 WGA in transitional or quiet sleep, in which the interburst activity voltage is higher than 25 µV and the interburst activity duration shortens to 1–2 s. Bursts consist of mixed-frequency activity with amplitudes between 50 and 150 µV.

Tracé continu Pattern seen in term infants in wakefulness and active sleep, consisting of irregular delta and theta activity of 50–100 µV during awake and activity sleep. This term is synonymous with activité moyenne.

Tracé discontinu Earliest known EEG pattern that is seen in neonates. Beginning as early as 30 WGA, trace discontinu pattern is seen in quiet sleep only. The pattern is characterized by bursts of 30–300 µV in amplitude with interburst activity typically less than 25 µV in amplitude with a duration shortening as neonate matures.

Transients Also termed graphoelements, these are sharp waves that may be normal for gestational age or if asymmetric may signify a region of abnormal dysfunction.

Transitional sleep The period between active sleep and quiet sleep, when clear sleep states cannot be identified. This is a type of transient indeterminant sleep.

Variability The natural, unstimulated change a neonate experiences between sleeping and wakefulness. At term, the neonate should show variability of all three stage, waking, active sleep and quiet sleep without external influences. Neonates as young as 25 WGA can show natural unprovoked state changes.

Voltage Amplitude, measured in volts. Most activity is in microvolt (µV) ranges.

White matter Axons of the neurons, which are not at the surface of the scalp and do not typically give a negative potential. However, abnormal white matter lesions can cause focal slowing on EEG.

References

1. Blume W, Kaibara M. Atlas of pediatric electroencephalopagraphy. 2nd ed. Philadelphia: Lippincott-Raven; 1998.
2. Britton J, Frey L, Hopp J, et al. Electroencephalography: an introductory text and atlas of normal and abnormal findings in adults, children and infants. Chicago: American Epilepsy Society; 2016.
3. Hrachovy RA, Mizrahi EM, Kellway P. Electroencephalography of the newborn. In: Daly D, Pedley TA, editors. Current practice of clinical electroencephalography. 2nd ed. New York: Raven Press; 1990. p. 201–41.
4. Pressler RM, Cilio MR, Mizrahi EM. The ILAE Classification of seizures and the epilepsies: Modification for seizures in the neonate. Position paper by the ILAE Task Force on Neonatal Seizures. Epilepsia; 2021. p. 1–14.
5. Mizrahi E, Hrachovy R. Atlas of neonatal electroencephalography. 4th ed. New York: Demos Medical; 2016.
6. Sansevere AJ, Harrar DB. Atlas of pediatric and neonatal ICU EEG. New York: Springer; 2021.
7. Tsuchuda T, Wusthoff C, Shellhaas R, et al. ACNS standardized EEG terminology and categorization for the description of continuous EEG monitoring in neonates. Report of the American Clinical Neurophysiology Society, Critical Care Monitoring Committee. J Clin Neurophysiol. 2013;2:161–73. https://doi.org/10.1097/WNP.0b013e3182872b24.

Index

A
Abnormal background patterns, 92–97, 113, 120, 124–126
Abnormal frontal sharp waves, 106
Abnormal neonatal sharp waves, 105
Abnormal rhythmic frequencies, 93
Active sleep, 27, 28, 66, 69–71, 74
Activite moyenne, 58, 61
Adjusted age, 26
aEEG, *see* Amplitude integrated EEG
Alpha frequency, 11
α-aminoadipic semialdehyde dehydrogenase (ALDH7A1) activity, 220
Alpha seizure, 141
American Clinical Neurophysiology Society (ACNS) guidelines, 85
Amino acidopathies, 160
Amplitude, 133
Amplitude integrated EEG (aEEG)
    algorithm, 194
    artifacts, 194, 201–204
    background activity, 197–204
    basics of, 194–196
    burst suppression pattern, 200
    CFM, 200
    continuous low voltage activity, 201
    discontinuous background pattern, 199
    dual-channel, 198, 201
    electrodes, 194
    functions of, 196
    intermittent seizure activity, 203
    isoelectric tracing, 202
    limitations, 194
    seizure characteristics, 200–201
    single channel, 198
    status epilepticus, 202

Amplitude of waves, 9
Anterior dysrhythmia (AD), 61, 106
Anti-epileptic medications, 145
Antiquitin, 220
Apnea, 216
    during seizure, 211
    hyperekplexia., 216
    persistent, 211
Apnea of prematurity, 210
Artifacts
    at time of jerking movements, 176
    causes of, 173
    decipher, 176
    ECG lead, 184, 185
    EEG headset adjustment, 191
    environmental /physiological, 173
    hiccough, 177, 178
    loose electrode, 190, 191
    movements of neonates, 173
    muscle, 174, 175
    oscillator, 186, 188
    pacemaker, 186
    patting, 188, 189
    pulse, 185, 186
    rocking, 190
    seizure, 182
    sucking, 178, 179
    superimposed fast muscle, 176
    tremor like movements as, 180
    ventilator, 187
Asymmetrical bursts, 100
Asymmetrical EEG waveforms, 99
Asymmetry, 82, 98
Asynchronous bursts, 101, 102
Asynchrony, 100, 101
ATP-ase pump, 130
Awake, 27

B

Background pattern, 36, 37, 45
   of maturity, 28
   premature neonatal, 46
   28-29 WGA neonate, 44
B12 deficiency, 160
Behaviors, 27
Benign familial neonatal seizures, 163
Benign idiopathic neonatal seizures, 164–172
Benign non-familial neonatal convulsions, 164–172
Beta frequency, 11, 42
Bilateral closed lip schizencephaly, 120
Bilateral waveforms, 37
Bilirubin encephalopathy, 158
Biotinidase (B7) deficiency, 159
Bipolar montage, 131
Brief rhythmic discharges (BRDs), 123, 134–138
Burst activity, 30, 80
Burst suppression pattern, 79, 82–84, 87, 199, 200, 223, 226

C

Central delta frequencies, 39
Central delta waveforms, 41, 42
Central region sharp waves, 107, 113, 114, 118, 119
Cerebral function monitor (CFM), 195, 196, 200
Cerebral voltages, 12
Chronological age, 25, 26
Conceptional age, 25, 26
Continuous background activity, 28, 45, 50
Continuous low voltage activity, 199–201
Continuous pattern, 31, 197, 198
Corrected age, 26
Cortical signals, 6, 12

D

Delta brushes, 50
   in neonates, 52
   premature *vs.* term, 52
Delta frequency, 11, 36
   low amplitude, 49
   in occipital regions, 40
   in temporal regions, 40, 42
Depolarization of neurons, 131
Developmental and epileptic encephalopathies (DEE), 166
Diffuse amplitude abnormality, 89, 92

Diffuse cortical dysfunction, 94
Diffuse delta frequencies
   25 and 27 WGA neonate, 44
   28 and 29 WGA, 45
Diffuse low amplitude activity, 89
Diffuse low frequency, 92
Diffuse neonatal EEG slowing, 92
Diffuse theta frequencies, 35, 45, 53
   25 and 27 WGA neonate, 44
   in 23-24 WGA neonate, 35, 36
Digital EEG recordings, 18
Digital technology, 16
Discontinuous background
   pattern, 28, 31, 51, 197–199
   appearance of, 58
Double banana, 6
Downward deflection, 130
Dual channel mode, 195
Dyschronism
   external, 78
   internal, 78

E

Early infantile developmental and epileptic encephalopathy (EIDEE), 166, 167, 225
Early infantile epileptic encephalopathy (EIEE), 166
Early myoclonic encephalopathy (EME), 166–169, 225
Electrical interference, 201
Electrocardiogram (ECG)
   electrodes, 5
   lead artifact, 184, 185
Electrocerebral inactivity, 86, 87
Electrode "pop" artifact, 190, 191
Electrode's voltage, 131
Electroencephalogram (EEG)
   electrodes, 2
   electrode montage, 7
   history of, 1
   neonatal, 1
   neurophysiology, 1
   principles of, 1
   signals responsible for, 2
   waveforms, 2
Electrographic seizures, 137
Electromyogram (EMG) electrodes, 5
Electrooculogram (EOC) electrodes, 5
Encephalopathy
   abnormal background patterns, 77–88

bilirubin, 158
early infantile developmental and
   epileptic, 166
early infantile epileptic, 166
early myoclonic, 166, 168, 169
epileptic, 166
hypoxic ischemic, 158
medication effects, 162
mild findings, 78
presence of, 77
Encoches frontales (EF), 58, 60, 106
   features of, 106
Epilepsies, with abnormal EEG background
   patterns, 166
Epilepsy in infancy with migrating focal
   seizures (EIMFS), 167
   characteristics, 169
Epileptic activity, 21
Epileptic encephalopathy, 222–227
Epileptogenicity, 33
Evolution, 133
Excessive discontinuity, 87
Excessively discontinuous EEG
   background, 80, 92, 100
Excitatory postsynaptic potentials
   (EPSP's), 131
Extracranial abnormalities, 97

F
Factor V Leiden, 227
Familial type epilepsy, 163–165
Filters, 13
Flat trace, 200–204
Focal abnormality, low/high
   amplitude, 89
Focal low amplitude activity, 91
Focal neonatal seizure, 218
Focal seizures, 170, 171
Focal slowing, 92, 93
Folinic acid (B9) deficiency, 159
Frequency, 133
Frequency of waves, 9
Frequency patterns, 33, 52
   location, 46
   in 34-35 WGA neonates, 61
Frontal delta activity, 36
Frontal delta waveforms, 39
Frontal region sharp waves,
   106–112
Frontal sharp transients, 33, 38, 41,
   44, 46
   23-24 WGA neonate, 33, 34
   32-33 WGA, 55

G
Gamma-aminobutyric acid (GABA), 130
Gestational age, 25
   asynchronous, 30
   at birth, 27
   normal and abnormal interburst
      intervals, 81
   symmetric, 30
   21-22 weeks, 31
   23-24 weeks, 32–36
   25-27 weeks, 36–44
   28-29, 44–49
   30-31 weeks, 50
   32-33, 55
   34-35 weeks, 58–61
   36-37 weeks, 61–64
   38-40 weeks, 64–68
   41-44 week, 68–70
   45-48 weeks, 70, 72, 73
   with less discontinuity, 29
Glut 1 deficiency, 158
Glutamate, 130

H
Hemisphere activity, 101
Hemispheric dysfunction, 30
Hiccough, 173
   artifact, 177, 178
High voltage waveforms, 13, 15
Holoprosencephaly
   alobar, 228
   centro-temporal seizure, 229
   definition, 228
   and EEG findings, 227–230
   EEG in infant with, 230
   EEG in neonate with, 227, 229
   findings, 228
   lobar, 228
   semilobar, 227, 228
Homunculus, 132, 157
Humunculus, with EEG scalp electrodes, 157
Hyperekplexia (HK), 215–217
Hypocalcemia, 159
Hypoglycemia, 159
Hypomagnesemia, 159
Hyponatremia, 159
Hypothermia
   with HIE, 205–208
   neonatal therapeutic, 208
   therapeutic, 205, 207, 208
Hypoxic ischemic encephalopathy (HIE), 158,
      162, 205–208
Hypsarrhythmia, EEG pattern, 231, 233

I

Ictal interictal continuum, 134, 135, 137, 138
Impedance, 5–6, 195
Inborn errors of metabolism, 159, 160
Indeterminate background activity, 31
Indeterminate sleep, 67
Infantile developmental
    encephalopathy, 222–227
Infantile spasms, 230–233
Inhibitory postsynaptic potentials
    (IPSP's), 131
Interburst intervals (IBI), 28, 29, 78
Interictal epileptiform abnormalities, 138
Intermittent seizure activity, 203
International League Against Epilepsy, 134
Intracranial abnormalities, 97
Intracranial hemorrhage, 158
    cause of, 158
    neonatal, 155
    types of, 158
Intraparenchymal hemorrhage, 98
Ischemic stroke, 158
Isoelectric tracing, 200, 202

J

Jerking movement, 59

L

L-arginine supplementation, 221
Lennox-Gastaut syndrome, 166, 232
Level of consciousness, 27
Lissencephaly, 120
Loose electrode artifact, 190
Low voltage
    in all leads, 88
    suppressed pattern, 85
Lysine, 221
Lysosomal storage disorders, 160

M

Magnetic resonance venogram (MRV), 223
Maturation, 25, 30
Metabolic abnormalities, 159
Monorhythmic delta activity, 45
Montage, 6–8
Morphology, 133
Motor seizures, 132
Movement artifact, 63
Myoclonic jerks, 81
Myoclonic seizures, 225, 226
Myoclonus, 173, 223

N

Negative discharge, 8
Negative phase reversal, 8
Neonatal apnea, *see* Apnea of prematurity
Neonatal behavioral assessment scale, 27
Neonatal EEG techniques, 4–7
Neonatal encephalopathy with focal
    abnormalities, 124
Neonatal epilepsies, 163
Neonatal epileptic seizures, 133
Neonatal epileptic syndromes, 162–172
Neonatal hypoxic ischemic encephalopathy,
    194, 197
Neonatal seizures, 194, 195
    rhythmic activity, 134
    WHO 2011 guidelines, 134
Neuronal depolarization, 131
Neurophysiology, 1–3, 129
Non-familial type epilepsy, 165
Non-ketotic hyperglycinemia, 160

O

Occipital delta frequency, 41, 48
Occipital sharp transients, 33, 34, 38, 44
    negative, 47
    23-24 WGA neonate, 34, 35
    32-33 WGA, 55
Occipital theta frequency, 49
Ohtahara syndrome, 167
Organic acidemias urea cycle disorders, 160
Oscillator artifact, 186, 188

P

Pacemaker artifact, 186
Paper speed, 18
Parameters, EEG waveforms, 9–12
Parietal region sharp waves, 109, 111, 121
Patting artifact, 188, 189
Periodic lateralized sharp wave discharges
    (PLDs), 111, 122, 123, 135, 136
Peroxisomal disorders, 160
Phase reversals in EEG, 8
Porencephalic cyst, 234
Positive discharge, 8
Positive phase reversal, 8
Post-anoxic myoclonus, 84
Post conceptional age, 26
Post gestational age, 26
Post menstrual age (PMA), 25, 26
Post term, 70
Potassium flow, 130
Premature (central) delta brush, 41

Index 249

Premature infants, 28
Premature neonate activity, 30
Primordial sleep, 71
Pyridoxal phosphate (PLP), 221
Pyridoxine
  dependent epilepsy, 159, 217–222
  supplementation, 221

Q
Quiet sleep, 27, 28, 65, 69, 74

R
Repetitive seizures, 200
Reports, 22
Respiratory belt, 5
Ripple, 10
Ripple of prematurity, 57
Rocking artifact, 190
Rolandic dips, 114
  28 and 29 WGA, 44
  in neonate, 47
Rolandic sharp waves, 56

S
Scalp electrodes, 3, 4, 131, 157
Seizure
  alpha, 141, 153
  burden, 137
  central, 145
  characteristics, 155–158
  clinical, 152
  definition, 129
  drug withdrawal, 159
  epileptiform, 129
  etiologies in neonates, 158
  frontal, 143
  GABA, 130
  glutamate, 130
  myoclonic, 149
  neonatal, 155
  occipital focal, 148
  origin, 158
  post-feeding, 160
  potassium, 130
  progressive, 160
  refractory, 81, 221
  semiology, 129
  in setting of encephalopathy, 162
  sodium, 130
  temporal, 150
  time of onset, 160
  types, 155, 170
  vitamin D deficiency, 159
  vitamin K deficiency, 159
  with ECMO, 158
Self-limited neonatal epilepsy, 166
Self-limited familial neonatal epilepsy (SELFNE), 163–165
Self-limited familial neonatal-infantile epilepsy (SELFNIE), 163
Self-limited neonatal epilepsies, 163
Self-limited non-familial neonatal epilepsy (SELNE), 163
Sensitivity, 12, 15, 16
Sharp transients, 32, 33, 57, 64, 67, 70, 72
  location, 46
Sharp waves, 32, 138
  abnormal, 105, 113
  abnormal central, 118
  abnormal frontal, 106
  abnormal left frontal, 111
  abnormal left fronto-temporal, 108
  abnormal left temporal, 118, 119
  abnormal right centro-temporal, 115
  abnormal right occipital, 121
  bilateral abnormal central, 114
  bilateral frontal, 110
  bilateral parietal, 119
  central, 113
  central positive, 116
  central region, 107
  definition, 105
  focal, 124
  focal right occipital, 113
  frontal, 106
  fronto-central, 107
  high amplitude, 125
  high amplitude (vertex) central, 127
  high amplitude abnormal, 126
  high amplitude occipital, 120
  left and right frontal, 126
  left central positive, 116
  left frontal, 109, 112, 127
  localized, 105
  neonatal frontal, 112
  normal, 105
  normal frontal, 107
  occipital region, 109
  parietal region, 109
  positive central, 107
  repetitive, 115
  right frontal, 109
  and spike waves, 105
  temporal, 120, 125
  temporal region, 109

Single channel mode, 195
Sleep criteria, 67
Sleep spindles, 46
Sleep wake cycling, 197
Sodium flow, 130
Spindle, 10, 46
Startle, 173
Startle disease, 215–217
Status epilepticus, 138, 202
Sucking artifact, 178, 179
Sudden infant death syndrome (SIDS), 217
Symmetric anterior dysrhythmia, 60
Symmetry, 98–103
Synchrony, 30

T
Technical aspects, EEG, 4, 6, 12
Temporal alpha, 56
    and ripple, 57
Temporal delta frequencies, 48
Temporal saw tooth waveforms, 45
Temporal sharp transients, WGA 32-33, 55
Temporal sharp waves, abnormal, 118
Temporal theta, 33, 35
    23-24 WGA neonate, 35, 36
    28 and 29 WGA, 46
Temporal waveforms, saw tooth, 48
Theta activity, 35
Theta frequencies
    in occipital regions, 43
    in temporal regions, 43
Thiamine (B1) deficiency, 159
Timeline, of specific disorders, 160

Tracé discontinu, 31, 32, 36

U
Upward deflection, 130

V
Venous thromboses, 226
Ventilator artifact, 187
Very high voltage activity, 12
Vitamin D deficiency, 159
Vitamin K deficiency, 159
Voltage suppressed pattern, 86

W
Wakefulness, 28, 70, 74
Week gestational age (WGA), 25, 26, 31
    after 44, 50
    21-22, 31
    23-24, 32–36
    25-27, 36–39, 41, 43
    28-29, 44–49
    30, 77
    30-31, 50–52
    32-33, 53–58
    34-35, 58–61
    36-37, 61–64
    38-40, 64, 66, 68
    41-44, 68–70
    45-48, 71
Weeks conceptional age (WCA), 25
West syndrome, 232

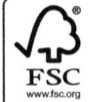

MIX
Papier aus verantwortungsvollen Quellen
Paper from responsible sources
FSC® C105338

If you have any concerns about our products,
you can contact us on
ProductSafety@springernature.com

In case Publisher is established outside the EU,
the EU authorized representative is:
**Springer Nature Customer Service Center GmbH
Europaplatz 3, 69115 Heidelberg, Germany**

Printed by Libri Plureos GmbH
in Hamburg, Germany